P E R I - I M P L A N T I T I S

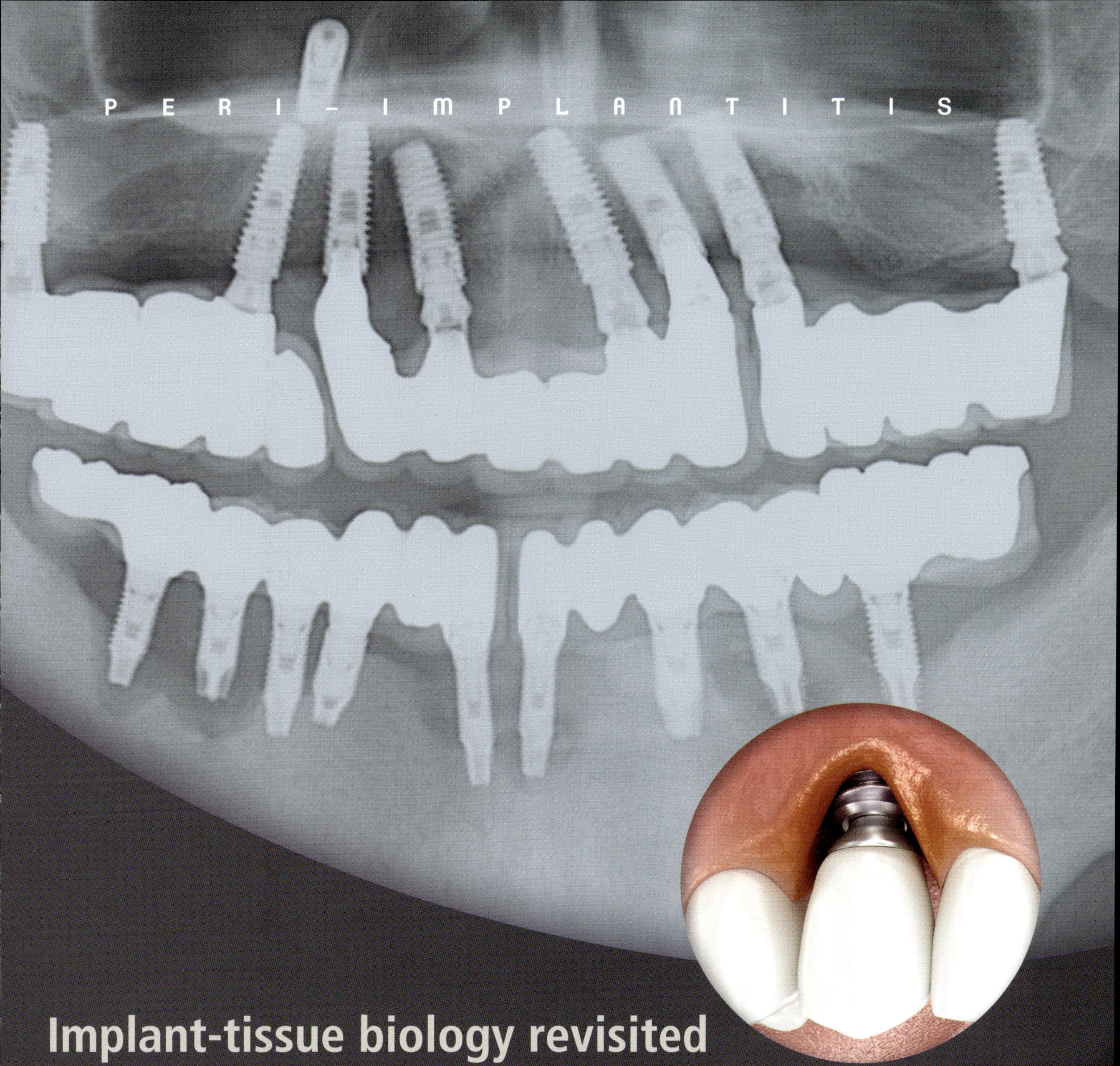

Implant-tissue biology revisited

Reality of Peri-Implantitis

Jeong-Chan Kim | In-Sung Yeo | Jung-Ju Kim

KOONJA

Reality of Peri-Implantitis
Implant-tissue biology revisited

1st Print 2025-09-30
1st Publication 2025-11-11

Author Jeong-Chan Kim, In-Sung Yeo, Jung-Ju Kim
Acquisition Editor Su-in Han
Developmental Editor Min-soo Kim
Designer Ji-won Shin
Illustrator Jung-Ju Kim, Yoon-ji Shin

Permissions may be sought at Koonja's rights department:
Tel: (82)-31-943-1888
Fax: (82)-31-955-9545
www.koonja.co.kr

Printed in South Korea
First Edition, © 2025 Koonja publishing, Inc.
ISBN 979-11-7068-360-5

USD 170.00

Reality of Peri-Implantitis

Implant-tissue biology revisited

Preface

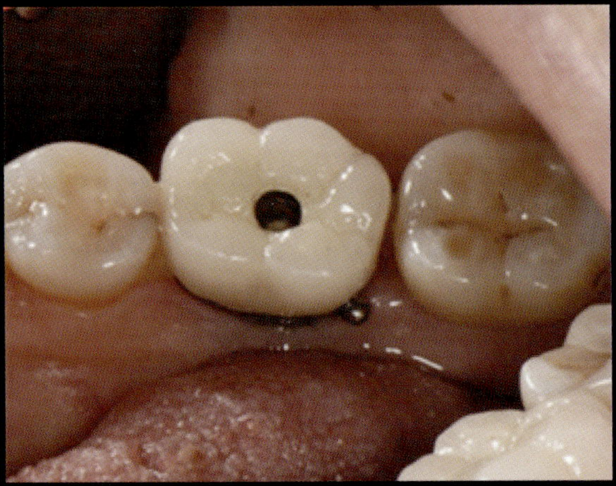
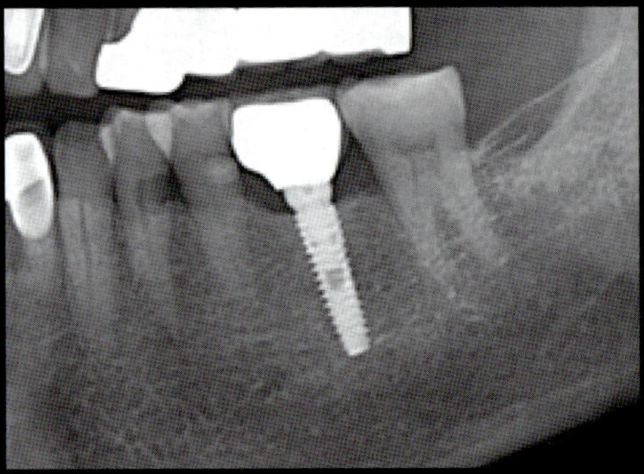

After dental implant placement, food impaction has traditionally been explained by the fact that implants remain stationary, whereas natural teeth exhibit mesial movement. However, certain clinical cases directly challenge this belief, which has long been accepted as a truth.

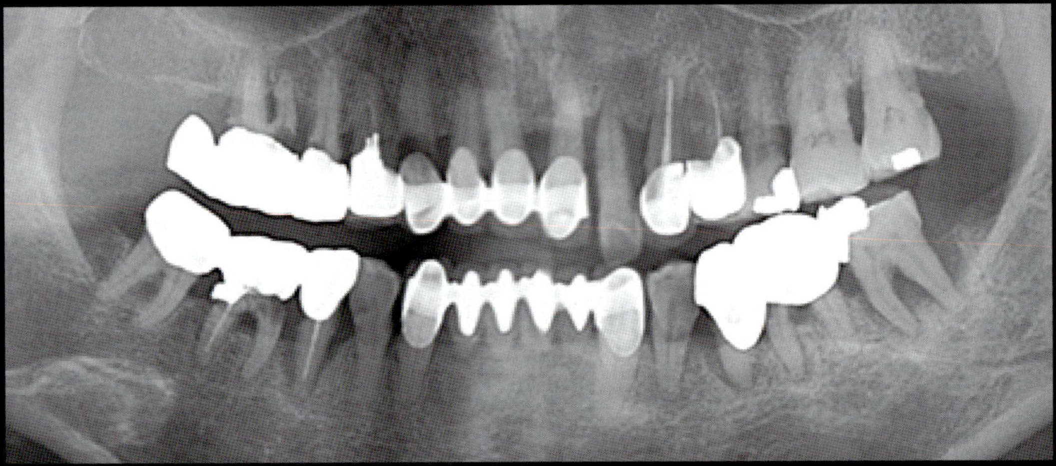

2014-02-24

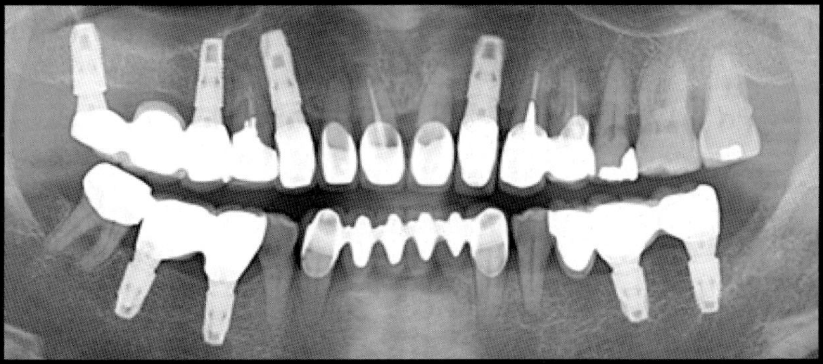

2015-09-11

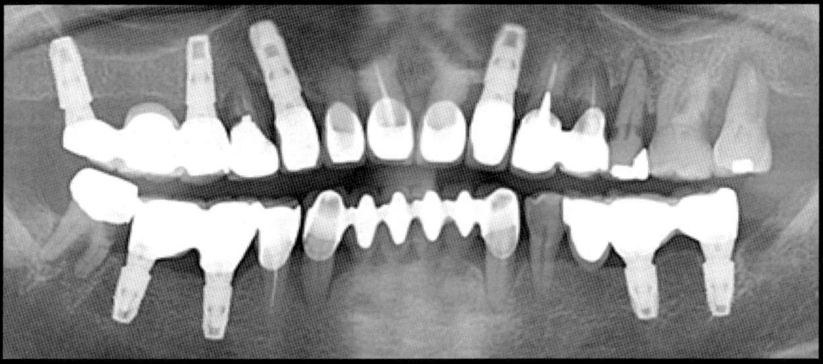

2022-01-08

In 2014, a patient with severe periodontitis underwent tooth extraction and implant surgery. Over the subsequent seven years, the patient's natural teeth showed progressive caries and worsening periodontitis, while the implants showed no issues whatsoever..

It has been widely taught that peri-implantitis is caused by bacteria and that the long-term prognosis of implants is contingent on the patient's oral hygiene. If this were entirely true, one might speculate that the patient only cleaned the implant sites, neglecting the natural teeth, which is an unrealistic scenario.

The essence of natural science lies in observing phenomena and discovering the laws governing them. These laws must comprehensively explain all phenomena occurring in nature. Yet, the clinical cases presented herein reveal discrepancies between established dental science and the natural processes observed in patients' oral environments. This raises critical questions: Either the natural science of dentistry is flawed, or the phenomena observed in patients are incorrect. Since natural phenomena take precedence over the definitions humans create in science, I believe there may be issues with our understanding of natural science. In other words, there is a strong possibility that there are errors within the natural science of dentistry. For over 25 years, I have contemplated this and continuously observed the natural phenomena within patients' mouths. I have strived to discover new natural laws. Now, the time has come for me to present the new natural science I have discovered.

We refer to individuals who can think beyond existing knowledge, authority, and conventions as geniuses. Many fields of human knowledge have developed thanks to such geniuses. There may also be errors in the new natural science I propose. Therefore, I eagerly await discussions with my fellow dentists and hope for a genius who can surpass me and correct my mistakes.

Summer 2025, Dongdaemun

Recommendation

The pace of development in dental implants has been so rapid that it has established itself as one of the most important fields in dentistry before a generation has even passed. Implants are among the treatments with the best prognosis and highest patient satisfaction in various clinical areas of dentistry. However, not all implants can be perfect, and statistically, some of the placed implants inevitably lead to complications.

Complications that arise after the completion of implant surgery and prosthetics include peri-implant mucositis, peri-implantitis, and prosthetic or mechanical complications. As the number of patients undergoing implant procedures increases each year, these issues have also risen significantly, posing challenges for clinicians.

In this context, I learned that Dr. Kim Jeong-chan is publishing a book titled "Peri-implantitis Not Taught in Textbooks." Dr. Kim is a senior and mentor with whom I have had a long-standing relationship. During a time when there were few methods of learning, I was able to start my foundation and clinical practice in implants thanks to Dr. Kim's teachings and support. Whenever I encountered difficult clinical cases, I could always rely on his assistance. Therefore, it is truly an honor for me to write this recommendation for his book.

In addition to his exceptional clinical skills, Dr. Kim possesses the insight to see beyond the surface of things, along with ingenuity and ideas. He has been actively engaged in numerous lectures over the years. It is a great pleasure that he is now publishing a book containing the valuable clinical data he has accumulated. Given the rapid increase in complications related to implants, I believe this book will greatly assist clinicians in problem-solving and prevention, serving as a stepping stone to broaden their perspectives.

Dr. Park Hwi-Woong, Seoul Ace Dental Clinic

Curriculum vitae

Jeong-Chan Kim

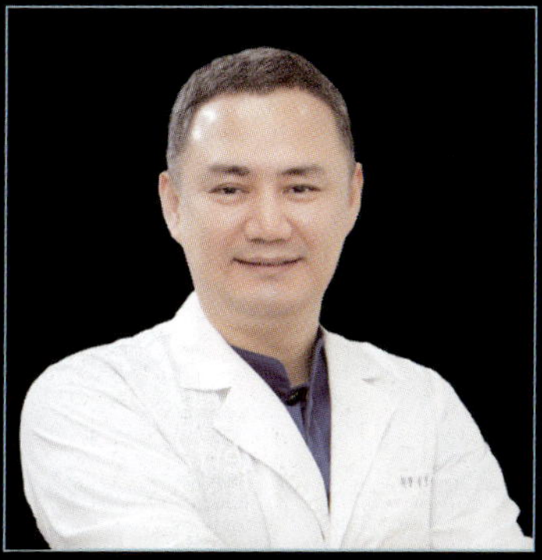

Bachelor, College of Dentistry, Seoul National University, Seoul, Korea

Residency, Department of Periodontology, Seoul National University Dental Hospital, Seoul, Korea

Adjunct Professor, Department of Periodontology, Seoul National University School of Dentistry, Seoul, Korea

Dongdaemun Dental Clinic, Seoul, Korea

In-Sung Luke Yeo

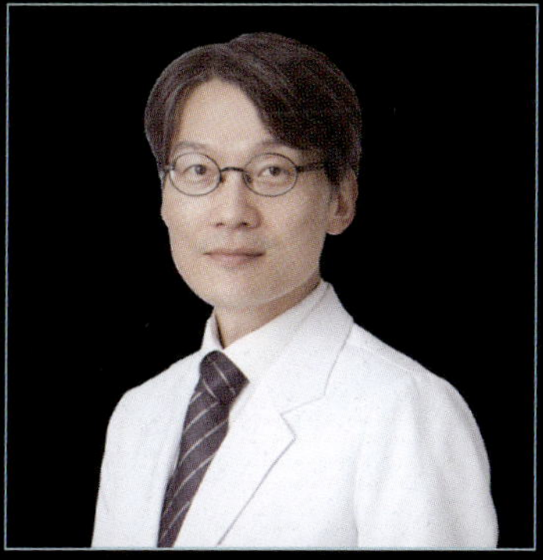

Bachelor, College of Dentistry, Seoul National University, Seoul, Korea

Board Certificate in Prosthodontics, Seoul National University Dental Hospital, Seoul, Korea, and Ministry of Health and Welfare, Korea

Master of Science and Doctor of Philosophy, Graduate School, Seoul National University, Seoul, Korea

Professor, Department of Prosthodontics, Seoul National University School of Dentistry, Seoul, Korea

Jung-Ju Kim

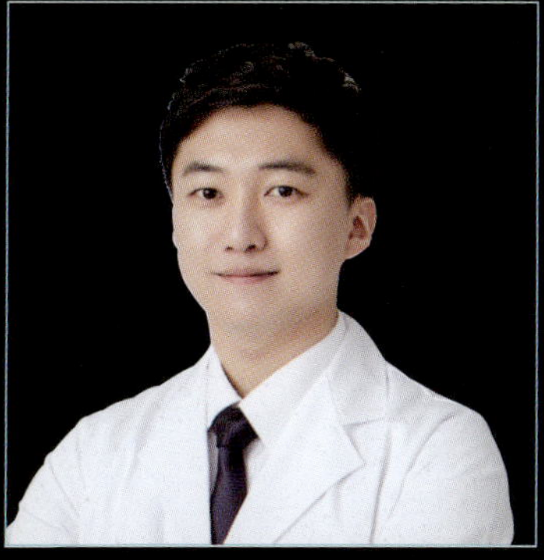

Master of Science and Doctor of Philosophy, Graduate School, Seoul National University, Seoul, Korea

Residency, Department of Periodontology, Seoul National University Dental Hospital, Seoul, Korea

Board Certificate in Periodontology, Seoul National University Dental Hospital, Seoul, Korea, and Ministry of Health and Welfare, Korea

Adjunct Professor, Department of Periodontology, Seoul National University School of Dentistry, Seoul, Korea

Meister Dental Clinic, Seoul, Korea

Contents

PART 1

PERI-IMPLANTITIS

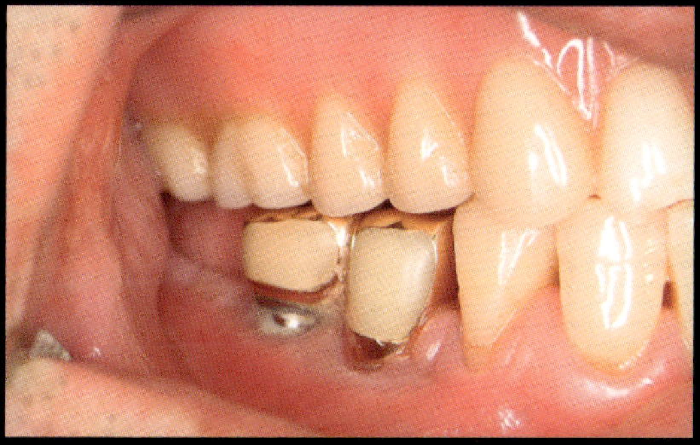

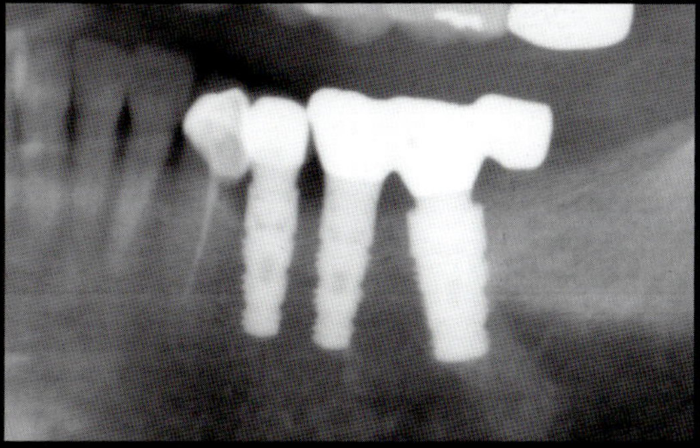

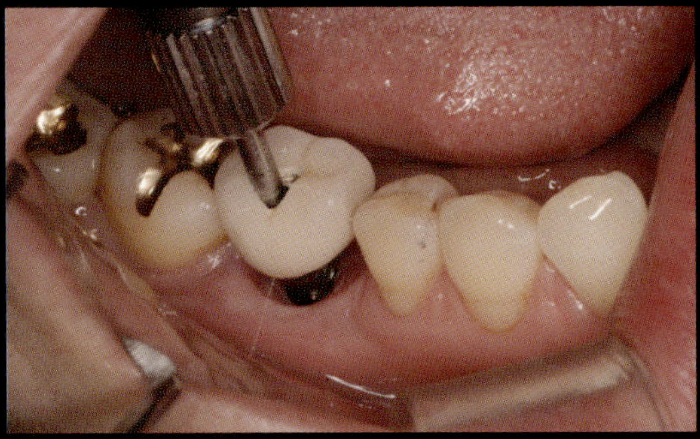

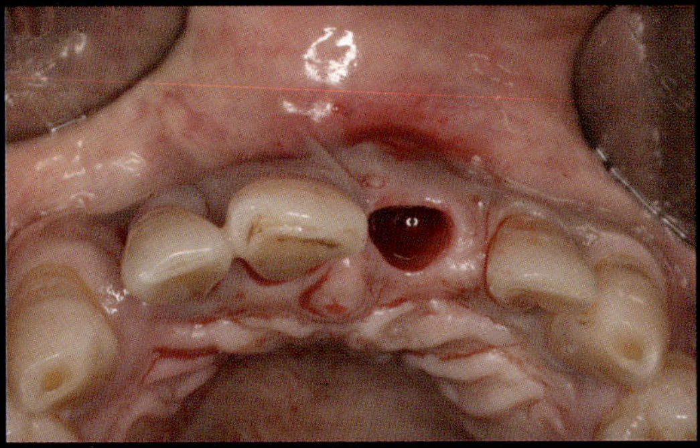

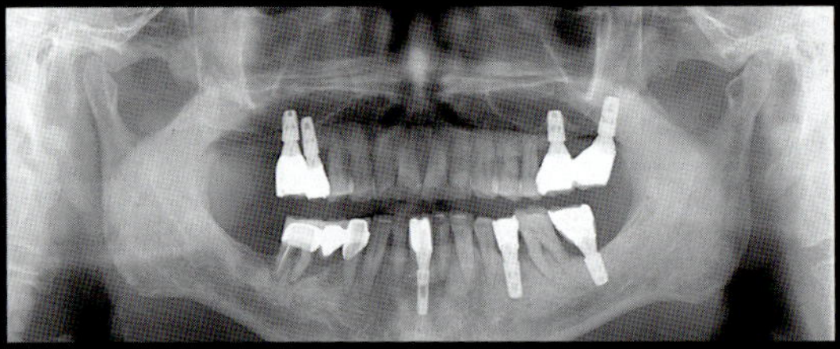

Contents

PART

2

PERI-IMPLANTITIS

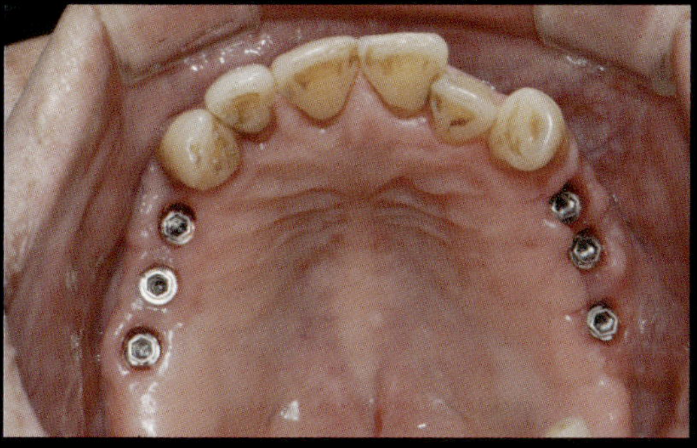

PERI-IMPLANTITIS

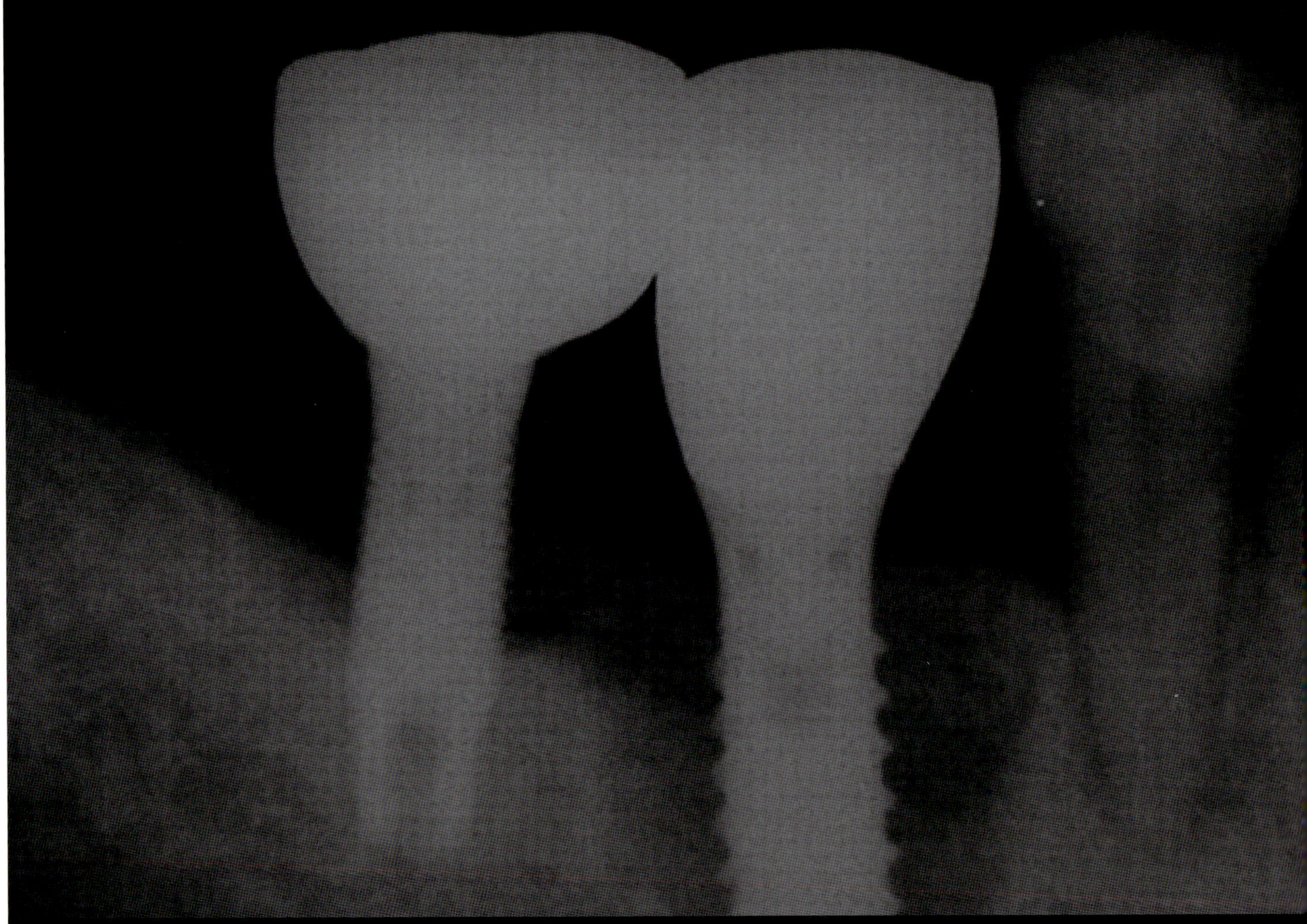

PART

1

PERI-IMPLANTITIS

Chapter 1

A Review of the Causes of Peri-implantitis

_ Regarding the Gingiva

Peri-implantitis is known to be caused by bacterial invasion, which is thought to result from poor oral hygiene in patients. Consequently, when we encounter peri-implantitis in clinical practice, we strive to educate patients about oral hygiene management, disinfect wounds with antiseptics, and prescribe antibiotics to control the invading bacteria. However, upon closely examining numerous clinical cases of implant placements, it becomes evident that not all implants are equally affected by peri-implantitis; rather, some are affected while others are not, and the degree of affliction varies among individual implants.

Just as teeth affected by periodontitis in natural dentition occur randomly, one might assume that peri-implantitis also arises randomly among implants. However, in science, natural phenomena should not be interpreted merely as random occurrences. As true scientists, we must explain why periodontitis and peri-implantitis occur randomly. It is difficult to believe that bacteria intentionally target specific implants for severe attacks. We need to understand why these phenomena occur. I believe that one of the reasons lies in the gingiva. Therefore, I would like to explore the relationship between the gingiva and peri-implantitis.

1. Peri-implantitis and the Gingiva

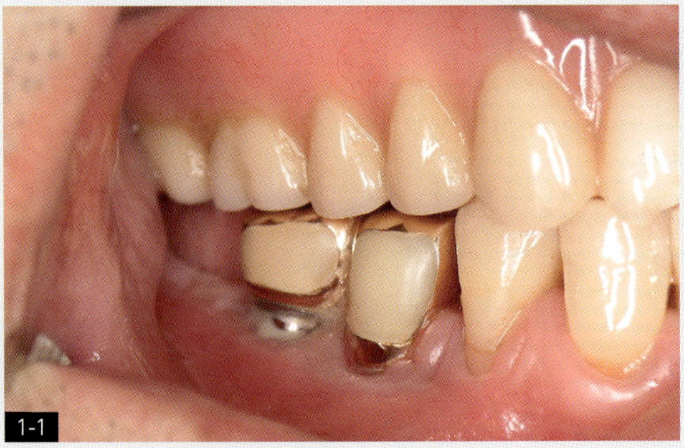

1-1

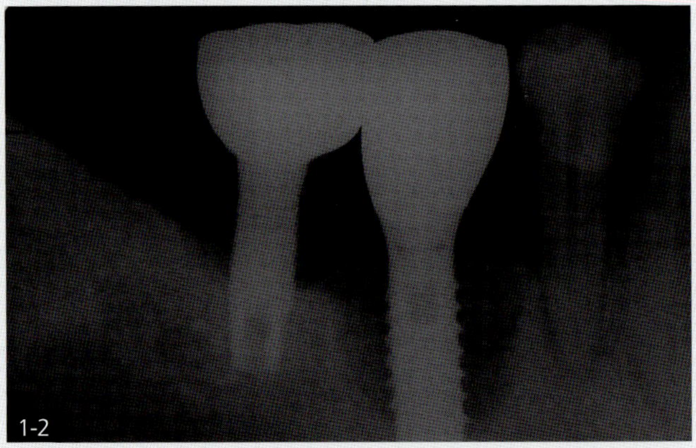

1-2

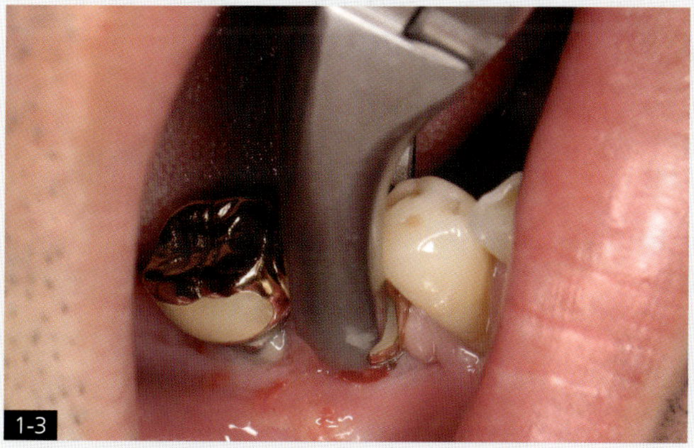

1-3

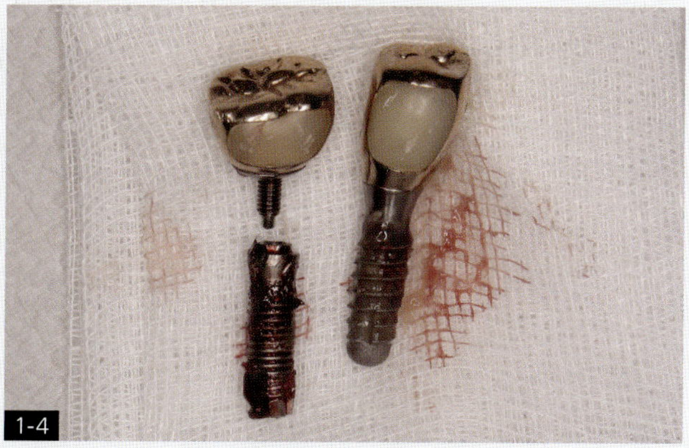

1-4

Peri-implantitis of unknown origin occurred around implants 45 and 46. Due to severe inflammation, both implants were ultimately removed. After the removal of the implants due to peri-implantitis, I pondered the causes. One of the suspected causes of peri-implantitis is excessive occlusal force. In this patient's case, the opposing teeth are dentures. While well-made dentures can exert significant force, they typically exert about one-fifth of the force of natural teeth, making it unlikely that excessive occlusal force was applied to the mandibular implant. If we assume a principle that all phenomena must be explained, then excessive occlusal force cannot be considered a direct cause of peri-implantitis.

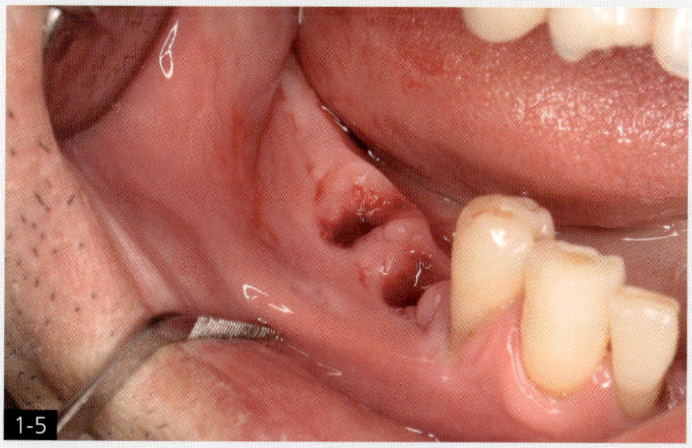

1-5

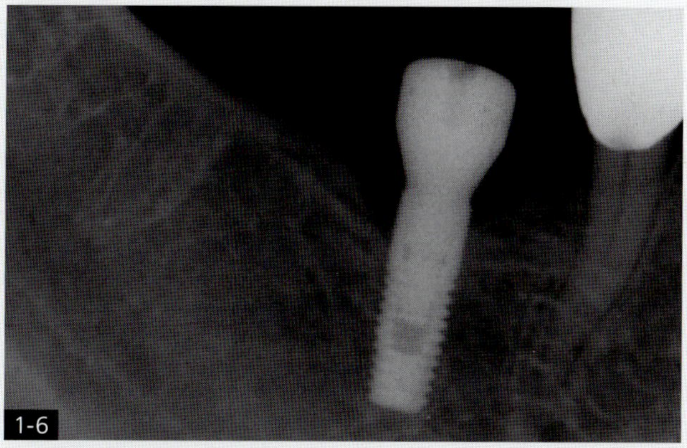

1-6

This was my first encounter with peri-implantitis, and I was quite perplexed, as my existing knowledge led me to believe that bacteria were the cause. I could not understand why bacteria would only attack these two implants. It was only after many years that I could begin to hypothesize the cause. In **Figure 1-5**, it can be observed that there is almost no attached gingiva on the buccal side. The absence of attached gingiva is likely associated with peri-implantitis.

Figure 1-6 shows marginal bone loss. Peri-implantitis occurred before the prosthetic process began. This clinical case raises questions about the relationship between occlusion and peri-implantitis.

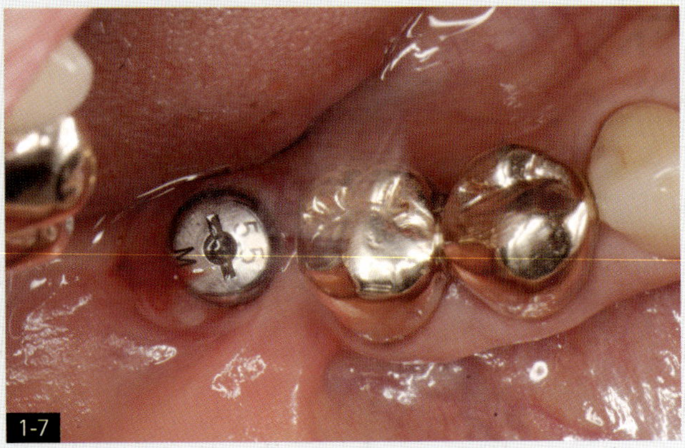
1-7

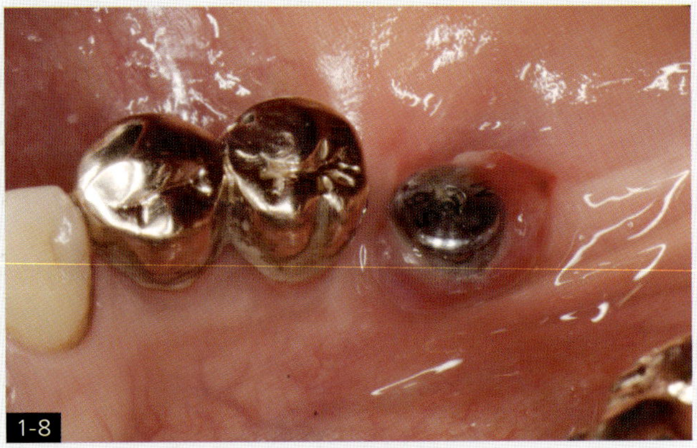
1-8

The oral condition before the application of load can be seen in the context of peri-implantitis. A senior dentist referred the patient to me, stating that since I specialized in periodontics, I should take good care of the treatment. I assumed the cause was bacterial, so I performed disinfection and prescribed antibiotics, but there was no change in symptoms **(Figures 1-7, 1-8)**.

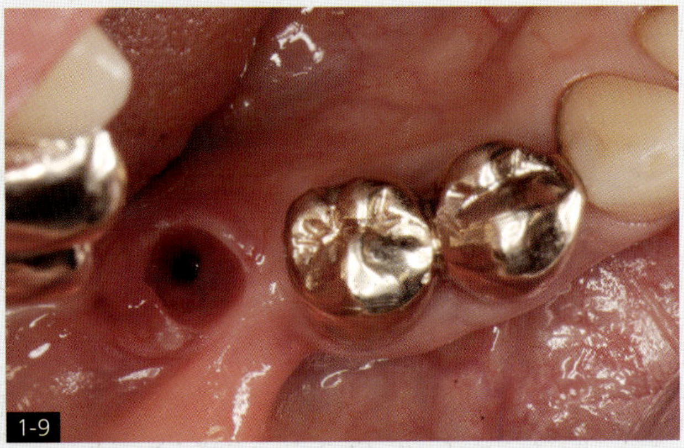
1-9

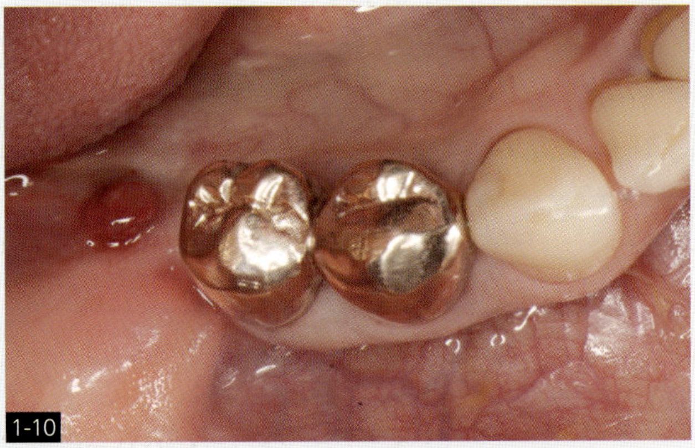
1-10

Consequently, I hypothesized a different cause. I considered that the absence of a defensive barrier preventing bacterial invasion, rather than bacteria itself, was the cause, and I decided to perform a gingival graft. The absence of attached gingiva on the buccal and lingual sides is evident **(Figure 1-9)**.

Since a gingival graft could not be performed on both the lingual and buccal sides, I removed the healing abutment as shown in **Figure 1-9** and placed a cover screw. Although the soft tissue covered the cover screw, an infectious source remained, leading to the observation of a gum boil in the soft tissue **(Figure 1-10)**.

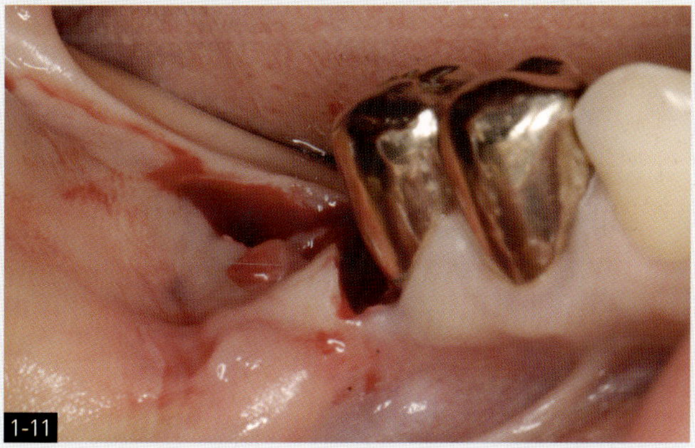
1-11

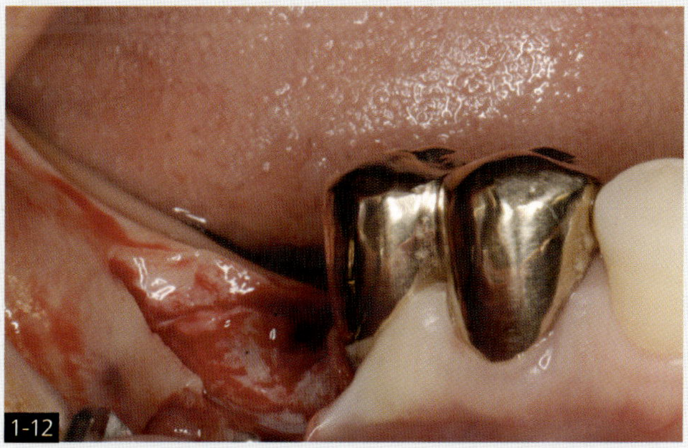
1-12

Preparation for the recipient site for the gingival graft is underway **(Figure 1-11)**. The buccal frenum also needed to be addressed, so it was incised and positioned buccally **(Figure 1-12)**.

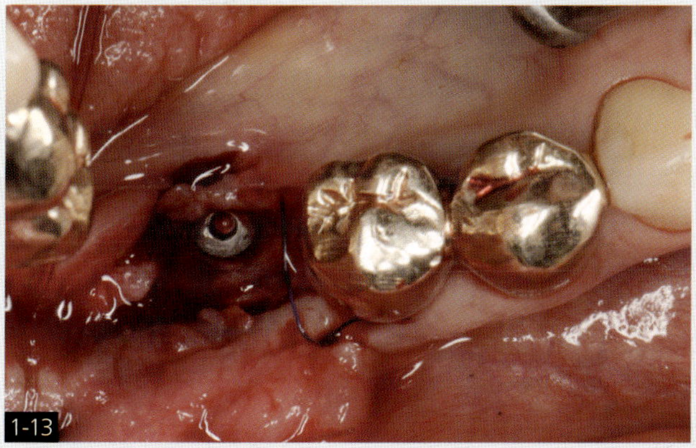
1-13

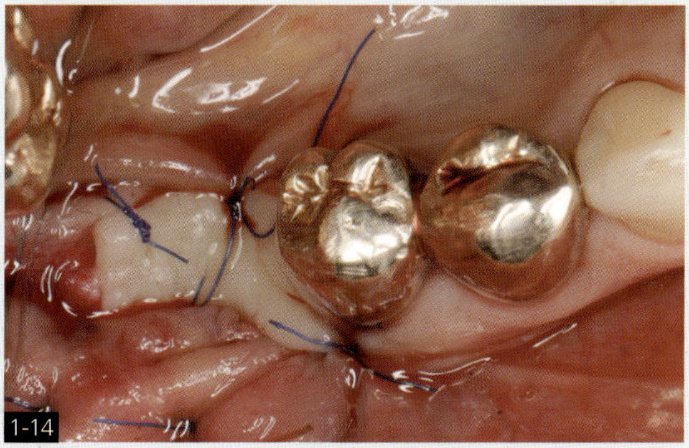
1-14

The soft tissue of the recipient site was moved buccally and sutured, and gingiva was harvested from the palate for grafting **(Figures 1-13, 1-14)**. The recipient site, excluding the cover screw, was vascular tissue, which significantly increased the success rate of the procedure.

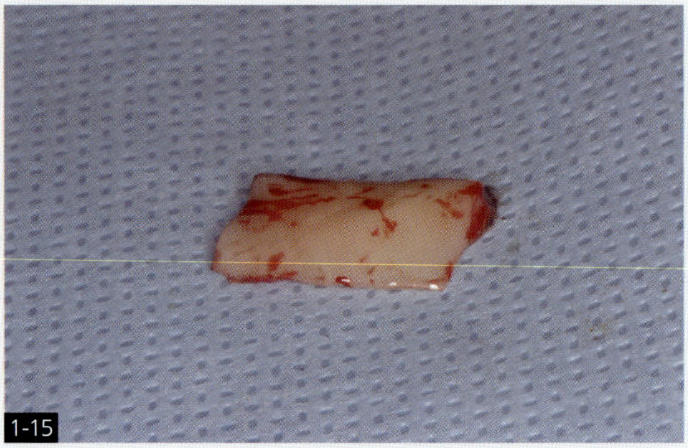
1-15

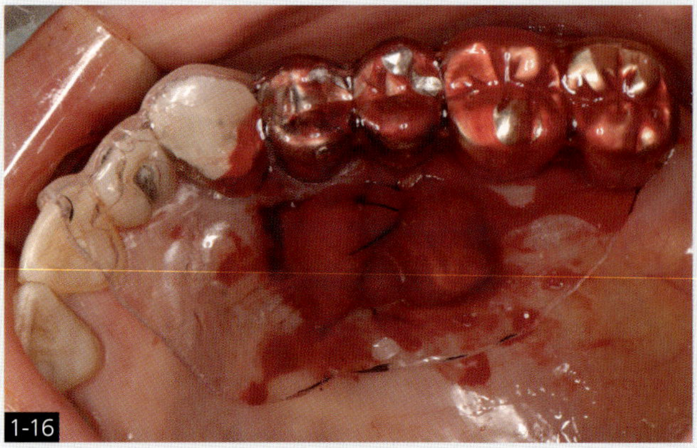
1-16

Gingiva was harvested from the palatal side using a surgical stent for hemostasis (Figures 1-15, 1-16).

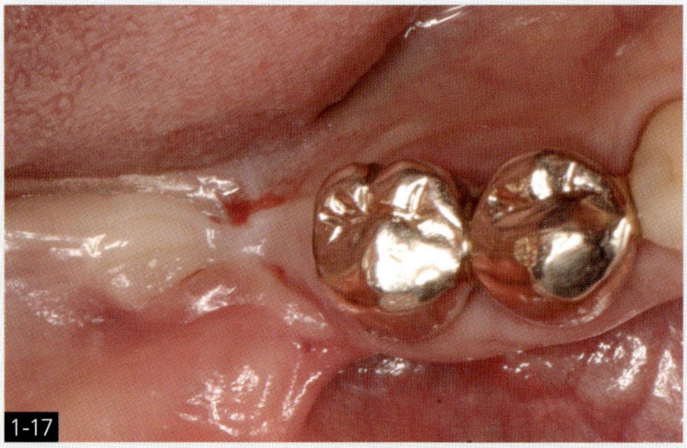
1-17

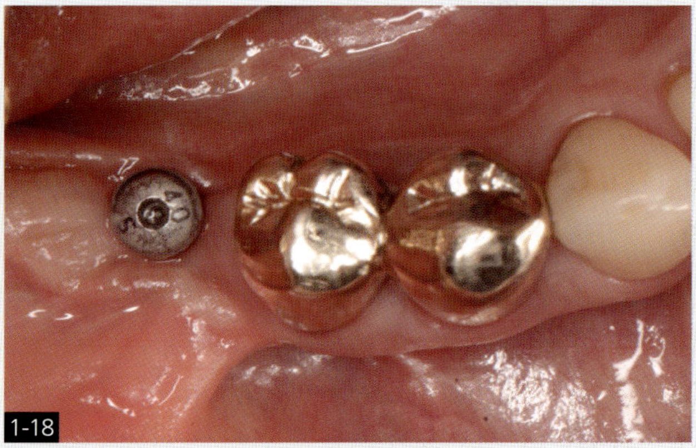
1-18

Six weeks after the soft tissue graft (Figure 1-17), a secondary surgery was performed. One week post-surgery (Figure 1-18), no further inflammation was observed.

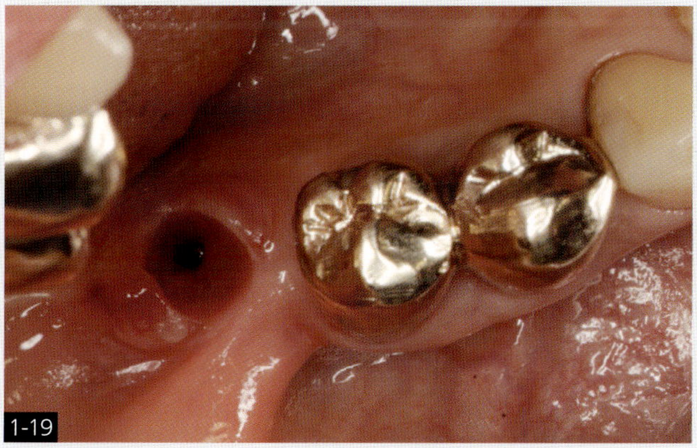
1-19

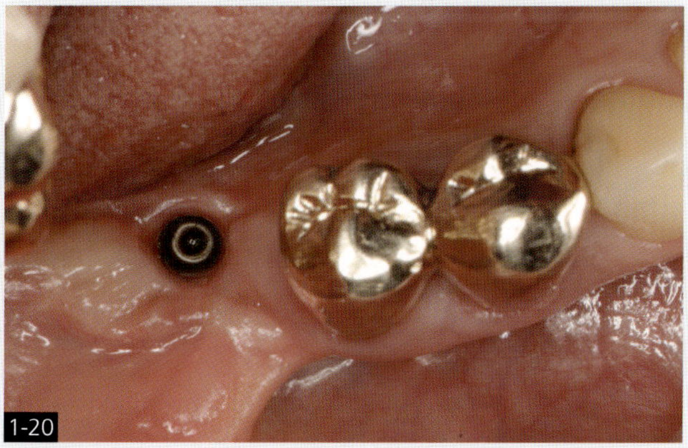
1-20

The condition of the implant before the gingival graft (Figure 1-19) and after the graft (Figure 1-20) shows that peri-implantitis has completely resolved. The treatment concept of creating a defensive barrier to prevent bacterial invasion was successful.

We, as dentists, are well aware that there are too many diverse types of bacteria in the oral cavity, and it is impossible and inadvisable to eliminate all of them. Therefore, in the treatment of peri-implantitis, we should apply the concept of creating a defensive barrier to prevent bacterial invasion rather than focusing solely on eliminating bacteria.

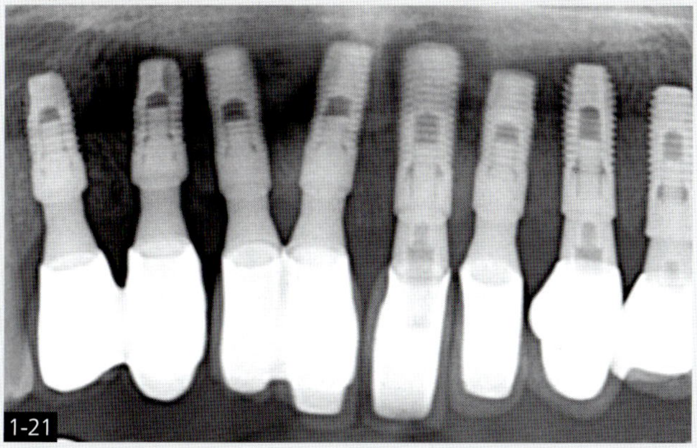
1-21

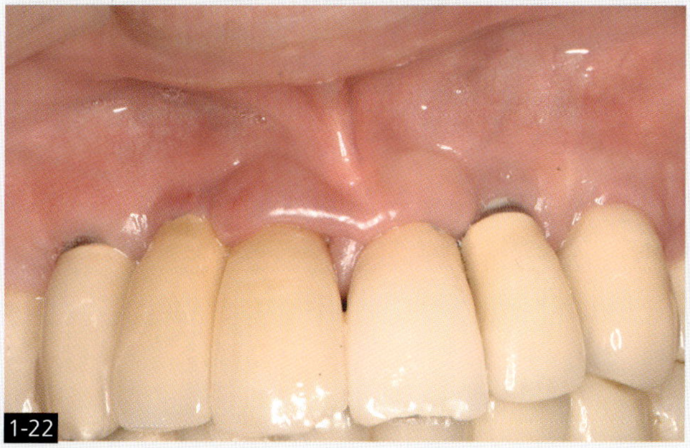
1-22

Based on my clinical experience, placing too many implants in close proximity can lead to poor clinical outcomes. However, when teeth are sequentially lost due to periodontitis, procedures like those shown in Figures 1-21 and 1-22 become necessary.

In the case of implant 11, administering antibiotics temporarily reduced inflammation, but once the antibiotic treatment ended, the inflammation recurred immediately. It is not feasible to administer antibiotics to a patient for life. Therefore, a fundamental treatment addressing the causes of inflammation, rather than merely controlling bacteria, is essential.

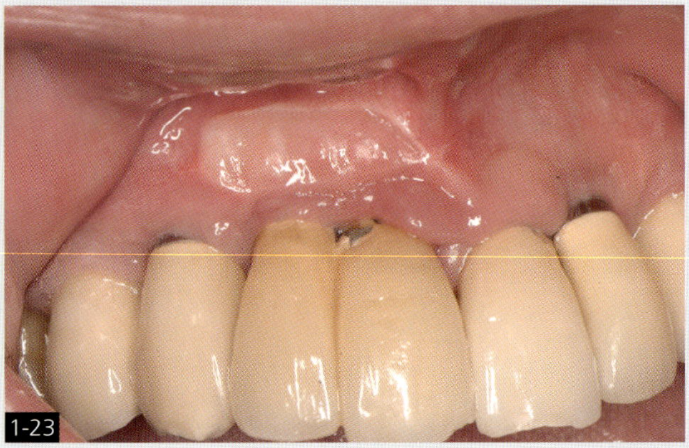

In this patient, the limitations of bacterial removal methods led to the decision to perform a gingival graft. Gingiva was grafted beneath the marginal gingiva to block bacterial invasion. Although the infection of the marginal gingiva did not heal, the spread of further infection was prevented by the grafted gingiva **(Figure 1-23)**.

2. Types of Implants and the Gingiva

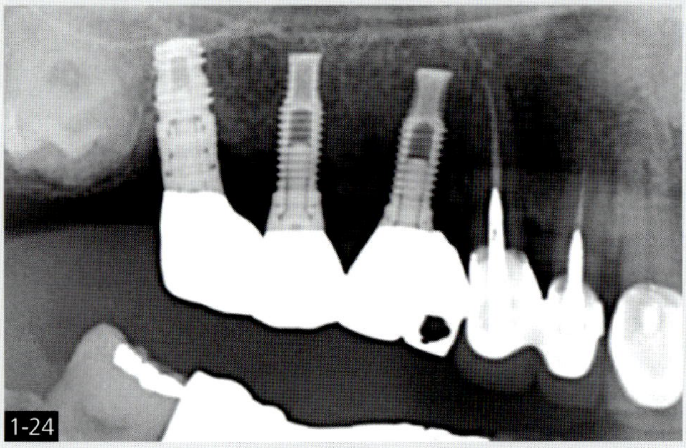

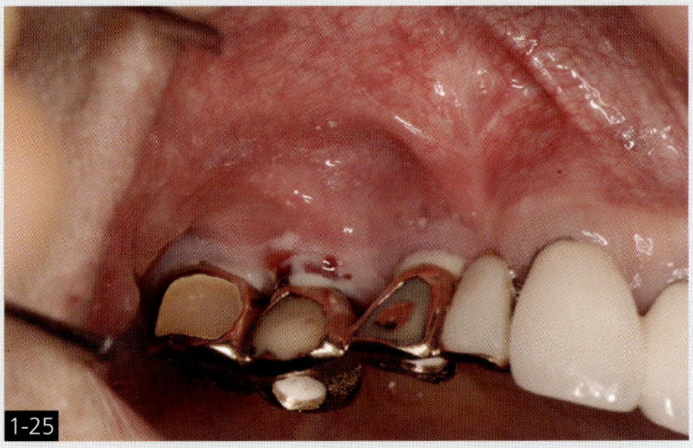

In the area where an external connection type implant was placed **(Figure 1-24)**, pus was observed being discharged **(Figure 1-25)**, indicating the presence of peri-implantitis.

Moving away from the assumption that bacteria invaded, it was noted that there was a lack of attached gingiva on the buccal side. I concluded that a gingival graft was necessary.

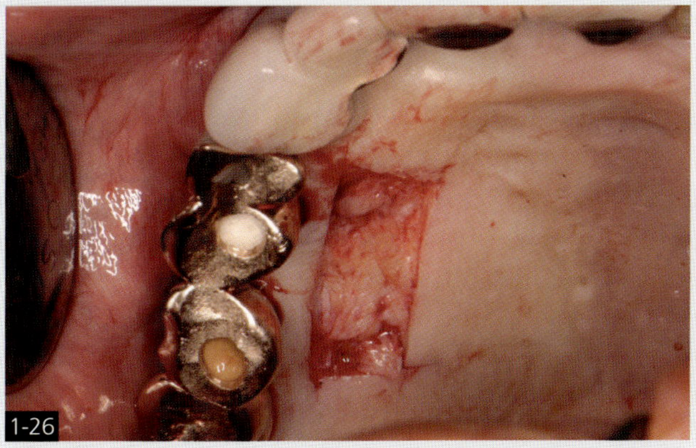
1-26

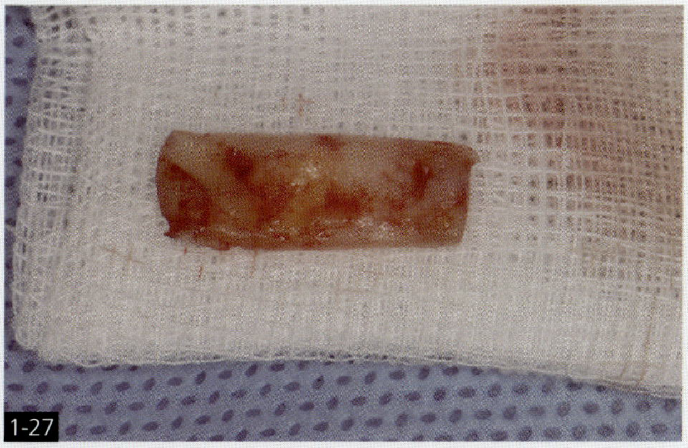
1-27

Gingiva was harvested from the palatal side. The harvesting site **(Figure 1-26)** and the harvested gingiva **(Figure 1-27)** are shown.

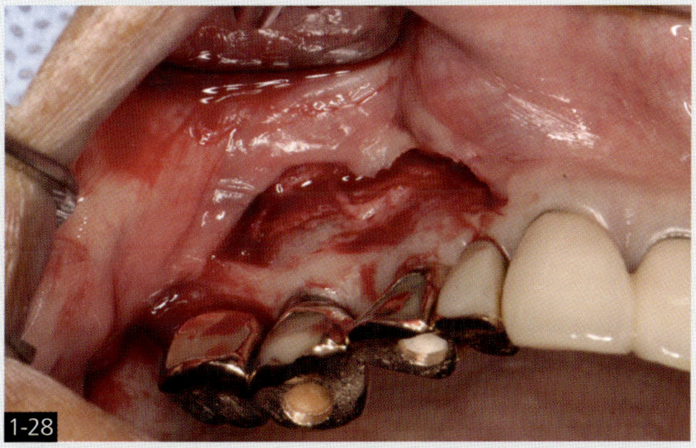
1-28

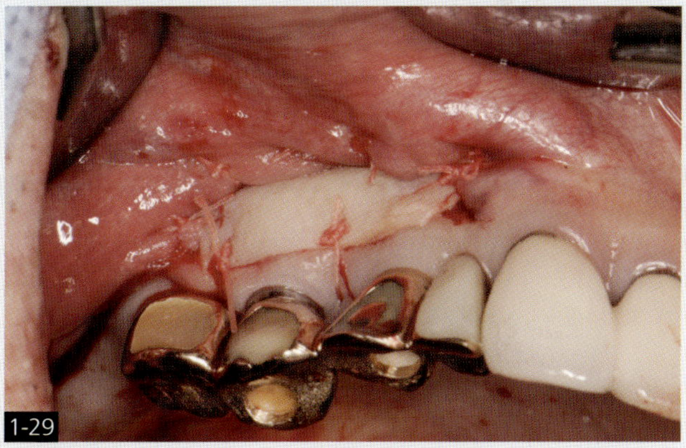
1-29

A partial layer of the recipient site was formed on the buccal side of the implant with peri-implantitis **(Figure 1-28)**, and gingiva was grafted **(Figure 1-29)**.

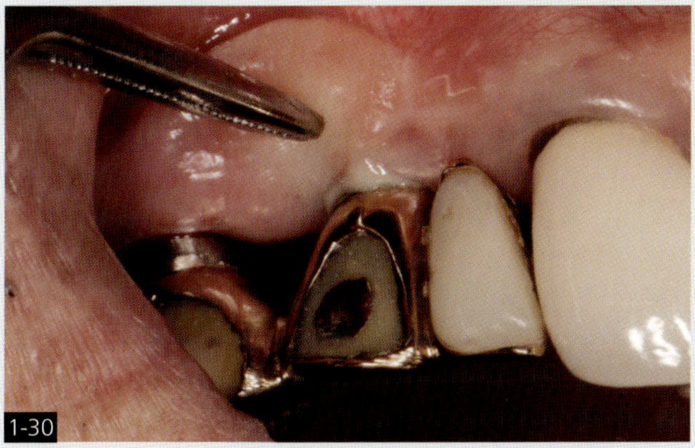
1-30

Despite a successful gingival graft, when the gingiva was lightly compressed, pus was observed being discharged, indicating that peri-implantitis was not completely resolved **(Figure 1-30)**.

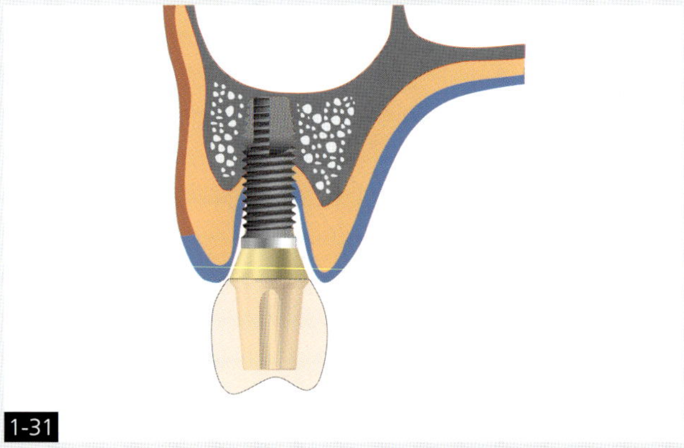

1-31

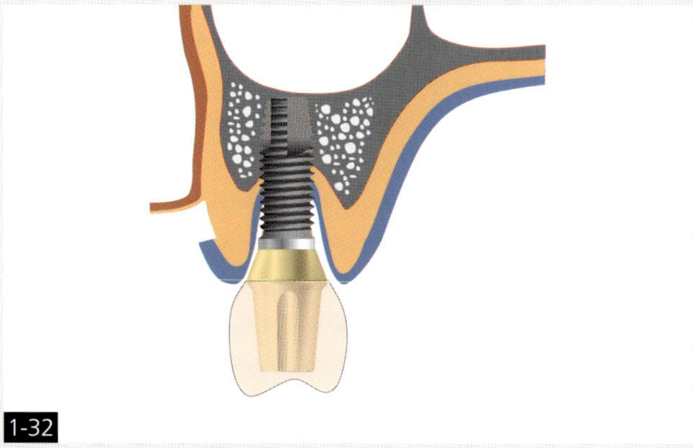

1-32

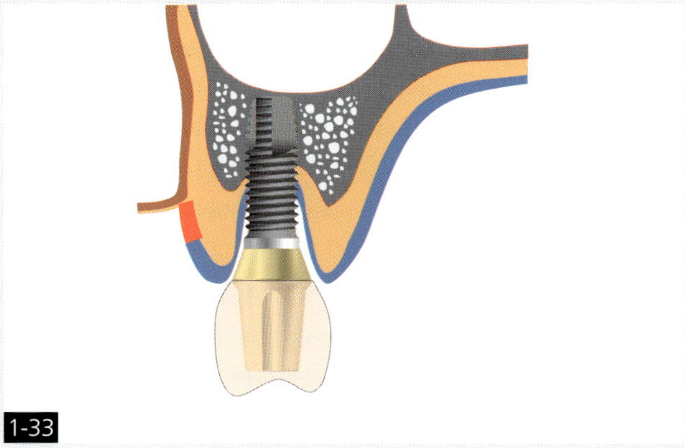

1-33

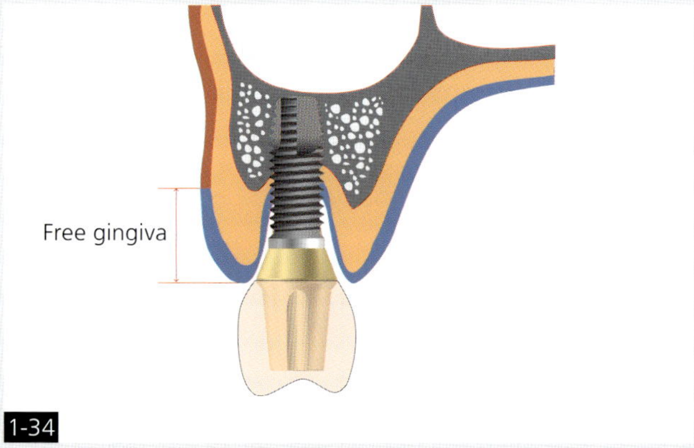

1-34

External connection type implants are associated with marginal bone loss. This marginal bone loss converts attached gingiva into free gingiva (this will be explained in detail later). Thus, although a gingival graft was performed in this case, the grafted tissue became free gingiva rather than attached gingiva, which presented some limitations. To aid in understanding this case, graphic representations are provided **(Figures 1-31~34)**.

Initially, there was no alveolar bone beneath the grafted gingiva. In other words, although mucosa was removed and gingiva was grafted, the absence of alveolar bone beneath the grafted tissue meant that the grafted gingiva could not effectively serve as a barrier against bacterial invasion, functioning instead as free gingiva, which is less effective at preventing bacterial encroachment. Implants should be surrounded by gingiva to defend against bacterial invasion. Attached gingiva provides the best protective effect, while free gingiva does not possess complete defensive capabilities.

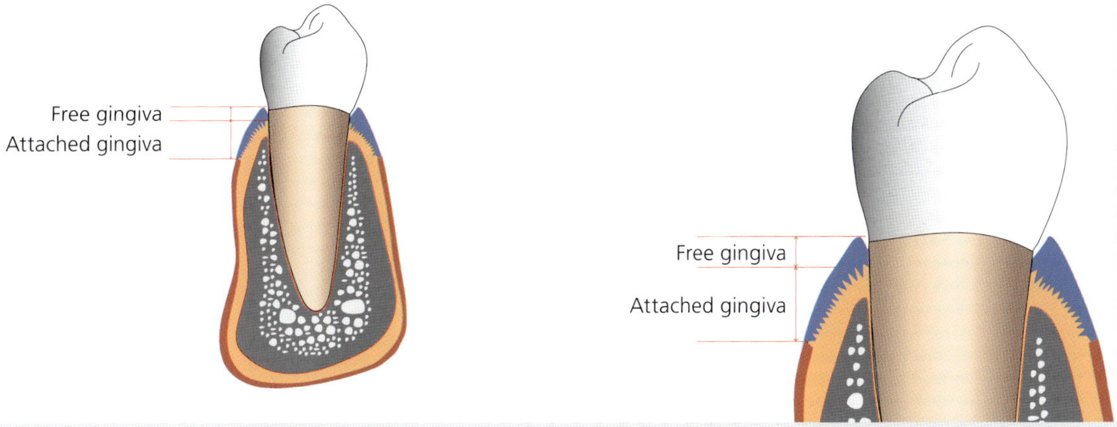

1-35

In natural teeth, the gingiva is histologically divided into free gingiva and attached gingiva **(Figure 1-35)**. Free gingiva indicates that it is separated, while attached gingiva means it is adhered to something. Specifically, as shown in **Figure 1-35**, attached gingiva is attached to the tooth root and alveolar bone.

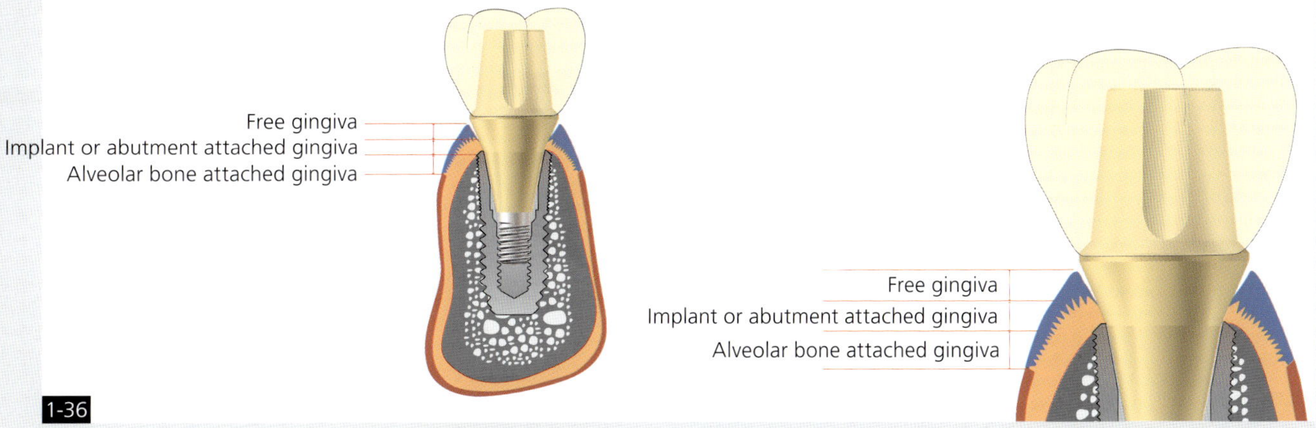

1-36

It is also necessary to examine the gingiva around implants. The gingiva around implants can be divided into attached gingiva and free gingiva **(Figure 1-36)**. Unlike natural teeth, the attached gingiva in implants is attached to the alveolar bone and the abutment or fixture **(Figure 1-36)**.

The part corresponding to the root of natural teeth is the upper part of the abutment and fixture. In natural teeth, the gingiva is strongly attached to the root via Sharpey's fibers, but such structures do not exist in implants. Therefore, the upper part of the attached gingiva (attached gingiva of the abutment or fixture) is mechanically vulnerable in protecting the underlying alveolar bone. For the attached gingiva to function effectively in its role, it must be bone-attached gingiva, which requires the absence of alveolar bone loss.

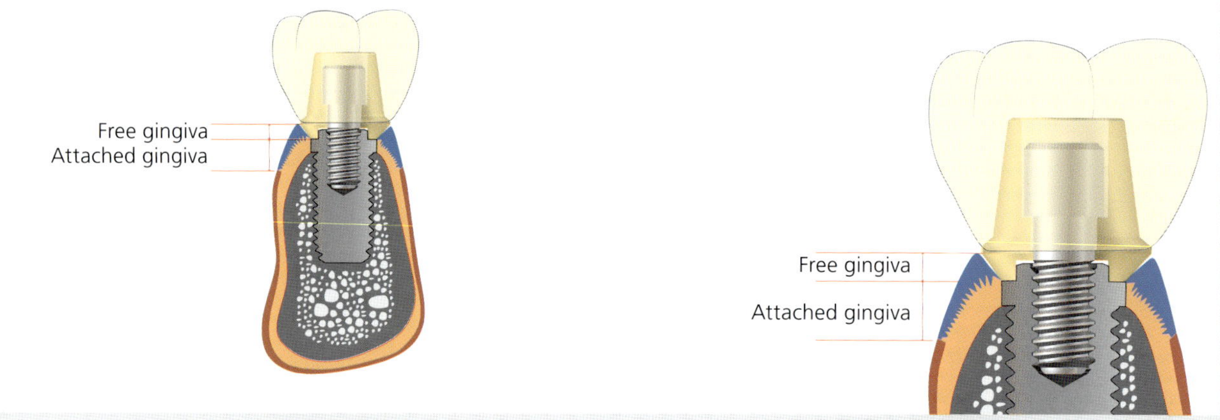

1-37

In the case of external connection type implants, as shown in the figure, the attached gingiva and free gingiva are distinguished, with attached gingiva further divided into bone-attached and implant (fixture) or abutment-attached portions **(Figure 1-37)**.

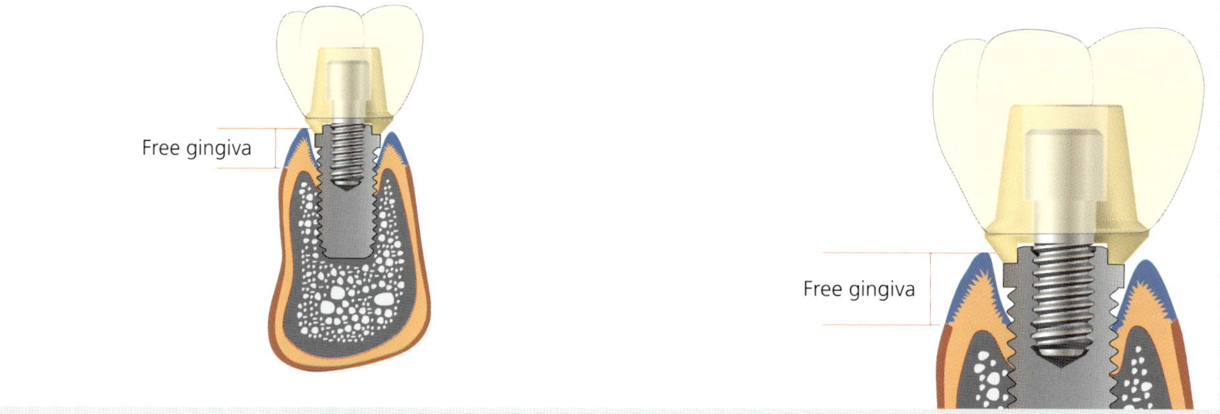

1-38

External connection type implants often exhibit marginal bone loss after being subjected to occlusal loading **(Figure 1-38)**. This phenomenon is frequently cited as a reason why excessive occlusal forces lead to alveolar bone loss and peri-implantitis. Marginal bone loss may stabilize after a certain point or may progress at a rate of 0.2 mm per year. Most experts consider this bone loss a physiological response.

However, marginal bone loss transforms attached gingiva into free gingiva, which diminishes its role in preventing bacterial invasion. Depending on the condition of the gingiva, marginal bone loss can lead to gingival recession and deepen periodontal pockets. Regardless of the outcome, marginal bone loss results in negative clinical consequences in peri-implant tissues.

3. Implant Bucco-Lingual Position and Gingiva

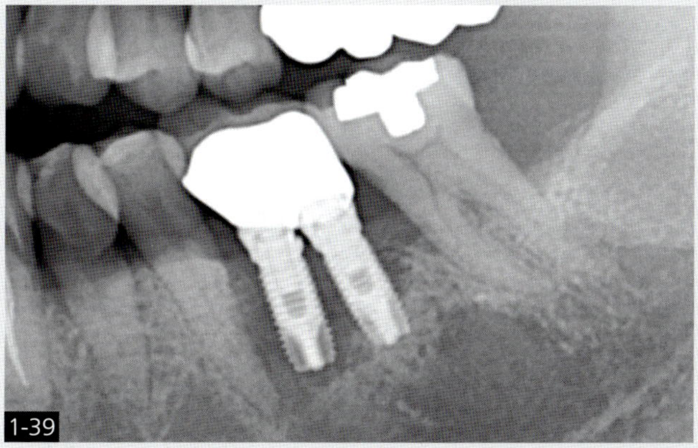
1-39

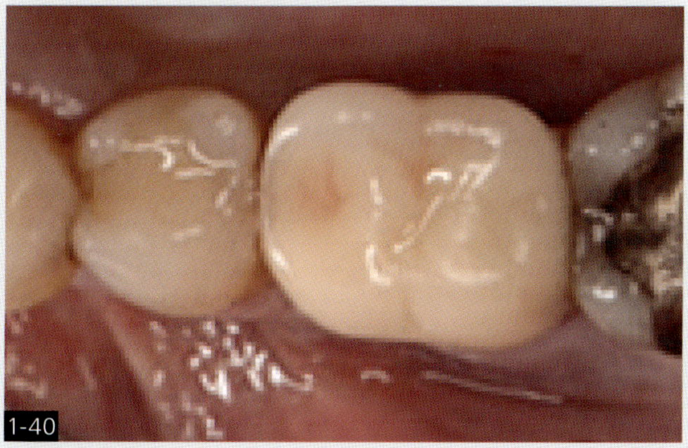
1-40

Two implants placed in the area of tooth 36 developed peri-implantitis **(Figures 1-39, 40)**. While it may be easy to attribute this to bacterial invasion, this explanation alone is insufficient. There are many clinical cases where peri-implantitis does not occur, despite the presence of bacteria.

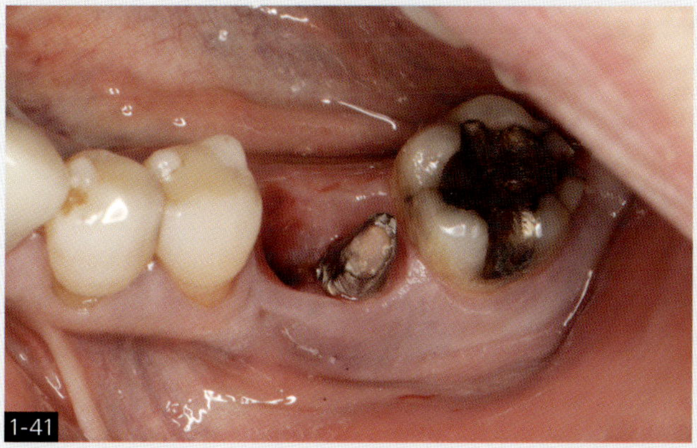
1-41

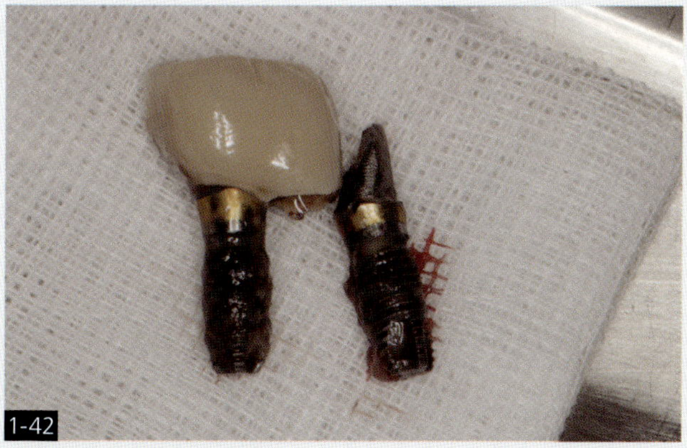
1-42

Due to severe peri-implantitis, the implants were removed. As seen in **Figure 1-41**, the implants were positioned significantly buccally. There is not much active discussion regarding the optimal positioning of implants in relation to the buccal-lingual axis. I believe that inflammation arises from implants positioned excessively buccally, which may seem like an absurd claim but warrants careful consideration.

The implant (fixture) can be likened to a boat floating in a river. If the boat drifts to the right side of the river, there will be less water on the right and more on the left. Similarly, if the implant is positioned buccally, the amount of buccal gingiva decreases. Conversely, if the implant is positioned lingually, the amount of lingual gingiva will decrease. Therefore, implants should ideally be placed in the center of the gingiva. In clinical practice, it is common for the center of the gingiva on the buccal-lingual axis not to align with the center of the alveolar bone. When implants are placed at the center of the buccal-lingual axis of the alveolar bone, they often end up being positioned buccally in relation to the gingiva, particularly in the maxilla.

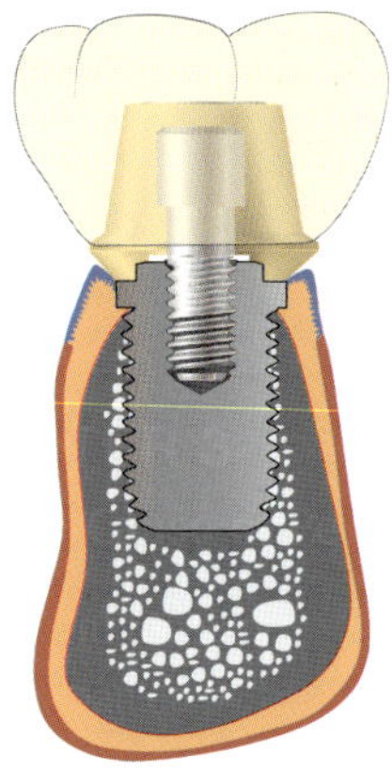
1-43

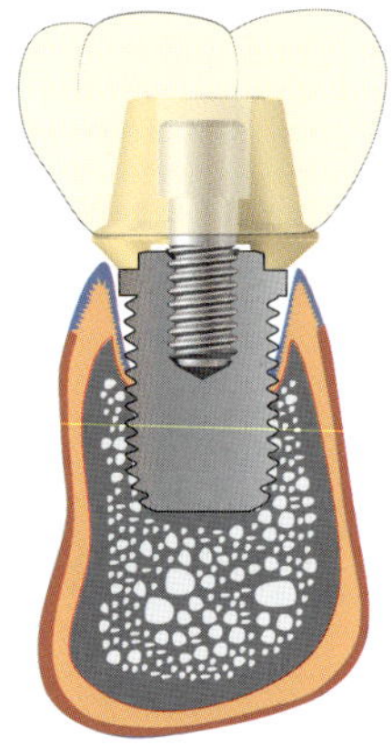
1-44

Wide implants (fixtures) have the advantage of being mechanically resistant to fracture. However, from a periodontal perspective, this can be detrimental. This complicates the decision-making process regarding the diameter of the implants to be placed during surgery. One of the potential complications that must be considered is mechanical fracture. To prevent mechanical fracture, the most effective approach is to place implants with a diameter above a certain threshold. However, this can lead to peri-implantitis. To accommodate larger implants, a larger hole must be created in the alveolar bone, which can result in a thinner remaining alveolar bone thickness. Postoperatively, this thinner alveolar bone tends to resorb rapidly. Such bone loss can convert attached gingiva into free gingiva or even lead to complete gingival loss. Additionally, it can shallow the vestibule depth **(Figures 1-43, 44)**.

While there is general agreement on the necessity of positioning implants within the alveolar bone, there is still ongoing debate regarding their placement within the width of the gingiva. In determining the diameter of the implant during surgery, it is essential to consider not only the width of the alveolar bone but also the width of the gingiva and the depth of the vestibule. Therefore, it is often advantageous to select abutments with a smaller diameter.

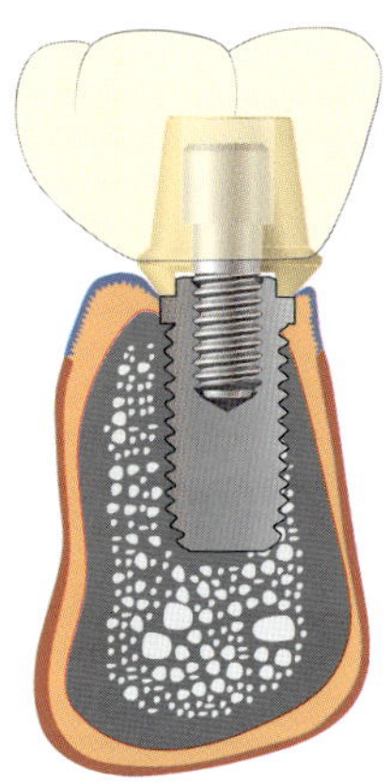
1-45

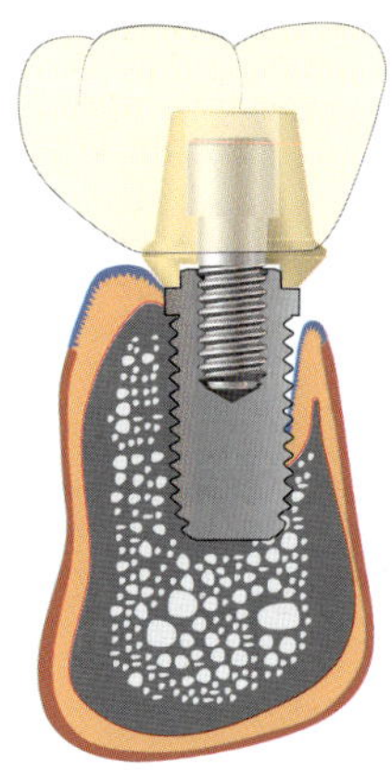
1-46

Similarly, implants that are placed off-center can lead to comparable outcomes. Implants positioned towards the buccal side can cause resorption of the buccal alveolar bone, resulting in the loss or conversion of the buccal attached gingiva into free gingiva, which compromises the protective barrier against bacterial invasion **(Figures 1-45, 46)**. The peri-implantitis observed in **Figure 1-41** is not merely a result of bacterial invasion but rather an iatrogenic consequence of the clinician placing the implant too buccally. From a preventive standpoint regarding peri-implantitis, dental practitioners should strive to position implants centrally within the gingiva. Two primary factors can be identified as causes of gingival issues: first, the use of implants that are prone to marginal bone loss; and second, the placement of implants that deviate significantly from the center of the gingiva, either towards the buccal or lingual sides, or the placement of excessively large implants.

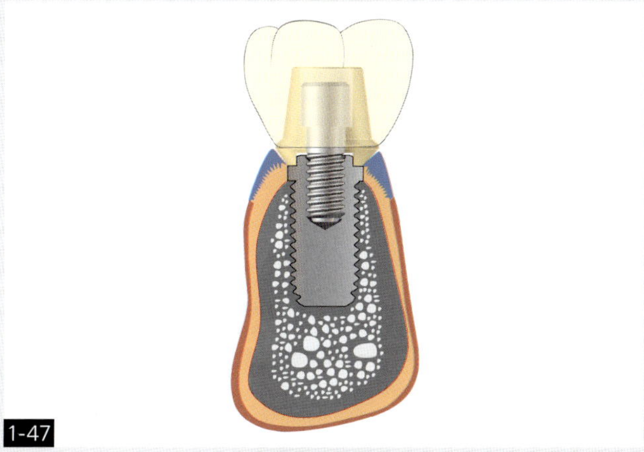
1-47

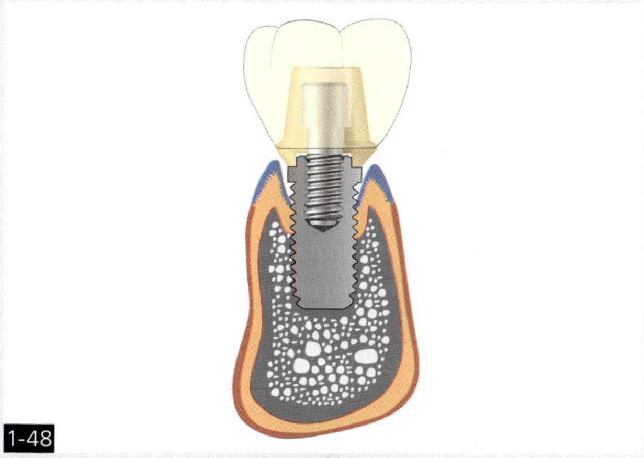
1-48

External connection type implants are generally associated with marginal bone loss. Even if this bone loss stabilizes after a certain extent, it can lead to significant damage to the gingiva, resulting in the loss of attached gingiva or its conversion to free gingiva, which is critical for preventing bacterial invasion. Therefore, I consider such marginal bone loss to be pathological rather than physiological **(Figures 1-47, 48)**.

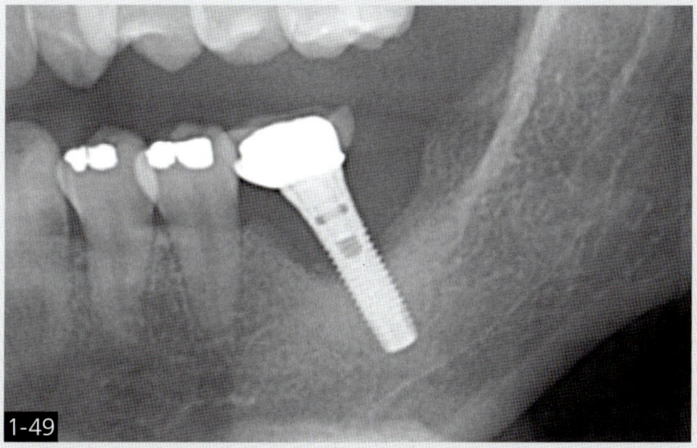
1-49

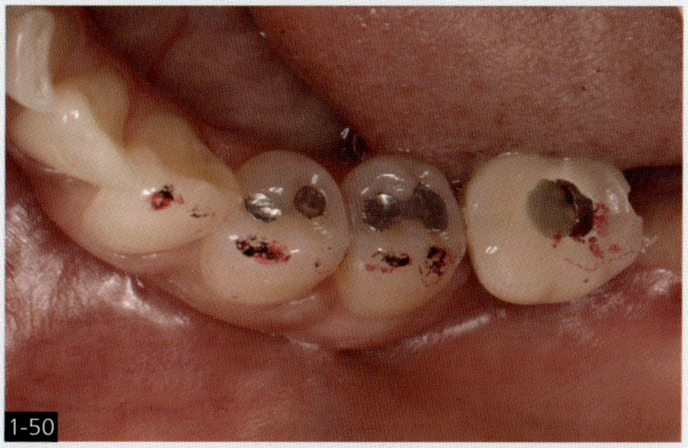
1-50

The clinical case presented shows that although the implant was centrally positioned in relation to the buccal and lingual aspects, the absence of buccal gingiva creates a scenario similar to that of an implant positioned buccally

(Figures 1-49, 50). Despite attempts to graft bone in the area of bone loss due to peri-implantitis, all grafts subsequently failed.

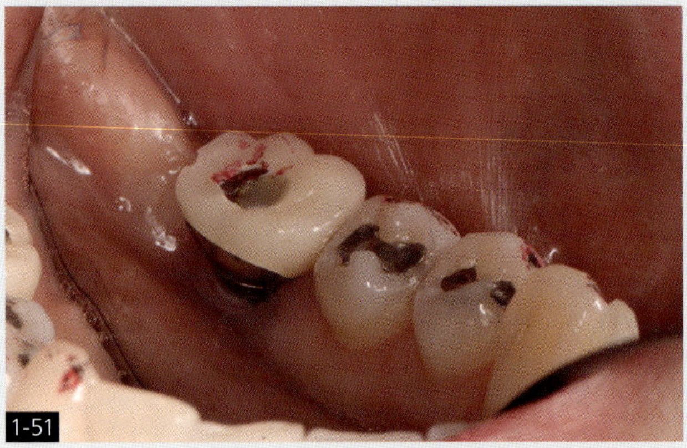

1-51

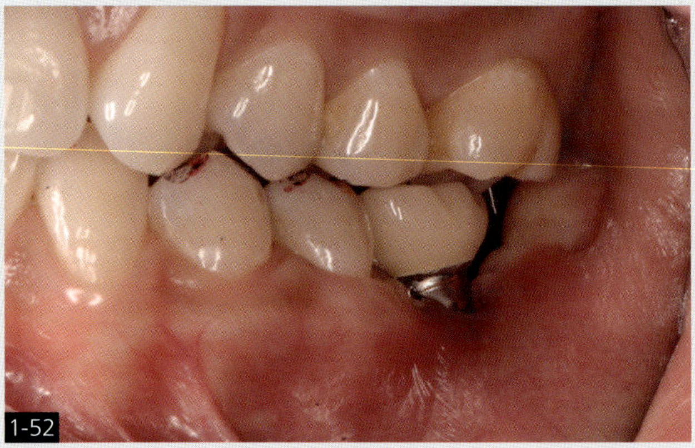

1-52

Observing the lingual and buccal aspects reveals the underlying cause **(Figures 1-51, 52)**. It is evident that there is no gingiva present on the buccal side of the implant. The loss of gingiva, which serves to prevent bacterial invasion, has allowed for the occurrence of peri-implantitis. Had there been an effort to establish attached gingiva to prevent bacterial invasion prior to bone grafting, it is likely that a better outcome would have been achieved.

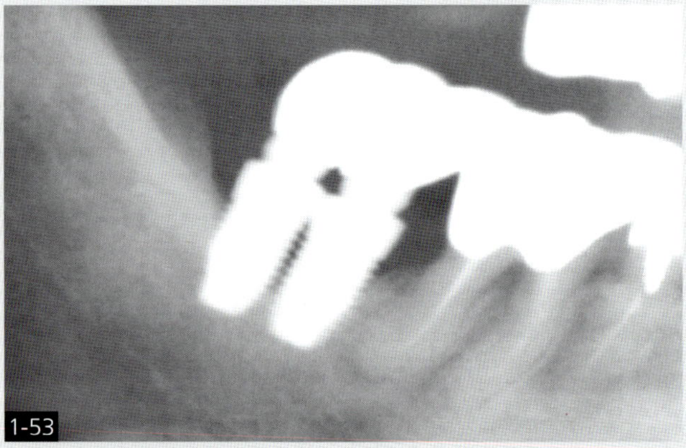

1-53

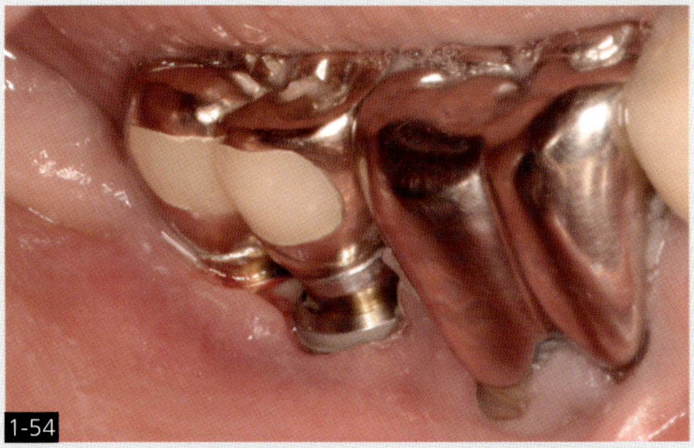

1-54

I believe that the readers' perspective has now expanded from a focus on bacteria to include considerations of gingiva. In cases of peri-implantitis **(Figures 1-53, 54)**, readers may now also observe the absence of attached gingiva and the shallow vestibule. It remains unclear whether the gingiva was originally absent or lost following the implant procedure, but it can be speculated that the placement of excessively wide implants is a significant contributing factor to gingival loss.

The placement of wide implants effectively displaces the implant both buccally and lingually, resulting in the loss of gingiva on both sides.

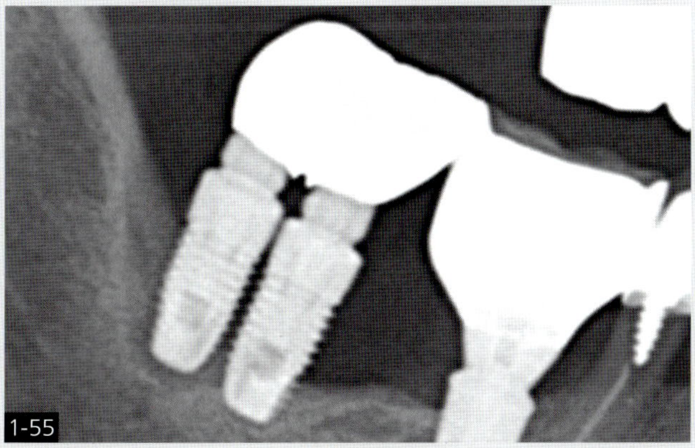

1-55

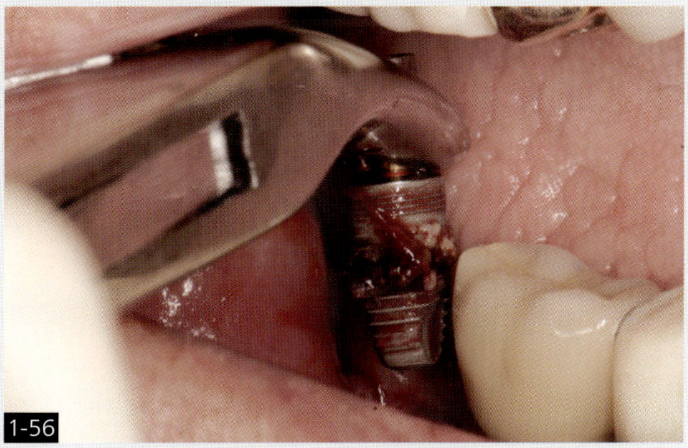

1-56

Peri-implantitis rarely resolves spontaneously and often leads to the removal of the implant **(Figures 1-55, 56)**.

The placement of excessively wide implants should be avoided. It is evident that wide implants cannot be placed when the alveolar bone is thin; however, caution should also be exercised regarding the placement of wide implants when the width of the gingiva is narrow. If it is essential to place a wide implant considering occlusal forces, I believe that in addition to alveolar bone grafting, gingival grafting should also be considered.

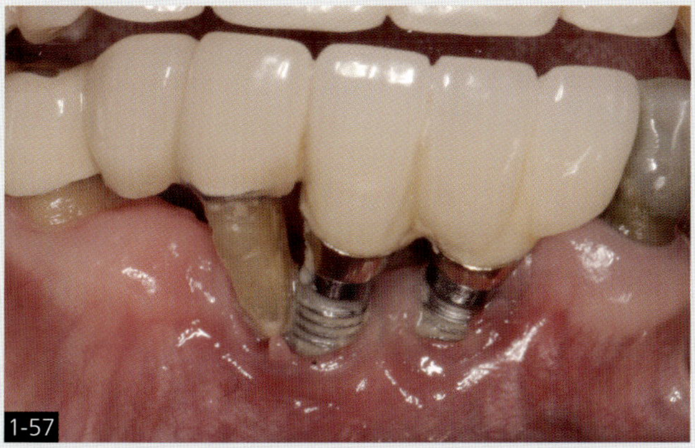

1-57

It can be observed that there is no gingiva on the buccal side, which suggests that peri-implantitis may have occurred due to bacterial invasion **(Figure 1-57)**. A product that causes marginal bone loss was implanted, and such marginal bone loss likely led to gingival loss, creating an environment conducive to bacterial invasion. It is also necessary to consider iatrogenic causes. The positioning of the implant on the buccal side is one of the contributing factors to this outcome.

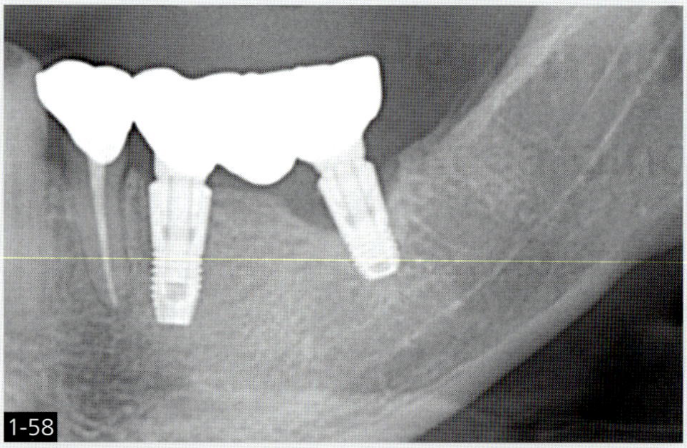

1-58

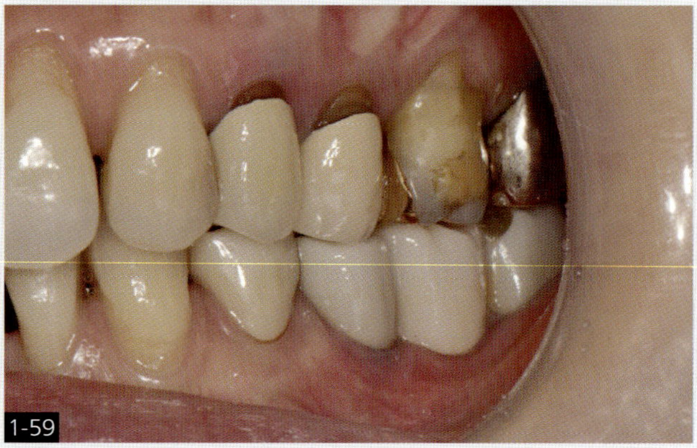

1-59

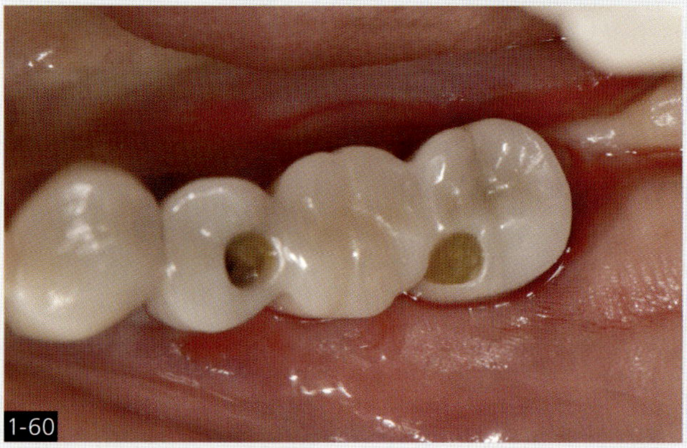

1-60

The patient is a relative of a well-known junior colleague who referred them to me **(Figures 1-58~60)**. As I specialize in periodontology, I was asked to resolve the issue of peri-implantitis that had arisen. The patient complained of mild pain and discomfort. While the cause can be attributed to bacteria and the patient's inadequate oral hygiene, blaming the patient does not resolve the issue. After contemplating the long-term prognosis of the implant, I would like to emphasize that the most critical factors in implant prognosis are not the patient's factors but rather the choice of product, the periodontal concepts applied during placement, and the prosthetic concepts used to complete the restoration—specifically, the product's factors and the dentist's factors.

As shown in **Figure 1-60**, it is evident that implant number 37 was placed excessively buccally. Given that nothing could be done with the implant in this position, I decided to remove it and re-implant it lingually.

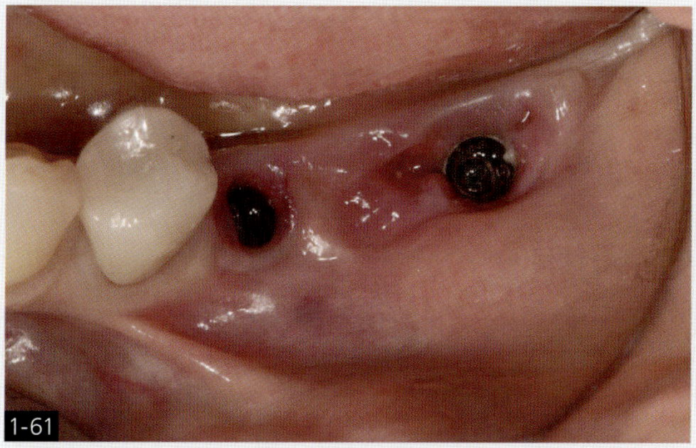

1-61

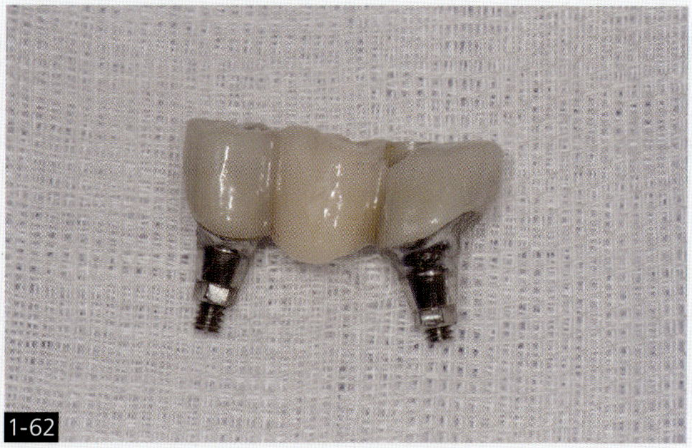

1-62

After the removal of the prosthesis, it can be seen that there is no gingiva on the buccal side of implant number 37 **(Figures 1-61, 62)**. This suggests that the cause of peri-implantitis was not due to bacterial invasion but rather the placement of the implant on the buccal side, which eliminated the buccal protective barrier. Alveolar bone grafting and buccal gingival grafting can create a protective barrier against bacterial invasion. However, such procedures are extremely challenging in the mandibular molar region. Grafting gingiva in the absence of a vestibule is nearly impossible.

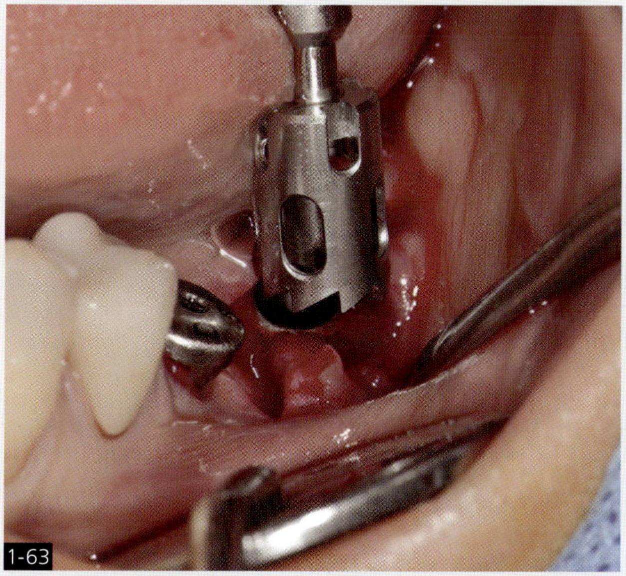

1-63

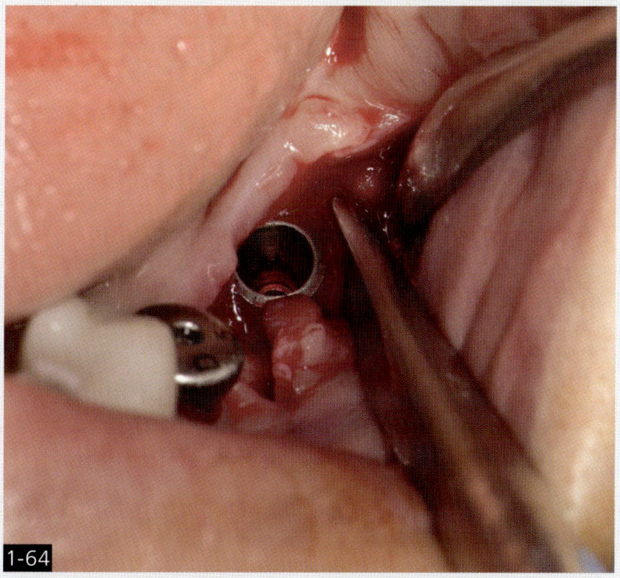

1-64

Implant number 37 is an Astra implant with a diameter of 5.0 mm and a length of 9 mm. Therefore, a trephine drill with an inner diameter of 5.0 mm and an outer diameter of 6.0 mm was prepared and used **(Figures 1-63, 64)**. When using a trephine drill, it is not necessary to remove alveolar bone for the entire length of the implant. Although the drilling did not reach the full length of the implant, if the extraction instrument can mobilize the implant, it can be sufficiently removed. Care must be taken not to drill too deeply and injure important anatomical structures. If the extraction instrument cannot mobilize the implant, it may be necessary to drill a little deeper **(Figure 1-64)**.

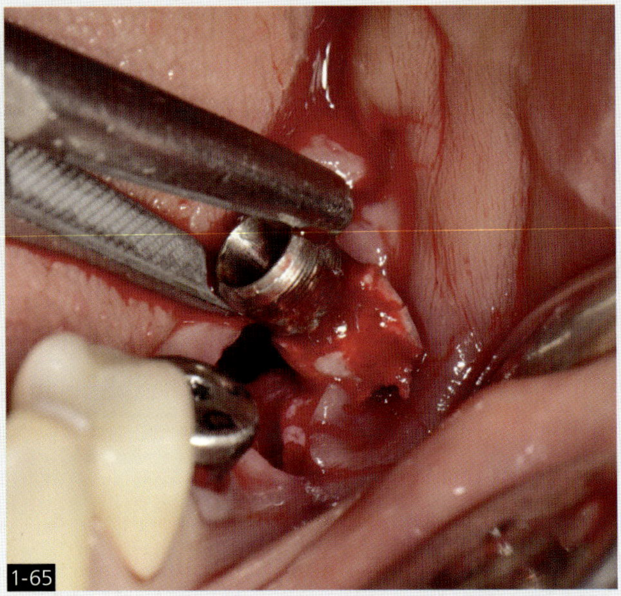

1-65

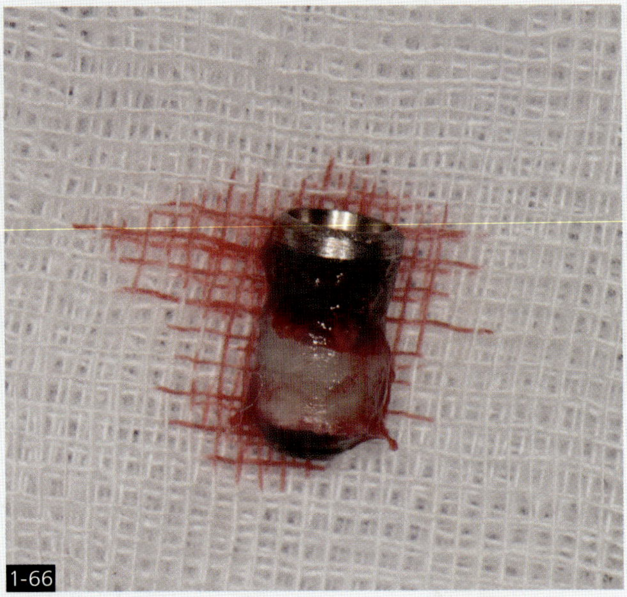

1-66

The images show the alveolar bone being removed with the trephine drill and the implant being extracted. Significant marginal bone loss can be observed **(Figures 1-65, 66)**.

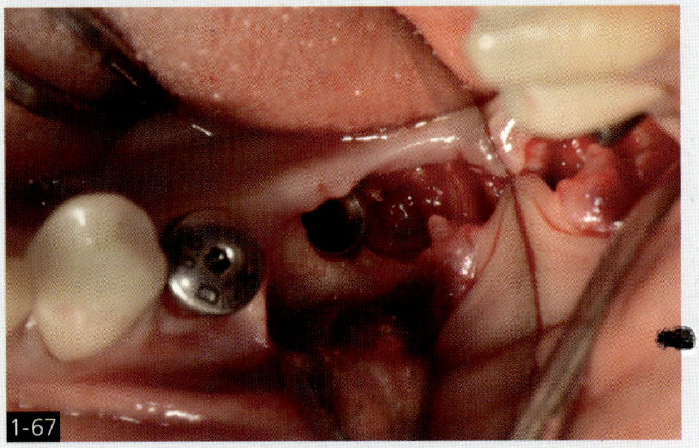

1-67

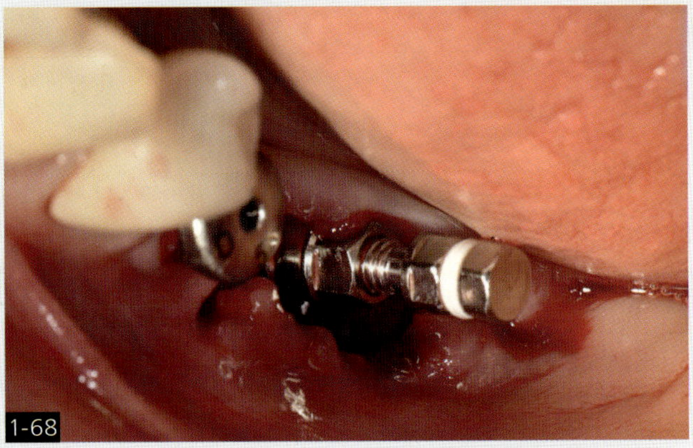

1-68

After drilling slightly mesially and lingually from the site of the removed implant, a new implant was placed. Since excessively wide implants negatively affect the gingiva, a domestic product with a diameter of 4.5 mm and a length of 8 mm was used for the new placement. As seen in **Figures 1-67 and 1-68**, the new implant was placed slightly more lingually than the removed implant (the slight buccal-lingual positioning can determine the occurrence of peri-implantitis).

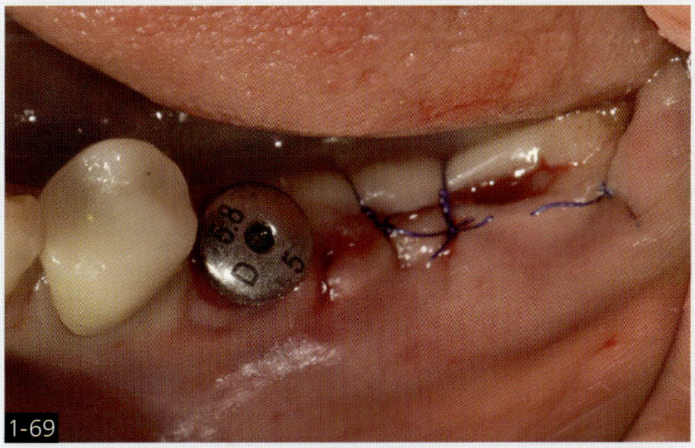
1-69

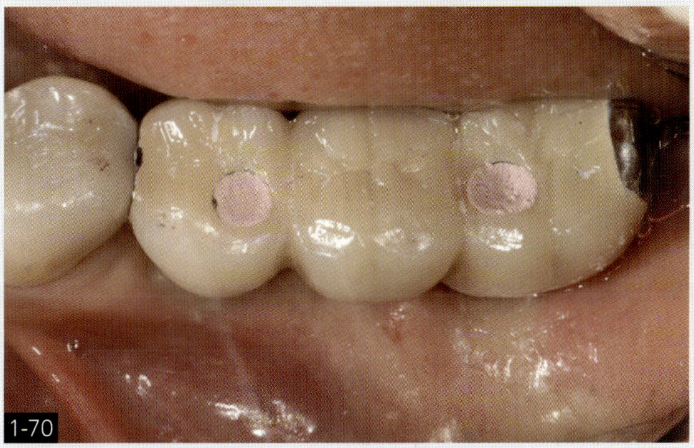
1-70

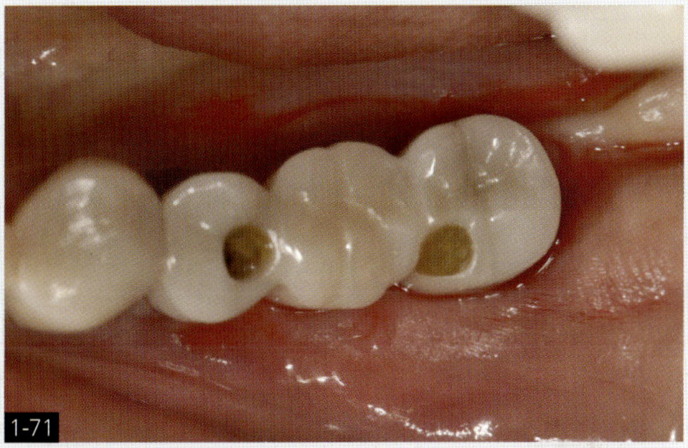
1-71

Compared to the previous prosthesis, it can be observed that the screw hole of implant number 37 has shifted significantly more lingually **(Figures 1-70, 71)**. The implant was also placed lingually, and the angle of the implant was inclined lingually to ensure that the screw hole of the prosthesis was centrally located.

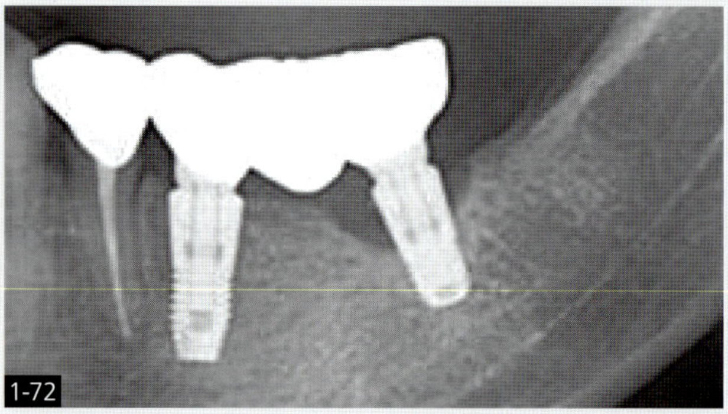

2019-10-21

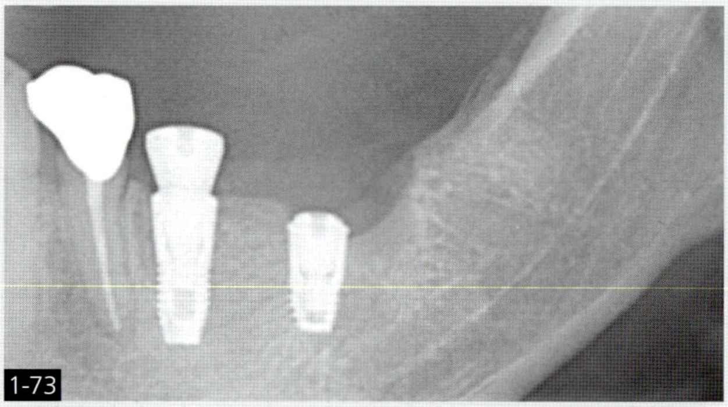

2019-10-31

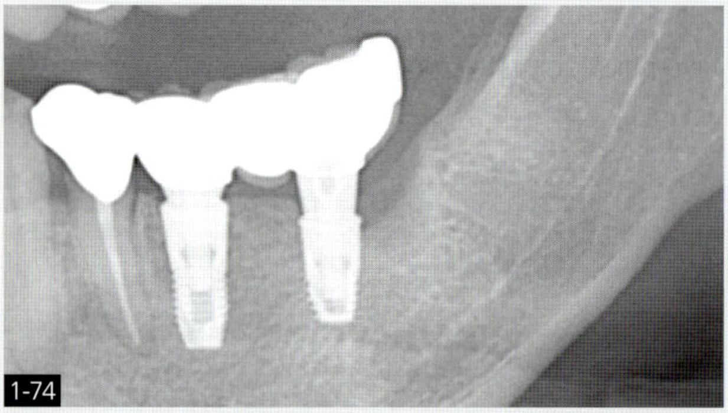

2020-1-9

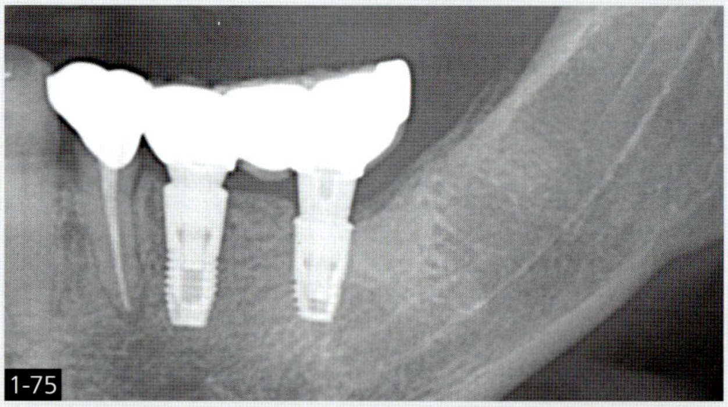

2020-10-15

Figures 1-72 to 1-75 illustrate the changes in alveolar bone throughout the treatment process. There are misconceptions that implants with micro-threads cause bone resorption. Although a micro-threaded implant was used, it can be observed that the alveolar bone gradually increased. (I believe that micro-threads significantly contribute to the increase of alveolar bone.)

The treatment of peri-implantitis typically involves the removal of inflamed tissue, cleaning of contaminants from the implant surface, and alveolar bone grafting. However, I resolved the issues simply by surgically relocating the implant to a more lingual position. Although the centrifugal portion of the newly placed implant number 37 was exposed, no alveolar bone grafting was performed. Remarkably, one year post-surgery, X-rays showed that the alveolar bone had completely recovered. I hope this case emphasizes to readers the importance of the buccal-lingual positioning of implants. I believe that most intraosseous defects will heal spontaneously, so there is no need to focus the surgery on bone grafting for the defect.

Another clinical case illustrates how crucial the buccal-lingual positioning of implants is. A patient who had undergone implant surgery at another clinic came to my office.

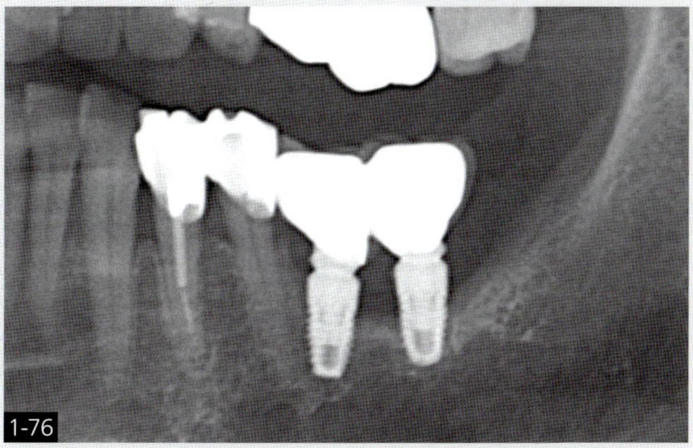
1-76

In the upper radiograph, significant alveolar bone loss can be observed in the areas of implants 36 and 37 **(Figure 1-76)**. Although Astra-type implants (fixtures) were placed, which typically do not result in bone loss or may even lead to increased marginal bone, peri-implantitis has developed.

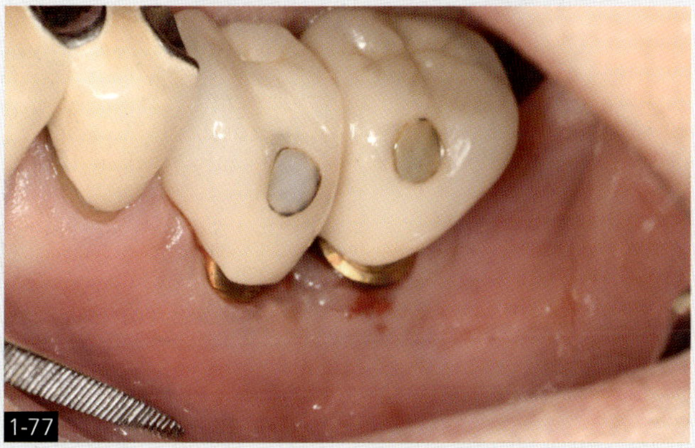
1-77

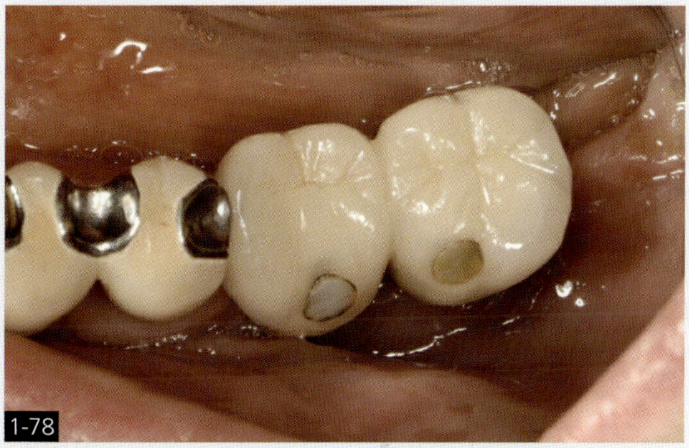
1-78

It is evident that the implants were placed buccally, and there is no attached gingiva on the buccal side **(Figures 1-77, 78)**. I have developed a habit of predicting that if I see marginal bone loss, the implant was likely placed buccally.

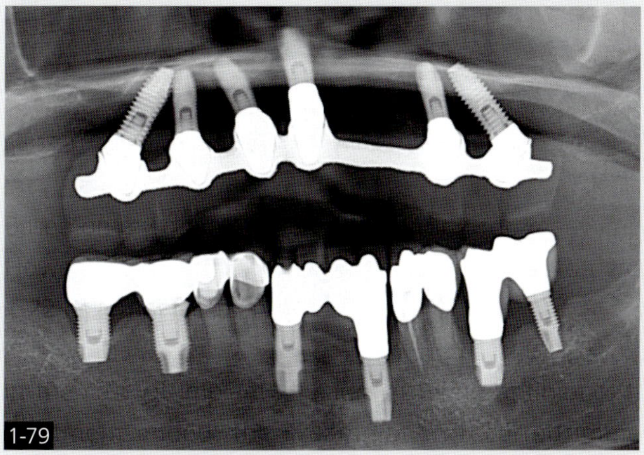
1-79

Let's examine another clinical case **(Figure 1-79)**. I continue to present similar types of cases to emphasize that the placement of implants buccally and the occurrence of peri-implantitis are not coincidental events.

Severe loss of alveolar bone around the maxillary implants can be observed. The mandibular area is also experiencing progressive marginal bone loss. While it may be tempting to attribute this solely to bacterial infection, the reality is more complex.

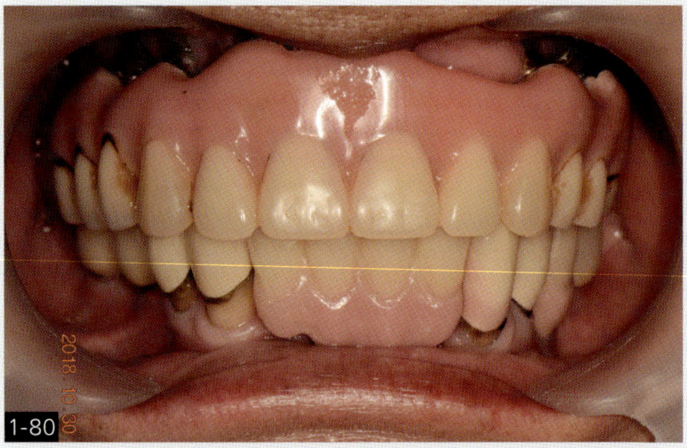

1-80

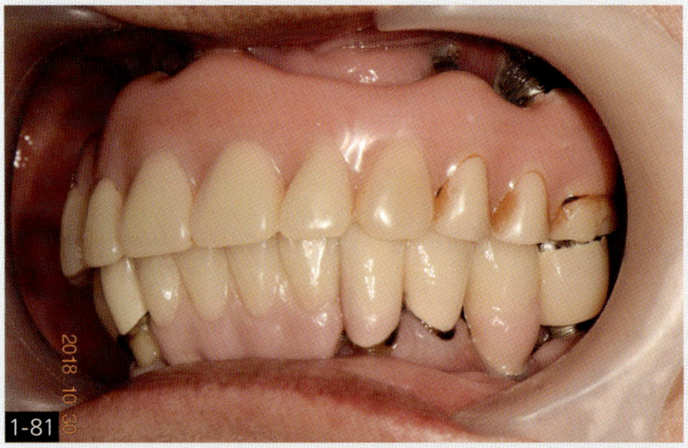

1-81

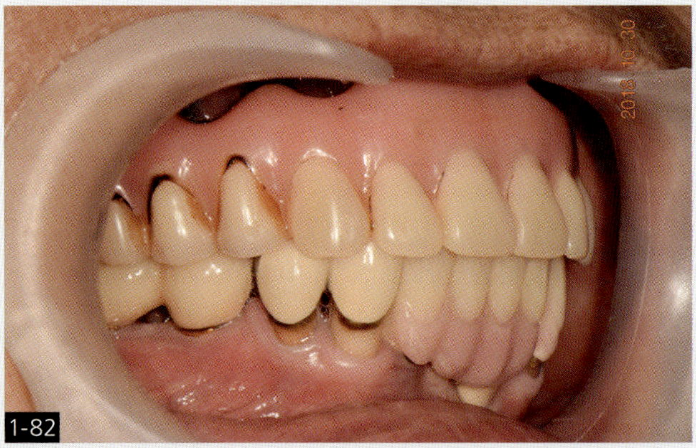

1-82

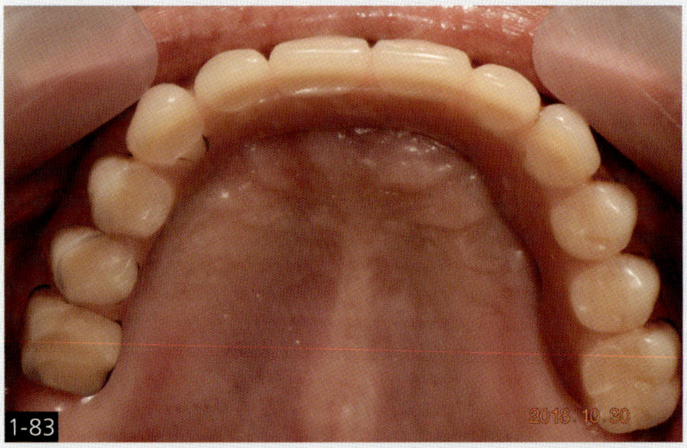

1-83

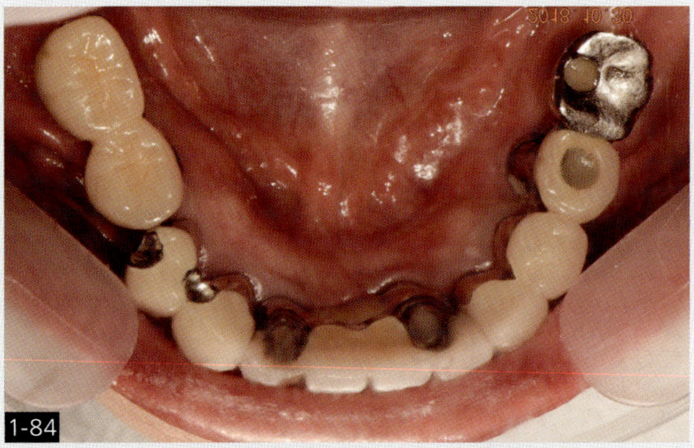

1-84

In the case of the maxilla, I believe there are also issues with the prosthetic design. If the implants in the maxilla had been splinted together with a denture placed on top, the outcome might have been better. Since the implants in the oral cavity were restored individually and then a denture was placed on top, the occlusal forces were not evenly distributed across all implants, which I believe contributed to the failure **(Figures 1-80~84)**.

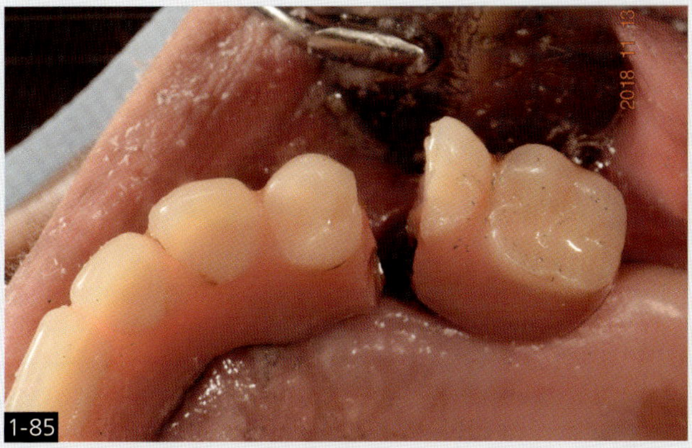
1-85

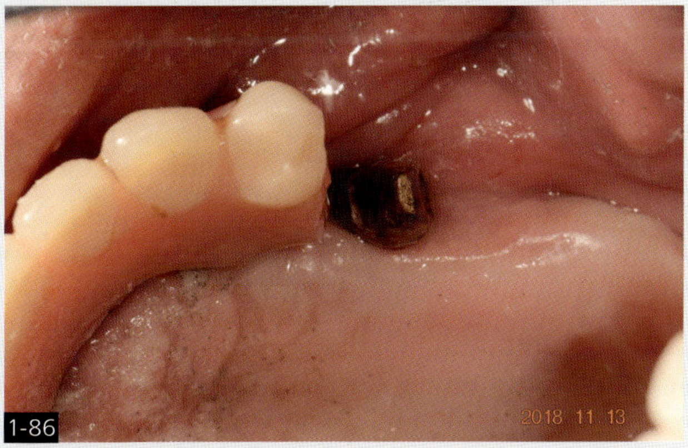
1-86

Since the patient needed to chew and engage in social activities, it was not feasible to remove all implants at once and perform simultaneous re-implantation surgery. Therefore, I proceeded by removing part of the denture and only the implants in that area for re-implantation **(Figure 1-85)**. It can be seen that the implants were severely placed buccally **(Figure 1-86)**. The hole created for implant placement was formed buccally, and the buccal bone was likely very thin, leading to the complete loss of that buccal bone and resulting in the clinical condition observed. If the implant is not placed centrally in relation to the gingiva but rather buccally, it may result in the absence of gingiva on the buccal side. The loss of the thin buccal bone and the resulting loss of gingiva likely allowed for bacterial invasion, leading to the observed outcomes.

It is hard to believe that the dentist responsible for this case intentionally placed the implant buccally. I consider two possible reasons for this. During implant surgery, when the soft tissue is retracted, it is difficult to assess the condition of the gingiva based on the alveolar bone. In other words, it is difficult to determine whether the buccal-lingual position of the implant being placed is within the range of the gingiva or outside of it. The second reason is that, in most cases, the lingual or palatal areas have a higher density of alveolar bone, while the buccal or facial areas have lower density. As a result, when drilling carelessly, the formed hole often shifts buccally or facially from the initially intended position. Therefore, we dentists must closely monitor whether the formed hole shifts buccally or facially during the surgery. This means that we must perform the surgery with care and check at every moment. Over a period of about a year, I placed implants one or two at a time starting from the posterior area, completing the process as shown **(Figure 1-87)**. I positioned the implants centrally in relation to the gingiva, leaving a sufficient amount of alveolar bone and gingiva on the buccal side. Additionally, I refrained from using excessively thick implants. As a result, there has been no further loss of alveolar bone over time. Although there is progressive loss of marginal bone in the mandible that may require re-surgery, the patient has postponed it due to the difficulties experienced during maxillary reconstruction. (I suspect that the excessive diameter of the implants is the cause of the mandibular alveolar bone loss.)

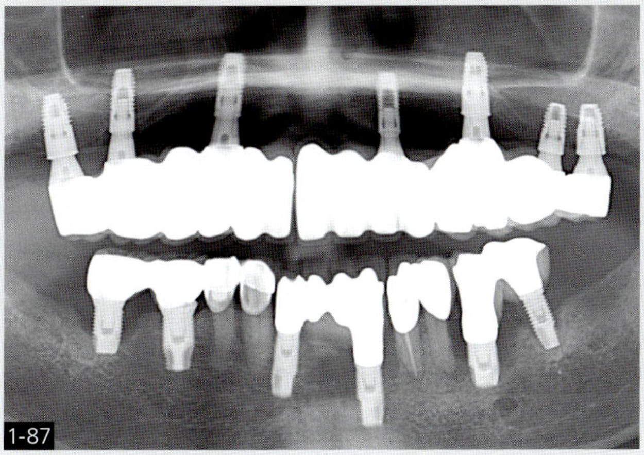
1-87

4. Immediate Implantation Considering Gingiva

I believe that immediate implantation is meaningful to patients for two reasons. First, it shortens the treatment period, and second, it preserves the alveolar bone (especially in areas like the anterior teeth where the width of the alveolar bone is thin).

Academically, it is known that alveolar bone loss occurs consistently regardless of whether immediate implantation is performed, but in actual clinical practice, I feel otherwise. Since it is difficult to predict how much buccal alveolar bone will recede in immediate implants, I strive to place the implant as far lingually as possible within the limits allowed by the lingual gingiva and alveolar bone, as well as the prosthesis. This is to ensure the formation of buccal gingiva and guarantee long-term prognosis.

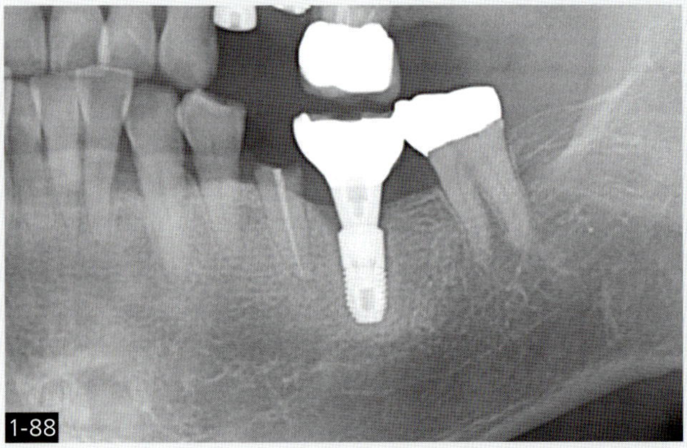
1-88

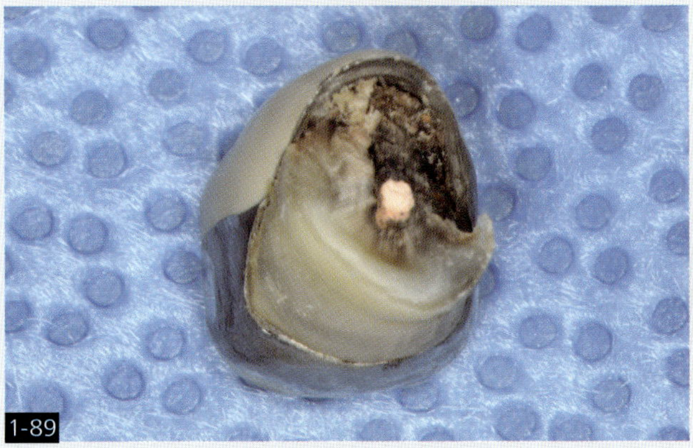
1-89

The patient's tooth number 35 had fractured **(Figures 1-88, 89)**. As seen in the clinical photos, the tooth is not positioned at the center of the gingiva but rather buccally, indicating that the width of the buccal gingiva is narrow **(Figure 1-90)**. Recently, with the widespread use of dental CT, it is possible to examine the relationship between the alveolar bone and the roots before treatment. In most cases, it is common to find that the roots are positioned buccally.

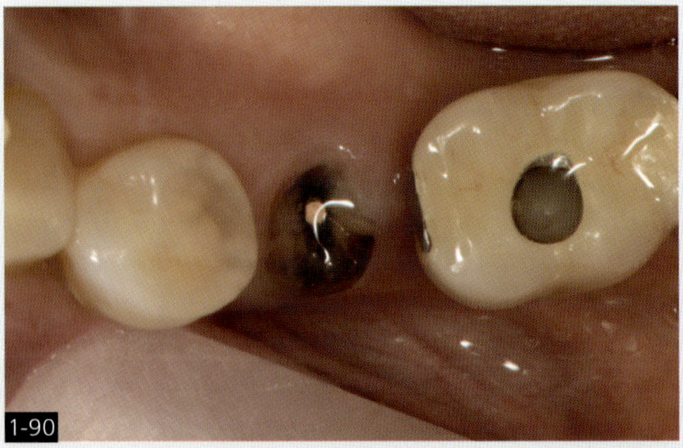
1-90

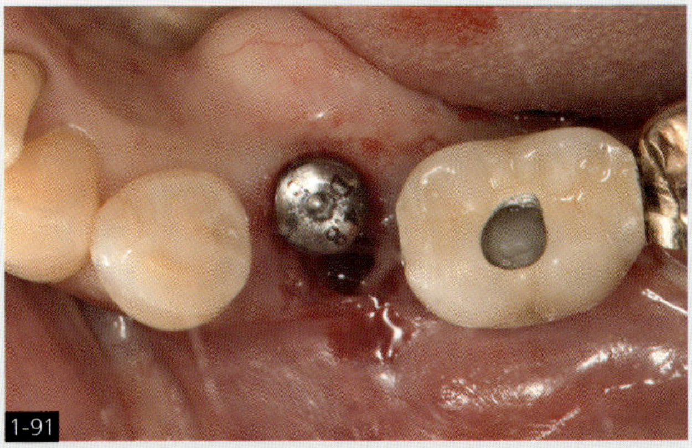
1-91

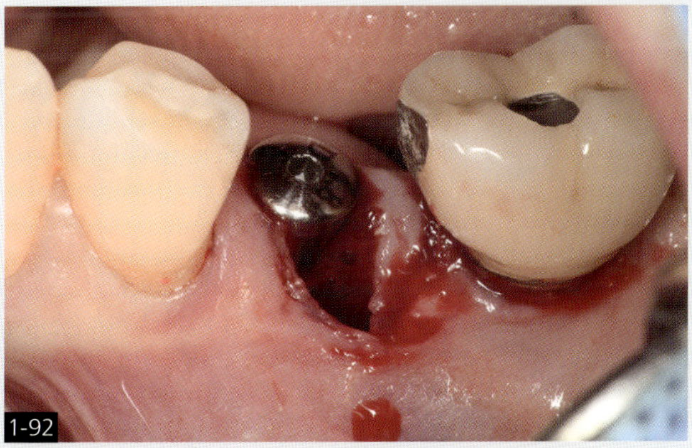

1-92

In such cases, if the implant is placed in the center of the extraction site, there may later be insufficient buccal gingiva, leading to peri-implantitis, so extreme caution is required during surgery. As shown in the figures, the implant should be placed as far lingually as possible within the limits allowed by the prosthetic design **(Figures 1-91, 92)**. The term "within the limits allowed by the prosthetic design" means that the abutment must fit within the crown to be restored. In this case, the angle of the implant placement should be slightly tilted buccally.

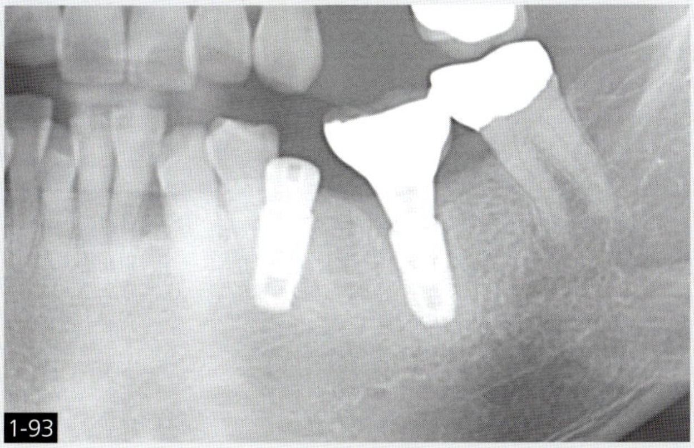

1-93

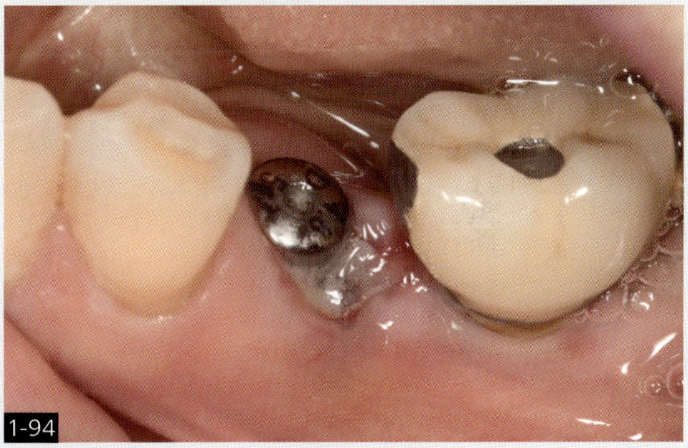

1-94

The implant is not placed in the center of the extraction site but as far lingually as possible, appearing to overlap with the natural tooth in the radiograph **(Figure 1-93)**. **Figure 1-94** shows the condition one week after placement. The space left by the buccal extraction is filled with a blood clot and is in the healing process. This area will eventually heal into gingiva.

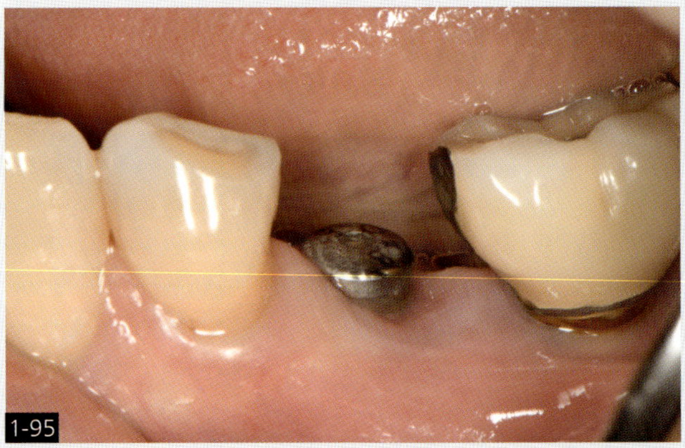

1-95

This is the appearance six weeks post-surgery **(Figure 1-95)**. As predicted, gingiva has formed in the area of the buccal extraction. When performing immediate implantation, the implant should not be placed in the center of the extraction site. As explained earlier, the center of the extraction site is actually shifted buccally within the alveolar bone. Even if it is at the center of the alveolar bone, it is often not the center of the gingiva but rather the buccal side, which increases the likelihood of peri-implantitis if the implant is placed buccally.

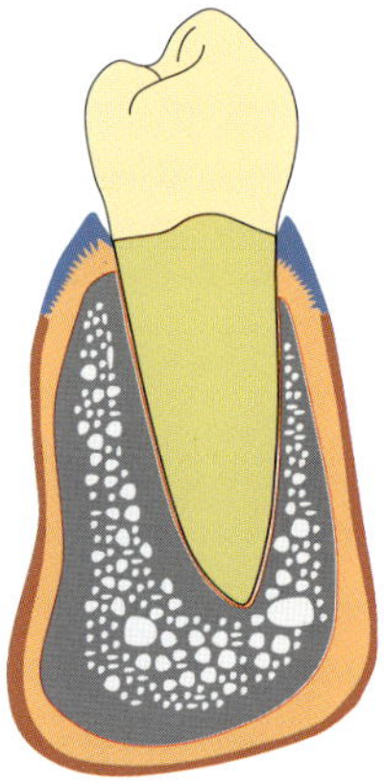

1-96

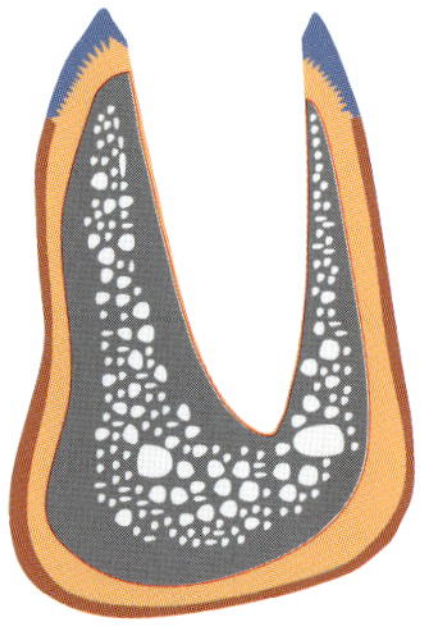

1-97

Even after performing immediate implantation following a CT scan, it is challenging to visualize the shape and position of the extraction site in three dimensions during surgery. In most cases, as shown in **Figure 1-97**, a buccal extraction site will exist.

1-98

If the implant is placed in the center of the extraction site, the buccal alveolar bone may gradually thin out during the healing process, leading to potential problems **(Figure 1-98)**. The loss of alveolar bone itself negatively impacts the long-term prognosis of the implant, but the loss of attached gingiva at the top of the alveolar bone can create even more serious issues in the future.

1-99

If drilling and placing the implant are done on the lingual side rather than in the center of the extraction site, sufficient amounts of alveolar bone and attached gingiva can be secured on the buccal side, thereby ensuring a better long-term prognosis. At this point, a strategy for drilling on the lingual side of the extraction site is necessary **(Figure 1-99)**.

In the preceding discussion, I have emphasized the importance of gingiva, particularly attached gingiva, and the significance of the buccal-lingual position during implant placement surgery. In many cases, practitioners recognize and pay attention to the importance of alveolar bone during implant surgery. However, when considering the long-term prognosis of the implant, gingiva (especially attached gingiva) may be even more critical than alveolar bone. In my practice, when the center of the alveolar bone does not align with the center of the gingiva, I prioritize the center of the gingiva over the center of the alveolar bone. This means that I accept a slight dehiscence in a specific area of the alveolar bone, placing the implant in the center of the gingiva.

Chapter 2

Treatment Surgical Methods for Peri-implantitis

Peri-implantitis is known to be caused by bacteria. These bacteria have been identified as being of the same species that cause periodontitis in natural teeth. Generally, these pathogenic bacteria are anaerobic, and they cannot survive unless a periodontal pocket is sufficiently deep. Therefore, I believe that it is not merely the invasion of bacteria that causes peri-implantitis, but rather that these pathogenic bacteria invade only after anaerobic conditions have been established.

In other words, it is not the bacteria that cause the formation of the periodontal pocket; rather, the pocket forms first, allowing pathogenic bacteria to inhabit and proliferate, leading to damage to the surrounding tissues.

1. Gingivectomy

If bacteria are the cause of peri-implantitis, then theoretically, treatment should be impossible. Additionally, since there are numerous bacteria in the oral cavity, one might expect that all implants would be affected by peri-implantitis, and any treatment would only result in recurrence. However, the reality in the oral cavity is different.

Among the many implanted implants, only a few develop peri-implantitis, and in many cases, treatment is successful without recurrence. Therefore, I believe we cannot simply conclude that the cause of peri-implantitis is bacteria.

We, as dentists, are well aware that we cannot and should not eliminate all the diverse bacteria present in the oral cavity. Thus, I consider not the effort to kill bacteria but rather the concept of a mucosal seal as a defensive barrier. If a lack of gingiva is the cause, then either a gingival graft should be performed, or the implant should be removed and replanted at the center of the gingiva. However, if the gingiva is normal, the situation may be different.

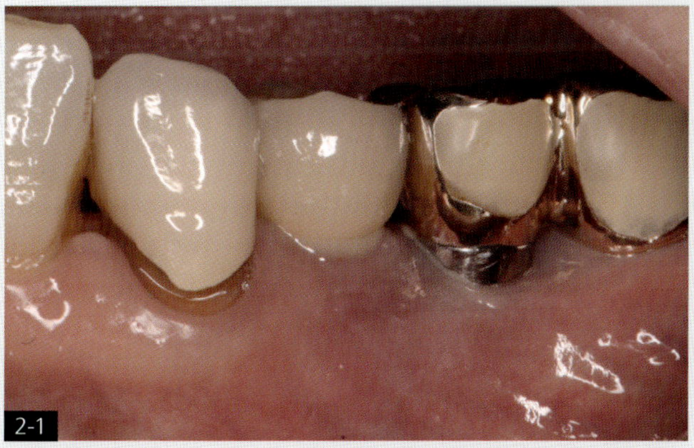
2-1

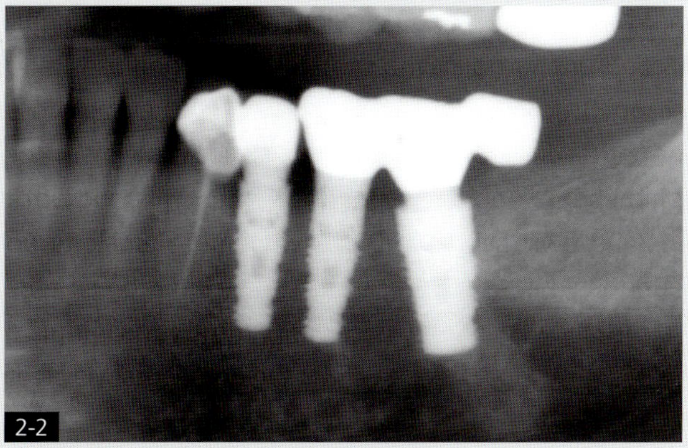
2-2

Peri-implantitis has occurred around implant number 34, with pus observed in the periodontal pocket **(Figures 2-1, 2)**. If we consider bacteria as the cause, we might think of prescribing antibiotics and disinfecting the periodontal pocket. However, such methods do not effectively reduce the bacteria. Once the effect of the medication wears off, pus begins to form again.

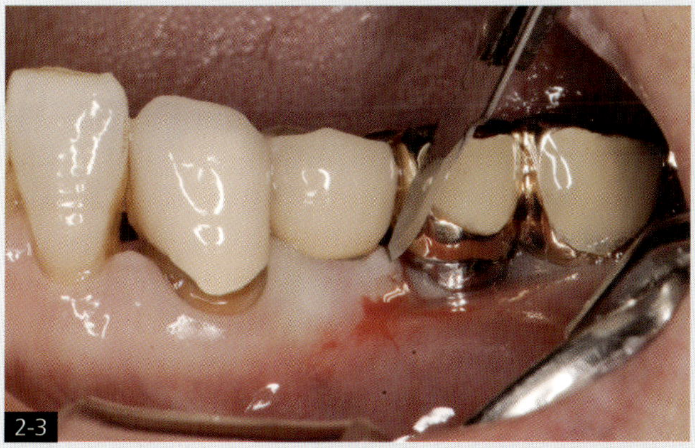
2-3

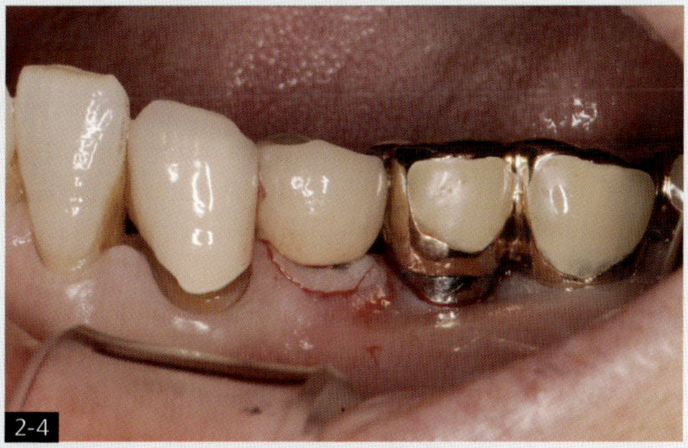
2-4

Since there is no method to eliminate all bacteria, we decided to eliminate the periodontal pocket, which serves as a habitat for pathogenic bacteria. A probing depth of less than 4 mm is referred to as a gingival sulcus, while a depth of 4 mm or more is referred to as a periodontal pocket. When the probing depth exceeds 4 mm, anaerobic conditions are enhanced, leading to an increase in the distribution of pathogenic bacteria. The increased pathogenic bacteria can cause periodontitis or peri-implantitis.

A method to suppress the proliferation of pathogenic bacteria without affecting normal bacteria is to reduce the depth of the periodontal pocket, converting it into a gingival sulcus. After anesthesia, an incision was made for gingival resection **(Figures 2-3, 2-4)**.

This procedure is possible even if some gingiva is removed, provided there is sufficient gingival width. If the gingival width is narrow, the procedure is not feasible.

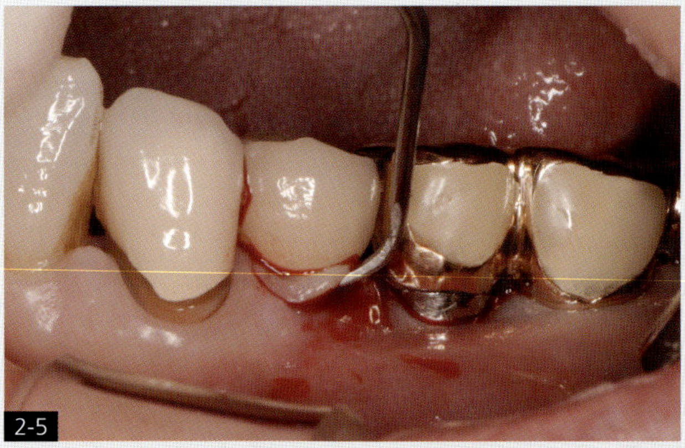

2-5

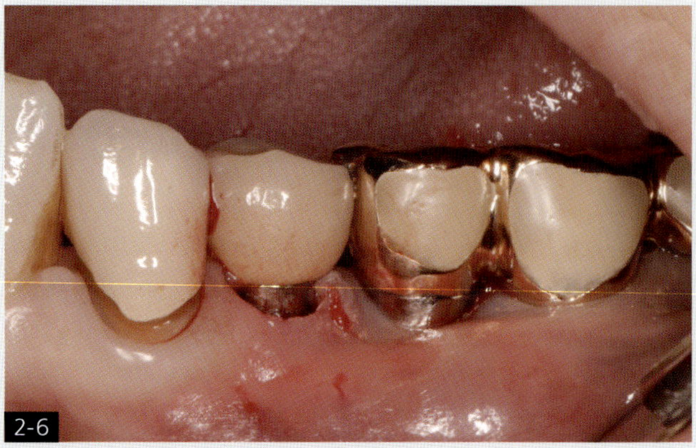

2-6

The incised gingiva was removed using a periodontal curette **(Figure 2-5)**. After the gingiva around implant number 34 was resected, the abutment was exposed **(Figure 2-6)**.

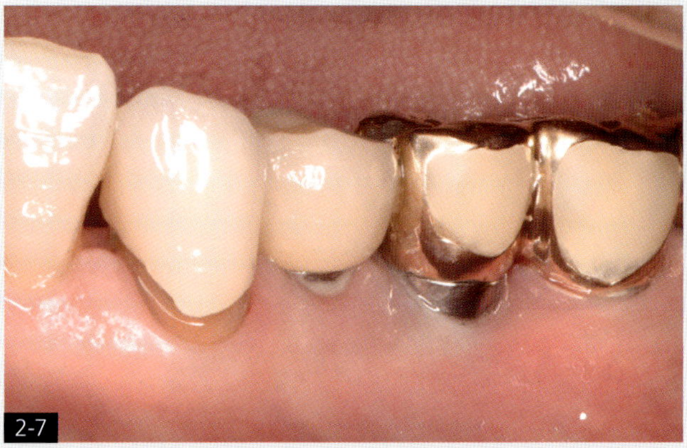

2-7

The healing appearance six weeks post-gingivectomy is shown **(Figure 2-7)**. After converting the periodontal pocket into a gingival sulcus, inflammation did not occur, and peri-implantitis was resolved. Over 15 years have passed, with only one instance of inflammation, and healthy gingiva has been maintained continuously.

I believe that reducing the depth of the periodontal pocket through gingivectomy to suppress the growth of pathogenic bacteria can be one method of treating peri-implantitis. However, this method should only be attempted when there is an abundance of gingiva.

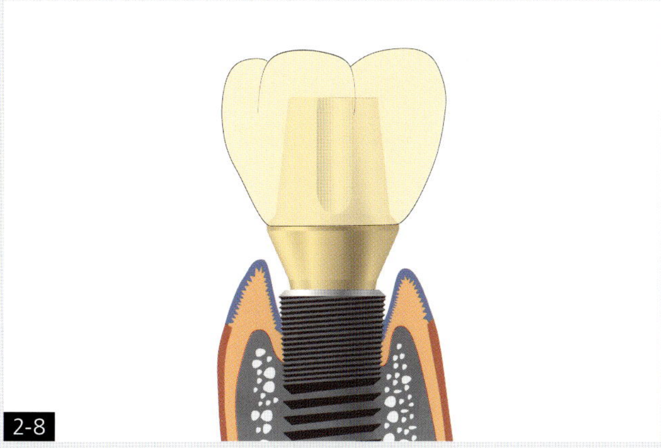
2-8

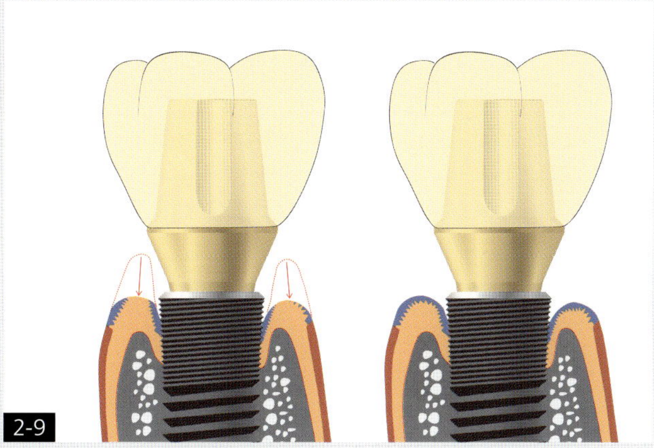
2-9

When the periodontal pocket is deep, there are two methods to reduce it: gingivectomy and re-attachment. Gingivectomy is a very simple method that involves cutting away the marginal gingiva in a state of deep periodontal pockets **(Figures 2-8, 9)**.

The resected marginal gingiva can heal and form and maintain a shallow gingival sulcus. However, in many cases, the resected gingiva may restore to its original appearance, leading to the reformation of the periodontal pocket. When the thickness of the gingiva and alveolar bone is substantial (thick bio-type) and vitality is high, certain patterns may emerge in the context of peri-implantitis.

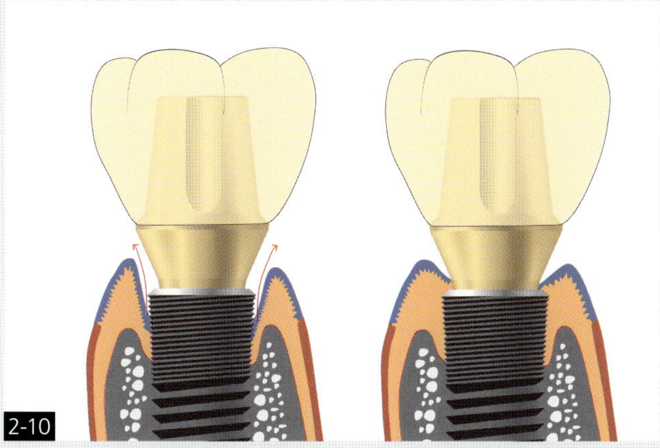
2-10

One method to reduce the depth of the periodontal pocket is to form a re-attachment **(Figure 2-10)**. Achieving re-attachment in natural teeth is nearly impossible because it requires the regeneration of cementum on the root surface, which is extremely challenging.

In contrast, in implants, if the contaminated implant surface is cleaned adequately, re-attachment can be achieved relatively easily, as there is no need for the regeneration of cementum, unlike in natural teeth. In **Figure 2-10**, the position of the epithelial cell attachment has moved from the bottom of the periodontal pocket to a higher position, which is referred to as re-attachment.

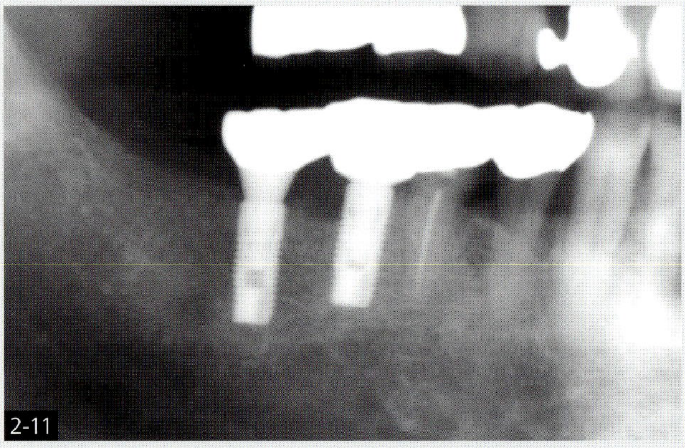
2-11

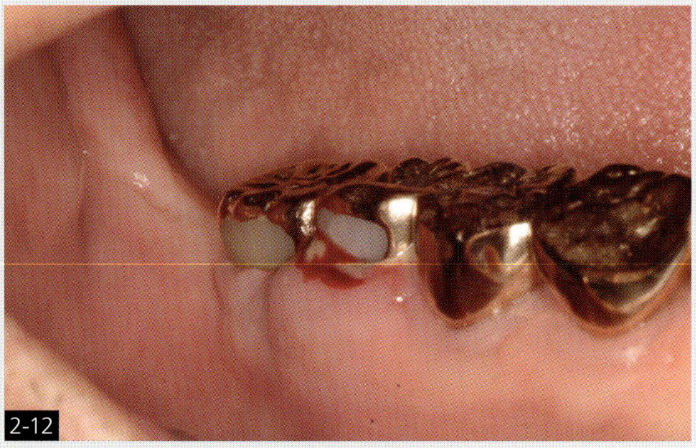
2-12

Peri-implantitis was observed around implant number 46, with loss of alveolar bone and swelling of the gingiva **(Figures 2-11, 12)**. It was diagnosed that a deep periodontal pocket had formed due to bacterial invasion, but instead of focusing on the treatment of the periodontal pocket, we decided to try a treatment method targeting the bacteria.

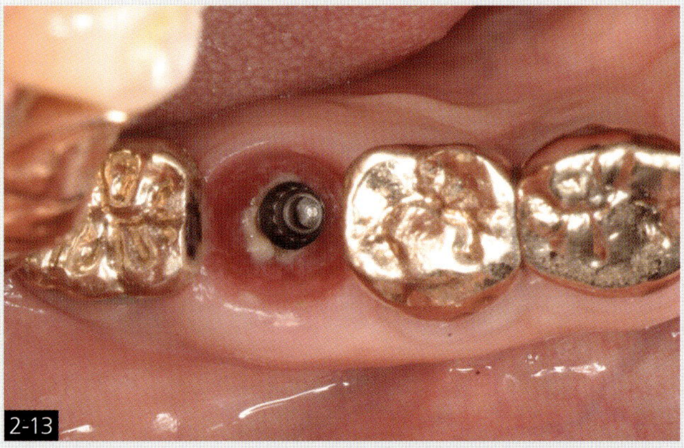
2-13

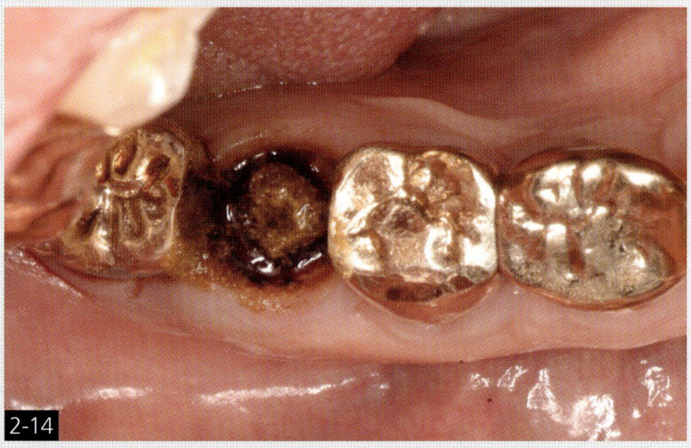
2-14

Based on the classical idea that bacteria are the cause, tetracycline, which can directly kill bacteria, was applied. Significant plaque accumulation was observed **(Figure 2-13)**.

After removing the implant prosthesis, the tetracycline capsule was opened, mixed with saline, and directly applied to the implant's periodontal pocket using a cotton pallet **(Figure 2-14)**.

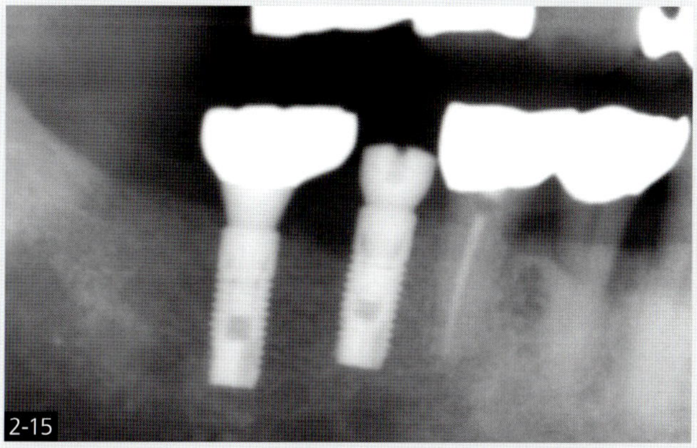

2-15

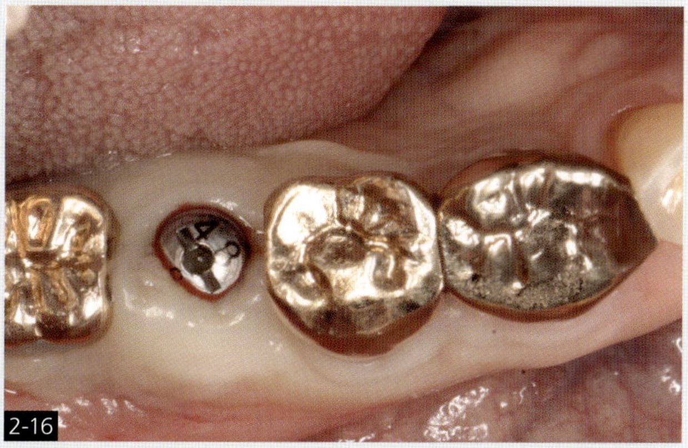

2-16

However, the problem was not resolved, and peri-implantitis recurred. The method of directly killing bacteria did not resolve the inflammation. The effect of the medication was temporary, and the gingival swelling persisted. Ultimately, it was determined that a method to reduce the periodontal pocket needed to be employed, leading to the preparation for gingival resection after anesthesia **(Figures 2-15, 16)**.

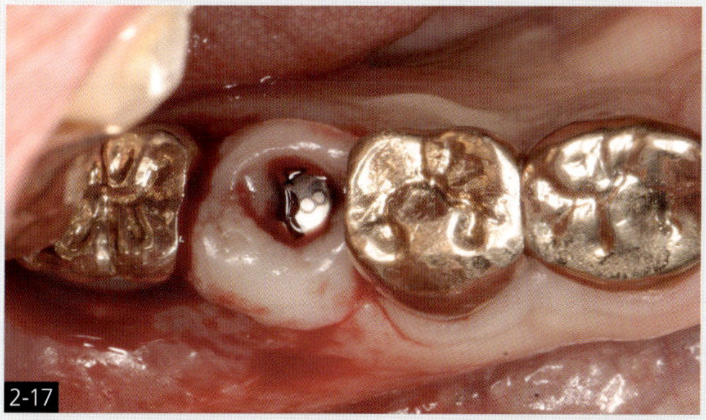

2-17

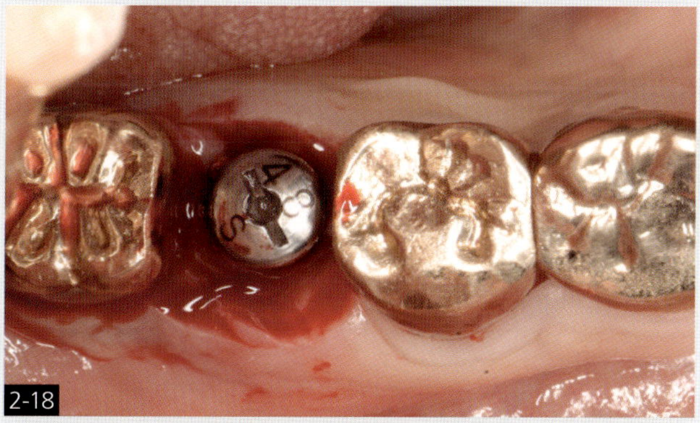

2-18

The marginal gingiva was incised and resected **(Figures 2-17, 18)**.

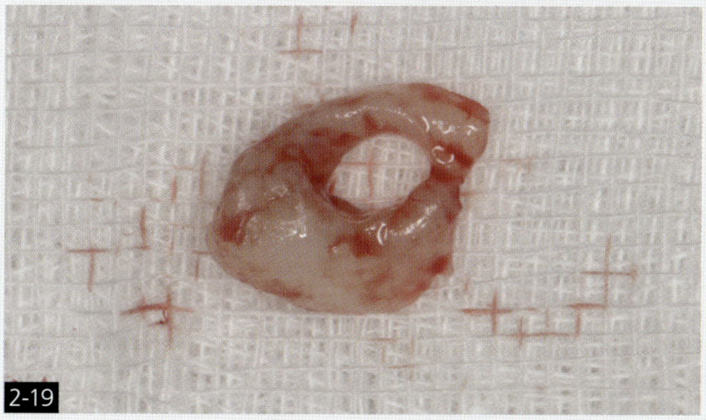

2-19

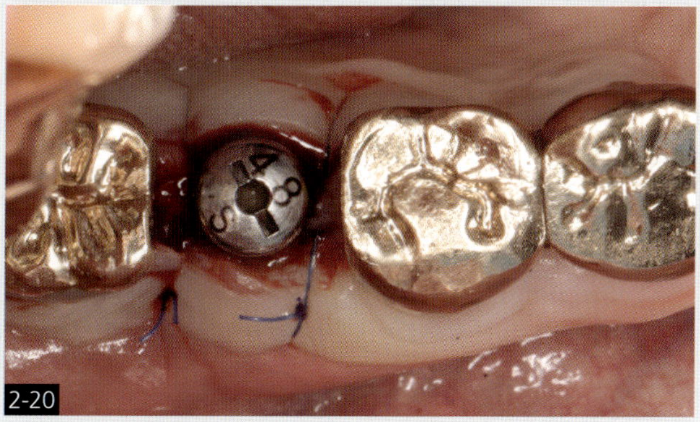

2-20

The resected gingiva was sutured to control bleeding **(Figures 2-19, 20)**.

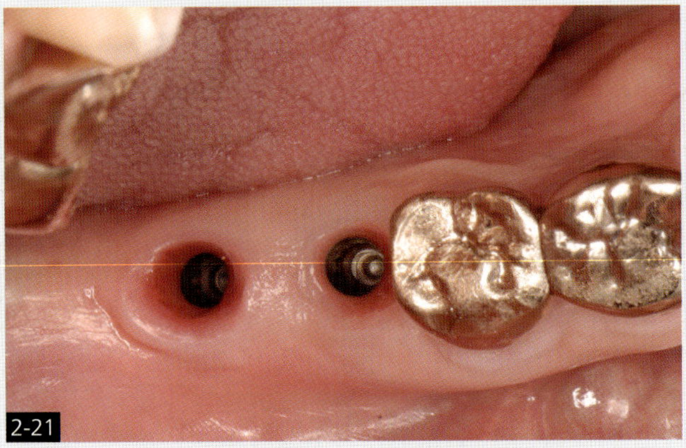

2-21

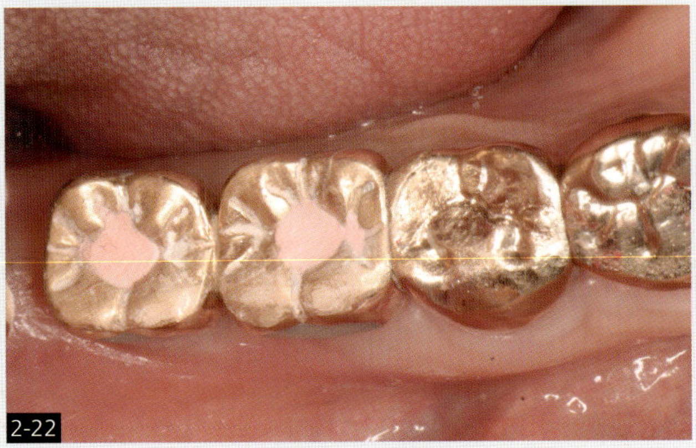

2-22

Despite the direct application of tetracycline, the gingival swelling was not resolved. However, the gingival resection effectively resolved the swelling, making it appear as though the peri-implantitis had been treated. As the peri-implantitis subsided, the gingiva regained a healthy appearance **(Figure 2-21)**. It was concluded that all issues had been resolved, and a new prosthesis was completed **(Figure 2-22)**.

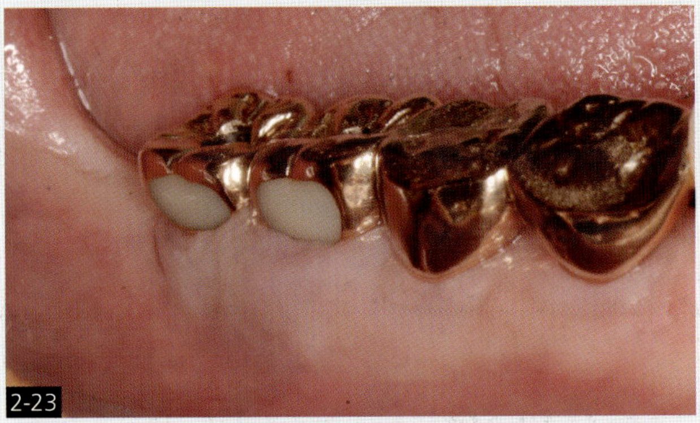

2-23

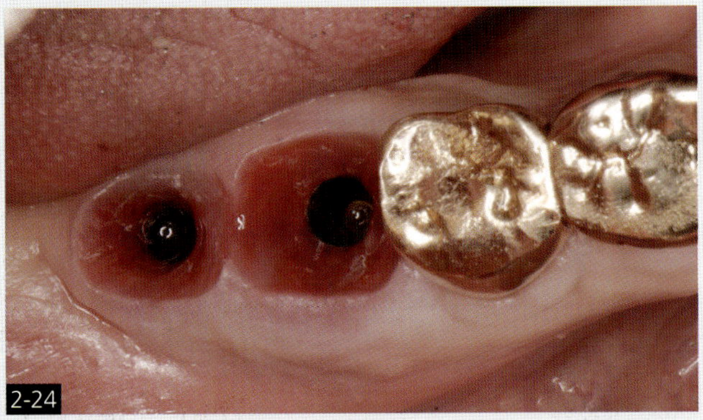

2-24

However, within a few months, peri-implantitis recurred. The gingival resection did not resolve the issue, and the gingiva swelled again, leading to the formation of a deep periodontal pocket **(Figures 2-23, 24)**.

This indicated that gingivectomy could not treat all cases of peri-implantitis, prompting further contemplation.

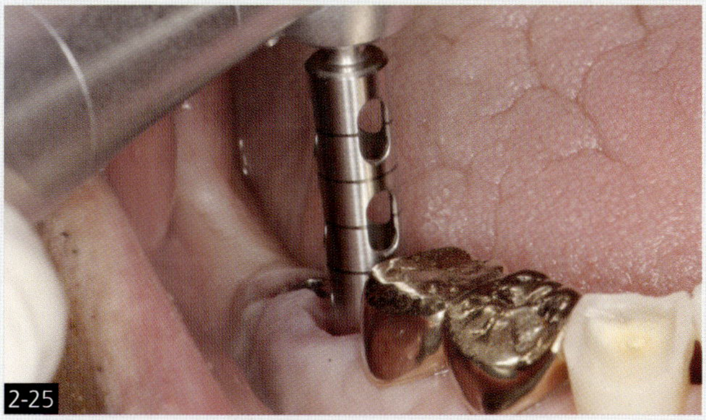
2-25

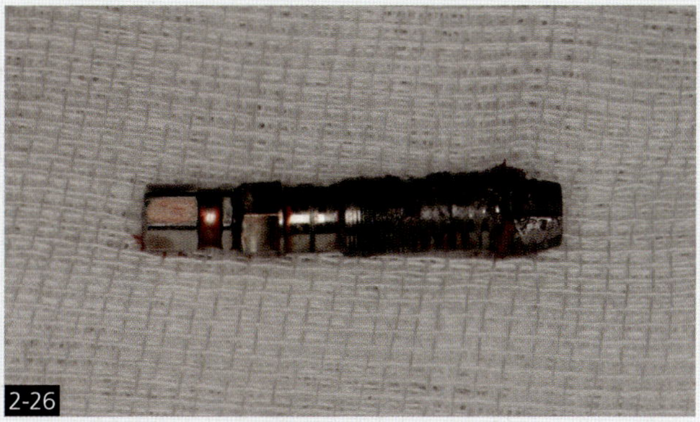
2-26

After the patient expressed frustration over the recurrence of peri-implantitis, a definitive solution was sought. While many attempts have been made to treat peri-implantitis, the most certain method is the removal of the implant **(Figures 2-25, 26)**. However, it is not feasible to remove the implant every time peri-implantitis occurs, and implant removal does not address the underlying causes or solutions for peri-implantitis. Therefore, we must continue to explore the causes and treatment methods for peri-implantitis.

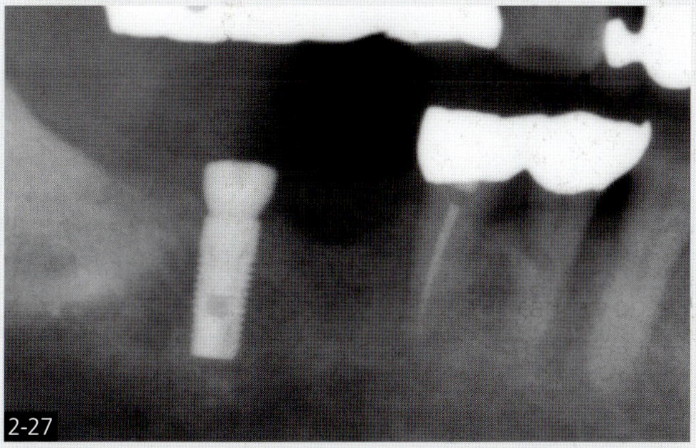
2-27

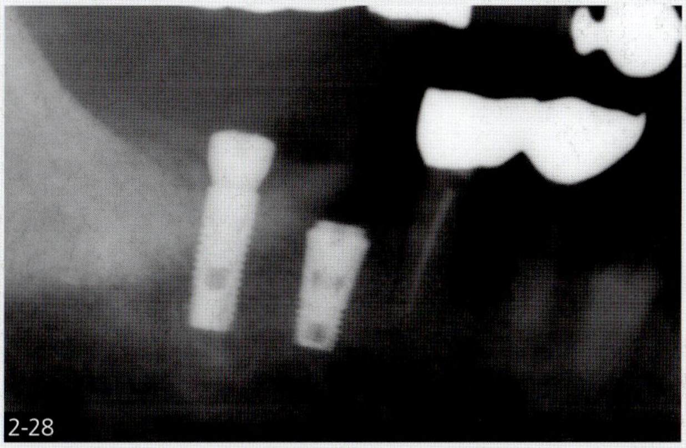
2-28

After removing the implant, we waited approximately three months for the alveolar bone to heal. Once sufficient healing had occurred, a new implant was placed **(Figures 2-27, 28)**.

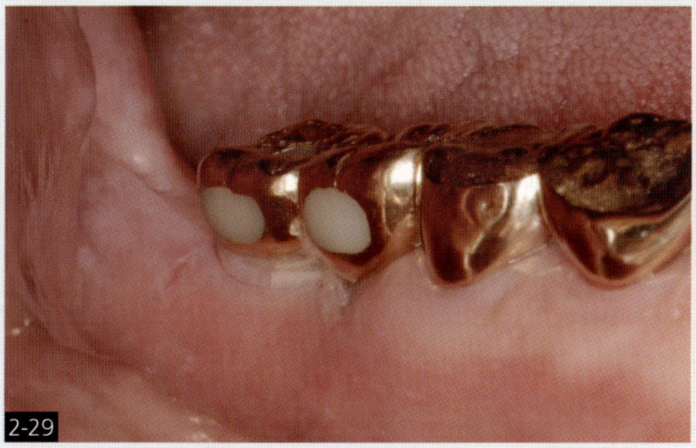
2-29

The placement of the new implant resolved all issues **(Figure 2-29)**. However, there is a need for the development of new surgical methods to reduce the depth of the periodontal pocket around implants.

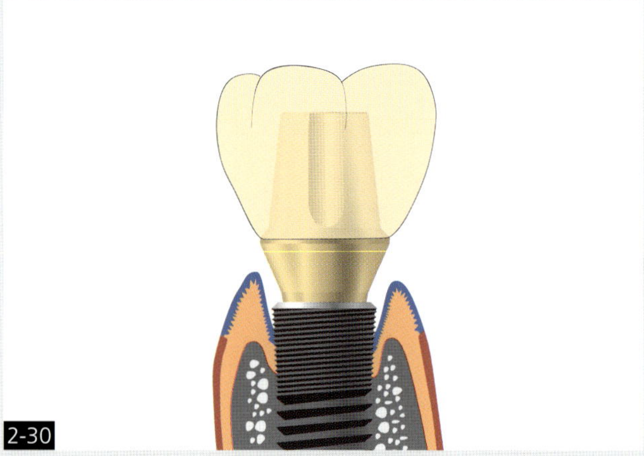

2-30

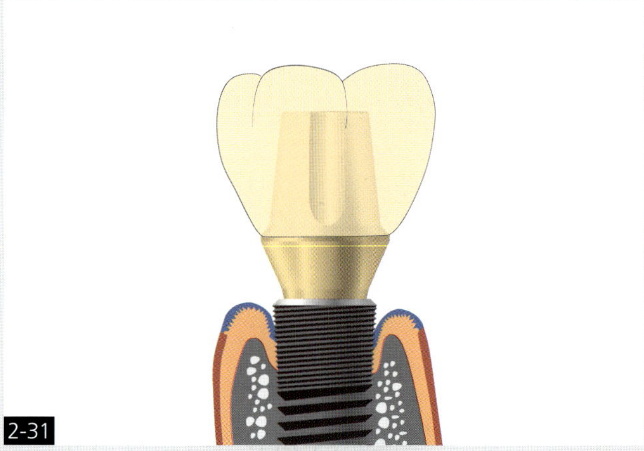

2-31

While it was imagined that resecting the marginal gingiva would reduce the periodontal pocket and that the reduced pocket would be maintained, this was not the case **(Figures 2-30, 31)**.

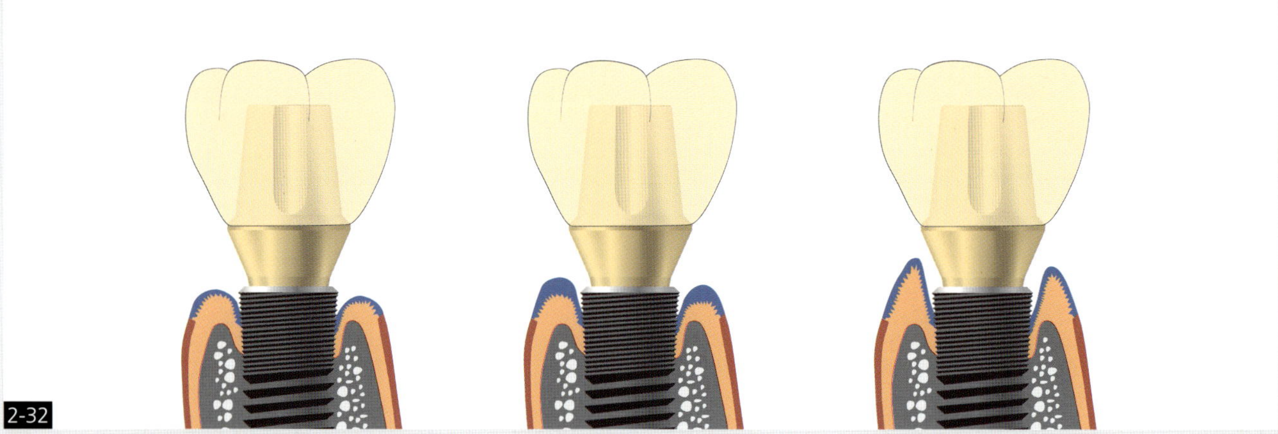

2-32

As the author observed, the resected marginal gingiva gradually returned to its original shape, and the periodontal pocket deepened again **(Figure 2-32)**. This prompted the need to find a method to reduce the periodontal pocket, which had not been encountered in any books or lectures, leading the author to creatively seek a solution. The following discusses the newly developed technique.

2. Epithelial isolation Technique

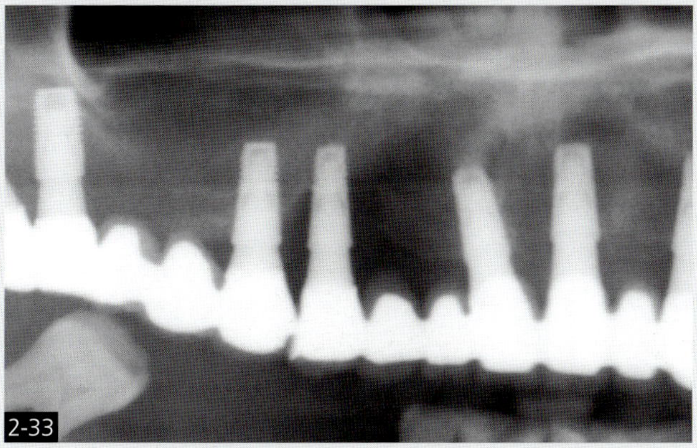
2-33

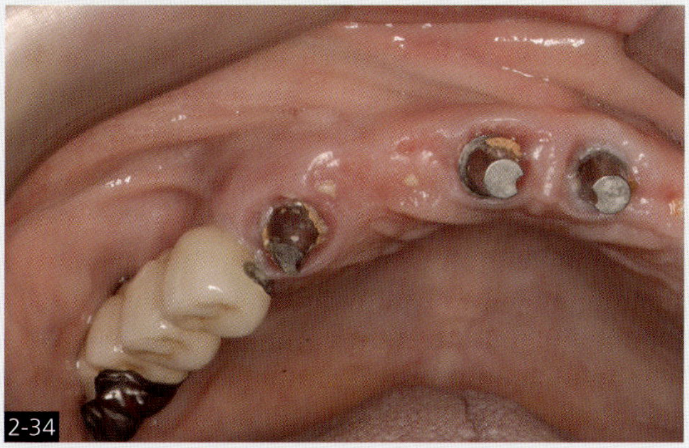
2-34

Peri-implantitis was observed around implant number 14. After much contemplation, the author decided to attempt a new surgical method aimed at eliminating the periodontal pocket (Figures 2-33, 34).

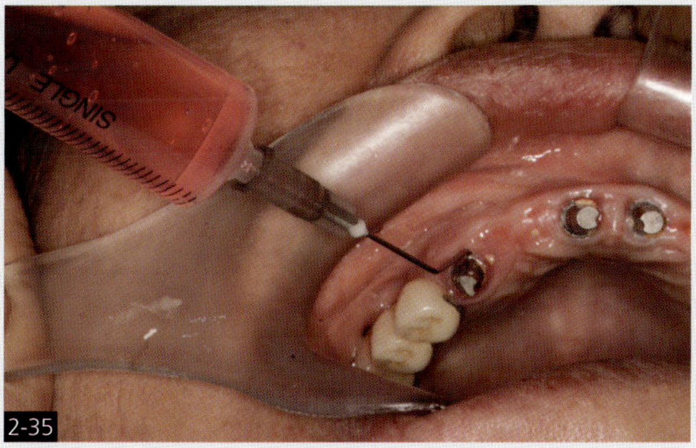
2-35

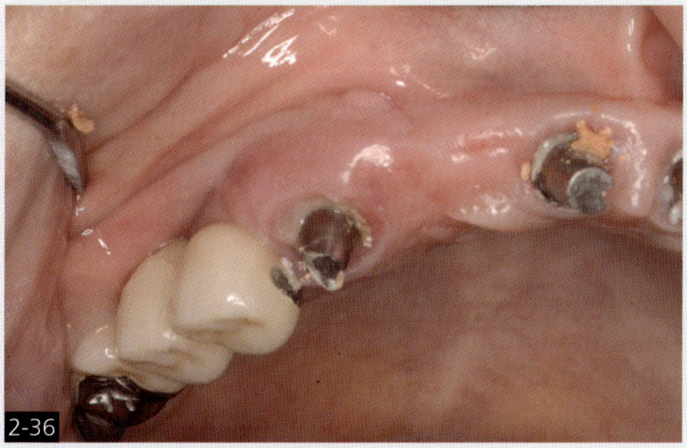
2-36

Initial attempts to eliminate bacteria were made, but they proved ineffective (Figures 2-35, 36). This confirmed the common understanding that peri-implantitis cannot be treated with non-surgical methods.

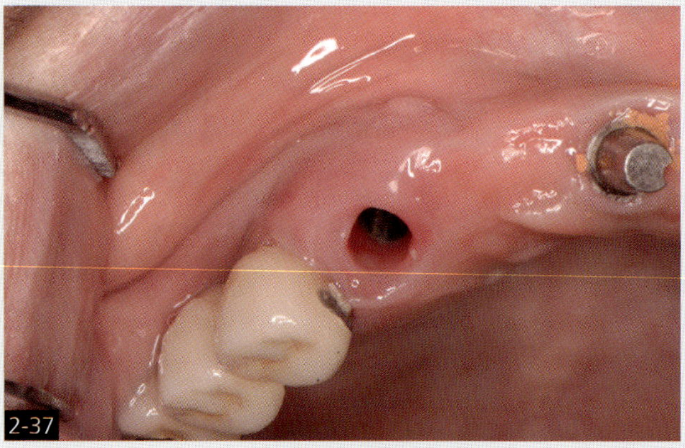
2-37

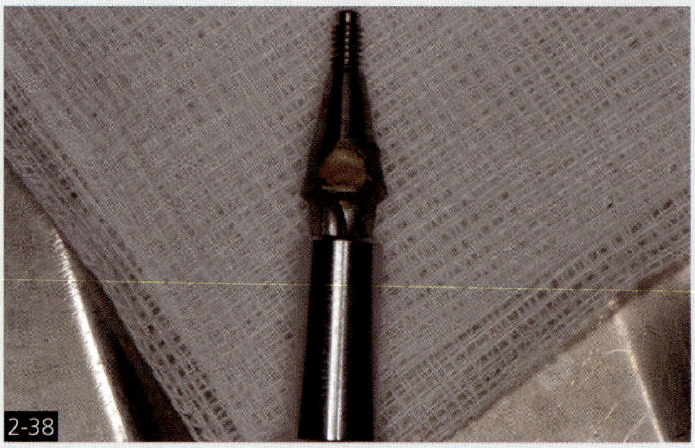
2-38

Curious about the cause of peri-implantitis, the abutment was removed. As seen in **Figure 2-38**, a significant amount of residual adhesive was found around the subgingival abutment. In this case, the residual adhesive was determined to be a contributing factor to the peri-implantitis. Therefore, consideration must be given to how to remove residual adhesive when planning implant treatment.

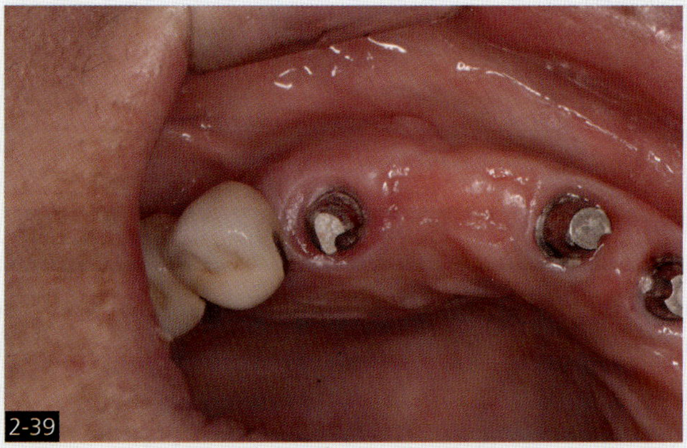
2-39

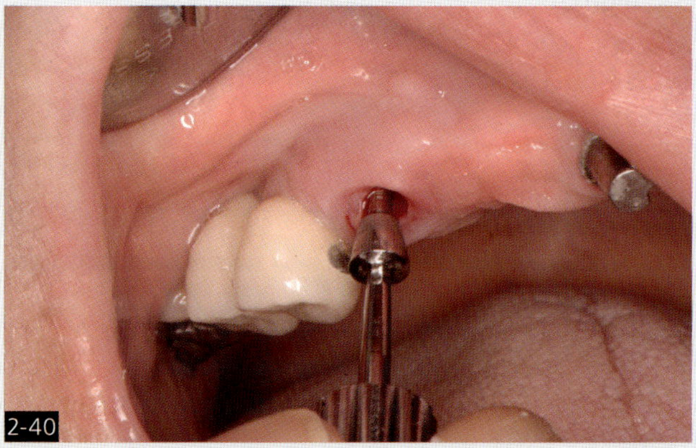
2-40

In natural teeth, removing calculus and plaque can eliminate gingival inflammation. Following this concept, the residual adhesive on the abutment was removed, but the gingival inflammation did not subside. This observation indicates that once peri-implantitis has formed, it does not heal spontaneously even if the cause is removed. The contamination of the implant surface by bacteria and the formation of a periodontal pocket around the implant are likely reasons for this **(Figure 2-39)**.

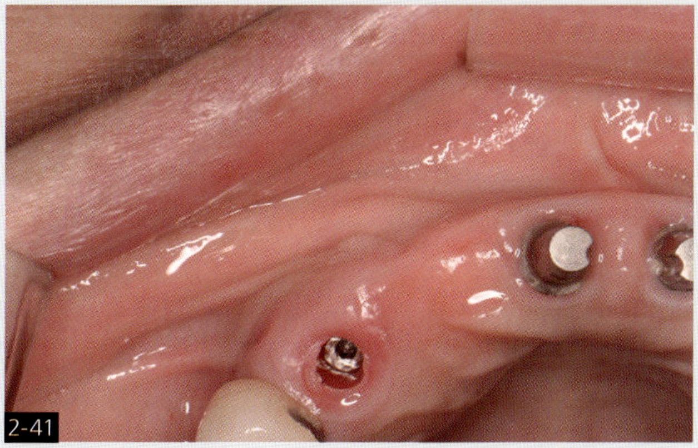

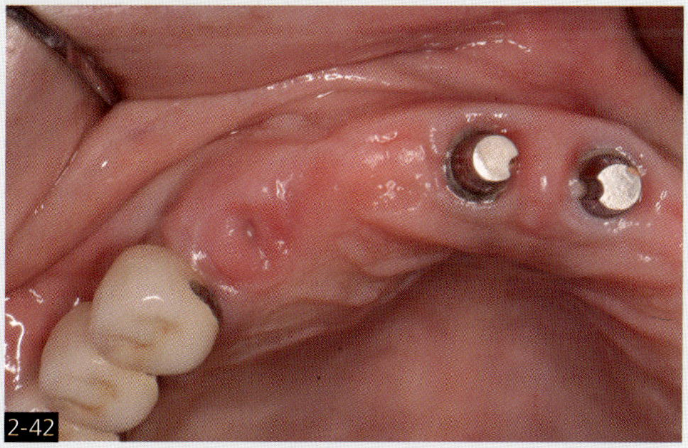

To utilize the new surgical method, the abutment was removed, and a cover screw was placed **(Figures 2-40~42)**. **Figure 2-43** shows the soft tissue covering the implant area approximately six weeks later.

When the abutment is removed and a cover screw is placed, this area is covered by soft tissue again, which depends on the position of the fixture top and the thickness of the soft tissue. If the fixture top is positioned too high, it will not be adequately covered by soft tissue. Additionally, if the soft tissue is thin, it tends to remain uncovered.

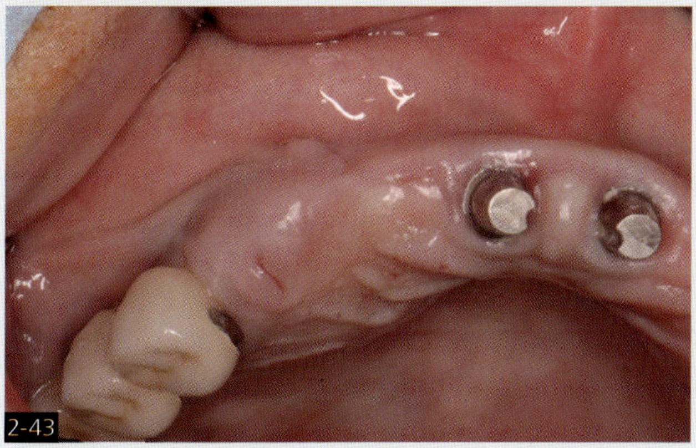

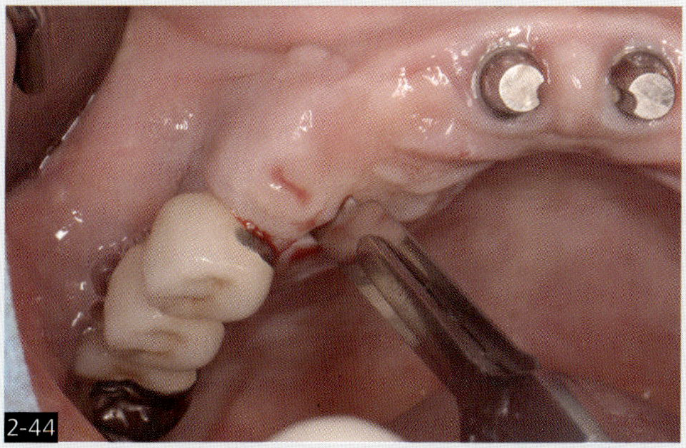

About six weeks after replacing with a cover screw, the surgical procedure was attempted **(Figure 2-43)**. It is advisable to avoid including the gingiva that the abutment penetrated during the incision **(Figure 2-44)**.

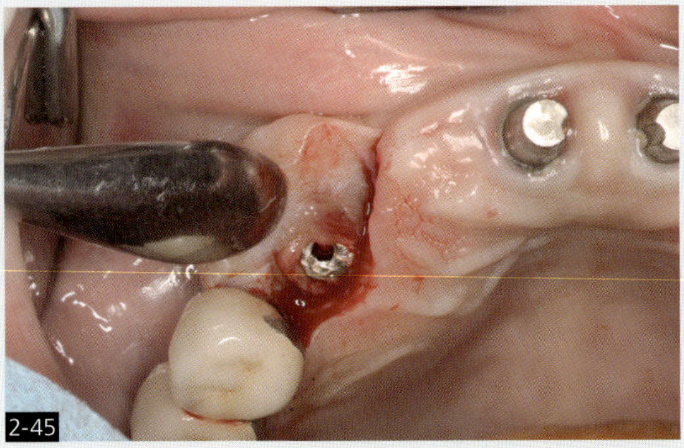
2-45

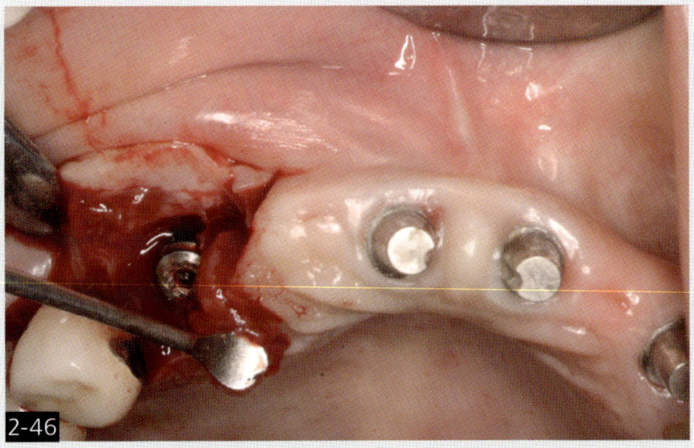
2-46

After elevating the gingival flap, granulation tissue was removed. Directly using a curette on the granulation tissue may not yield a single mass removal, so it is better to scrape it off gently, as if scraping the alveolar bone **(Figures 2-45, 46)**.

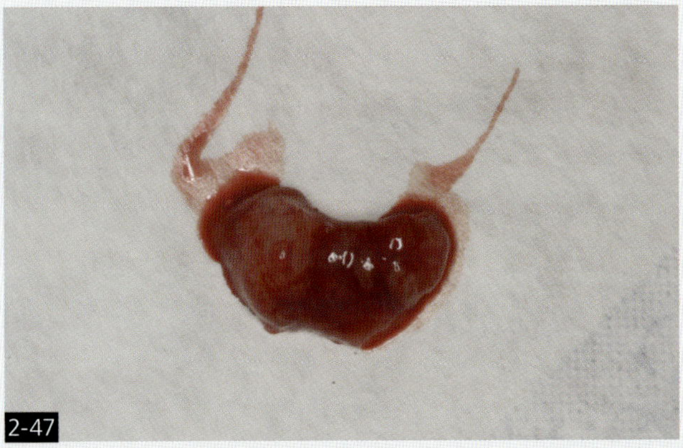
2-47

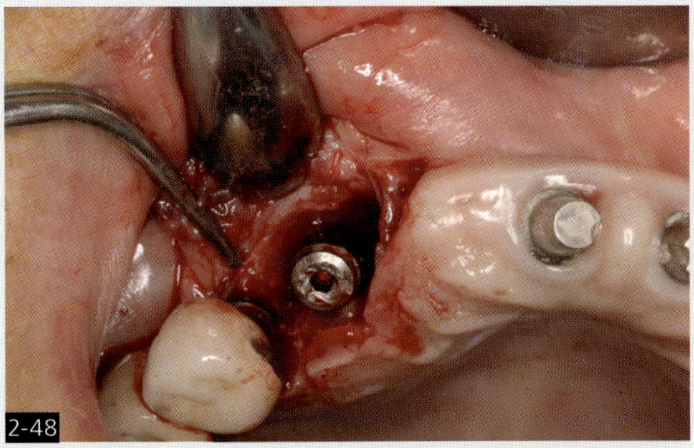
2-48

The granulation tissue was successfully removed as a single mass. Bacteria exist within the granulation tissue, and these bacteria form a biofilm, rendering antibiotic treatment ineffective. Therefore, it is advisable to surgically remove the granulation tissue **(Figure 2-47)**.

The implant surface is believed to be contaminated by bacteria, and if the implant surface is located within the periodontal pocket, contamination by bacteria cannot be avoided **(Figure 2-48)**.

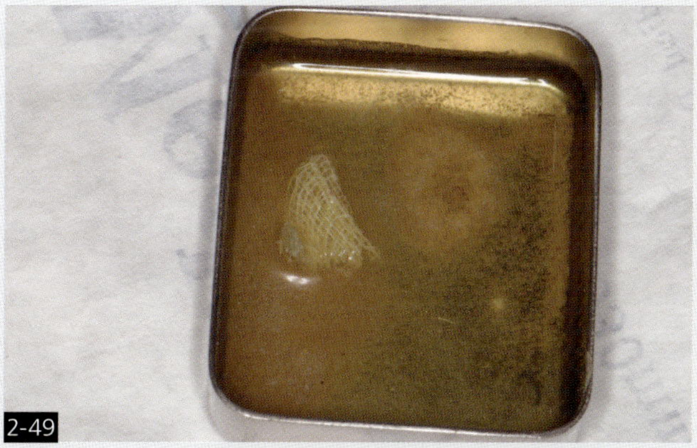
2-49

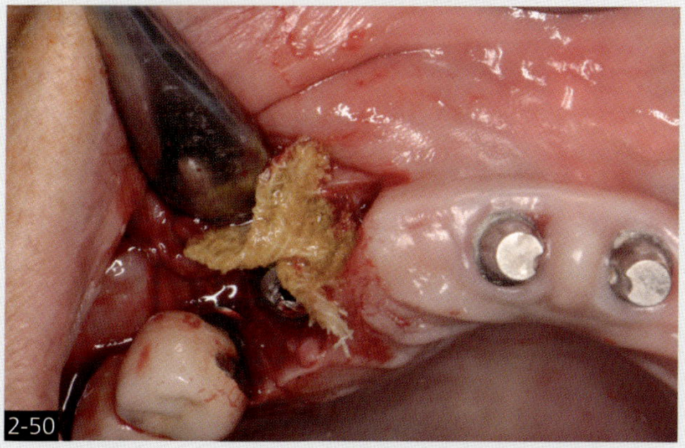
2-50

Cleaning the implant surface is crucial. A sanded surface without etching can be adequately treated with tetracycline alone. The tetracycline capsule is opened, and a solution is prepared by mixing it with saline **(Figure 2-49)**. A small piece of gauze is soaked in the tetracycline solution and applied for about five minutes **(Figure 2-50)**.

Tetracycline is manufactured in the form of a salt, which releases hydrochloric acid in solution. This acid lightly etches the implant surface while simultaneously removing contaminants and reducing surface roughness.

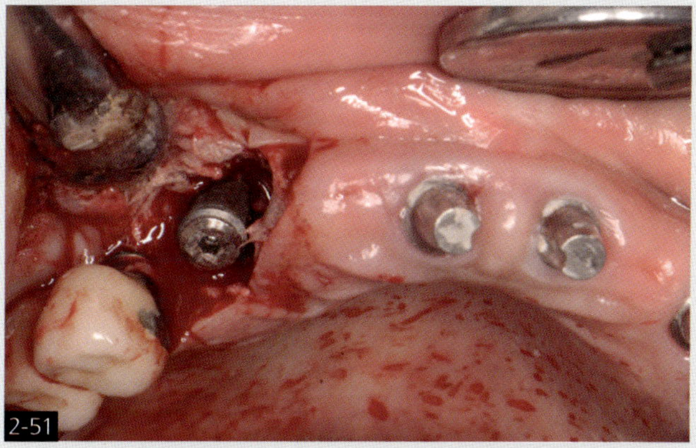
2-51

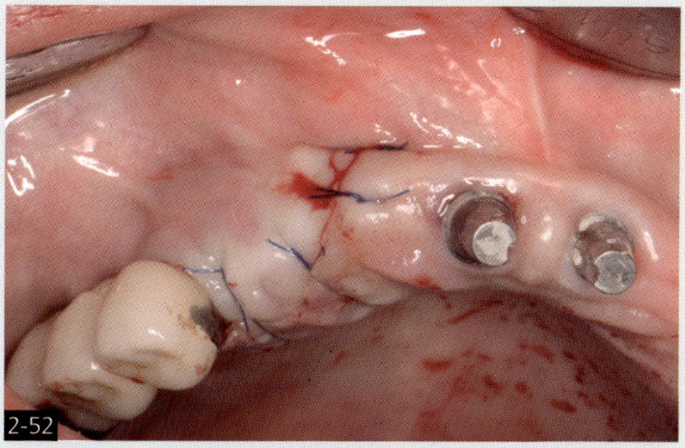
2-52

The tetracycline solution not only acts on the titanium implant but also affects the surrounding biological tissues, potentially causing chemical burns. As seen in **Figure 2-51**, there are signs of burns in the gingival tissue. Clinically, these chemical burns do not hinder the healing process.

As shown in **Figure 2-52**, the procedure was sutured without bone grafting. The reason for not performing a bone graft is to closely observe the healing process of this surgical method. When a bone graft is performed, it becomes challenging to determine through X-rays whether the graft is integrating well or if it is merely the appearance of the grafted bone, complicating the assessment of surgical success.

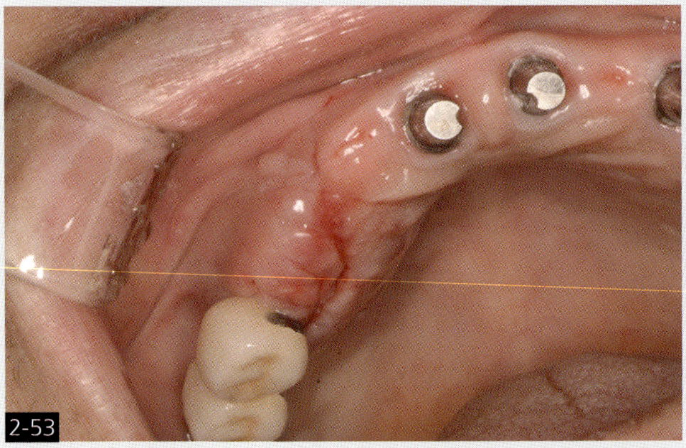
2-53

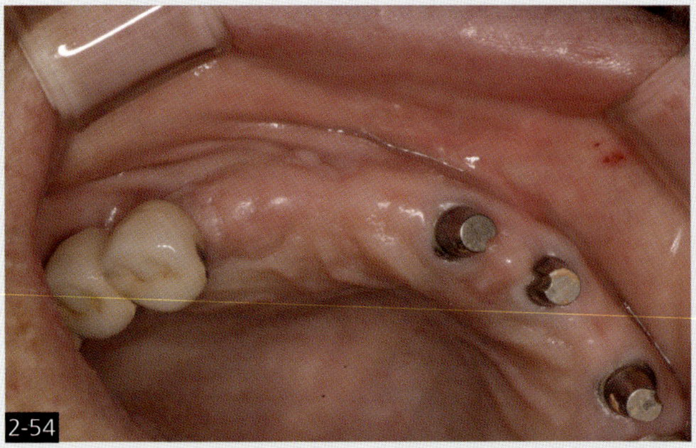
2-54

Healing is progressing well, as evidenced by the images taken two weeks **(Figure 2-53)** and six weeks **(Figure 2-54)** post-surgery. It is impossible to completely eliminate the bacteria that cause peri-implantitis. Therefore, the goal of this surgery is to reduce the depth of the periodontal pocket to a level where pathogenic bacteria cannot survive.

In cases where the periodontal pocket is eliminated through gingivectomy, recurrence is common. This is believed to occur because epithelial cells migrate deeply into the alveolar bone, leading to the recurrence of the periodontal pocket.

To prevent the recurrence of the periodontal pocket, it is necessary for the epithelial cells that have grown into the alveolar bone to undergo degradation. After removing the granulation tissue, cleaning the implant surface, and covering it with a flap, any remaining epithelial tissue is expected to degrade and disappear.

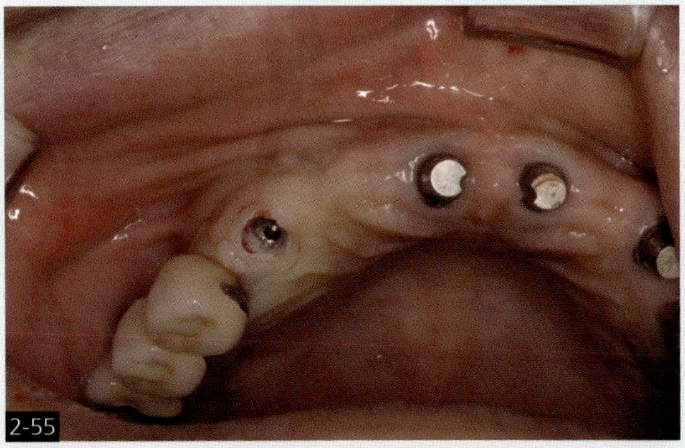
2-55

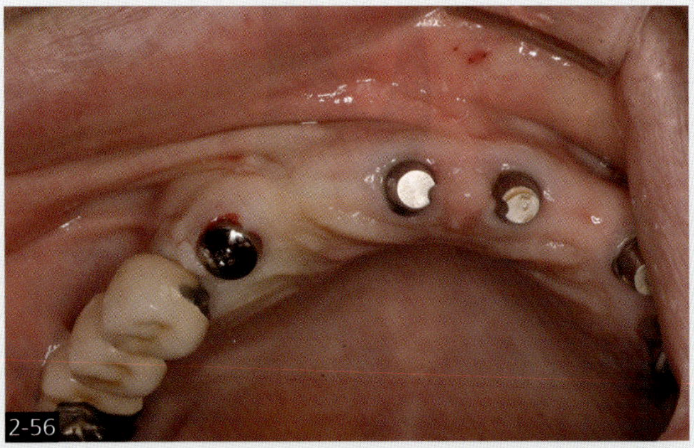
2-56

In the early stages of healing, the voids in the alveolar bone caused by peri-implantitis are filled with connective tissue. Even when a healing abutment is connected during a secondary surgery, there is no inflammation in the internal connective tissue, preventing the downward proliferation of epithelial cells. This means that the periodontal pocket is eliminated, and epithelial attachment forms on the abutment rather than the implant fixture. If contaminants remain on the implant surface, inflammation can develop in the connective tissue, leading to downward proliferation of epithelial cells and subsequent deepening of the periodontal pocket, resulting in a recurrence of peri-implantitis. Thus, cleaning the implant surface is crucial.

The epithelial tissue that formed the periodontal pocket within the gingiva is believed to have degraded and disappeared, allowing for a secondary surgery to place the healing abutment **(Figures 2-55, 56)**.

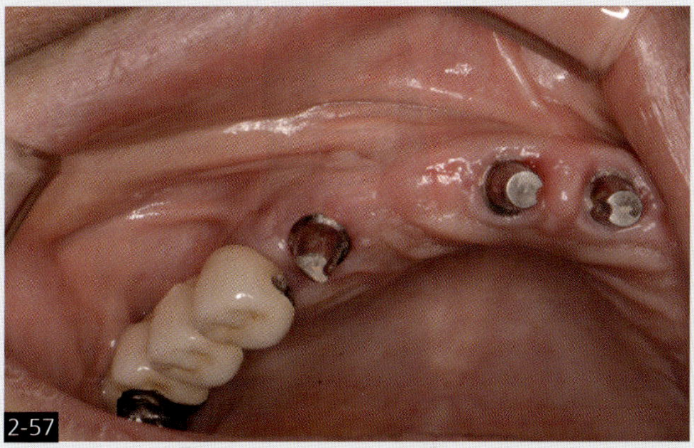
2-57

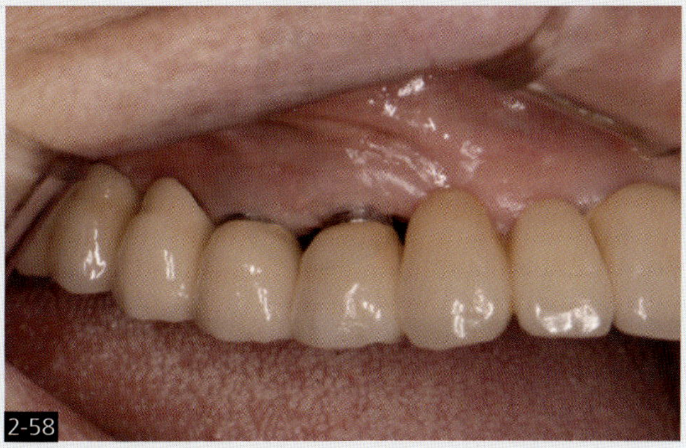
2-58

Peri-implantitis has been resolved, and the gingival inflammation has subsided, allowing for the reattachment of the existing prosthesis. The abutment used was the same as that previously employed with the prosthesis **(Figures 2-57, 58)**. This represents a successful reattachment, similar to what is attempted with natural teeth, by moving the epithelial attachment of the periodontal pocket towards the crown and reducing its depth.

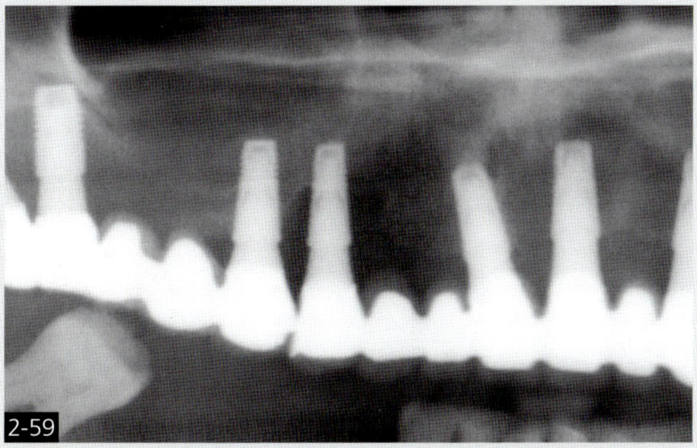
2-59

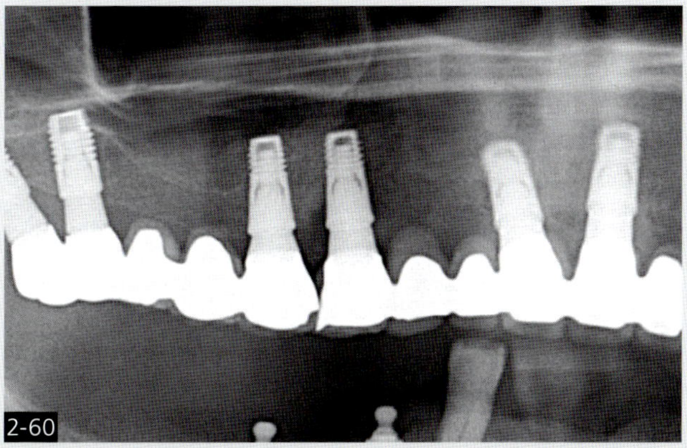
2-60

Figure 2-59 shows the initial occurrence of peri-implantitis, while **Figure 2-60** displays the radiographic appearance 11 years post-surgery, indicating significant regeneration of the alveolar bone. As confirmed in the surgical images **(Figure 2-51)**, considerable bone loss occurred due to peri-implantitis, but the defect was characterized as a contained defect. The natural biological response is for the defect surrounded by autogenous bone to fill with autogenous bone.

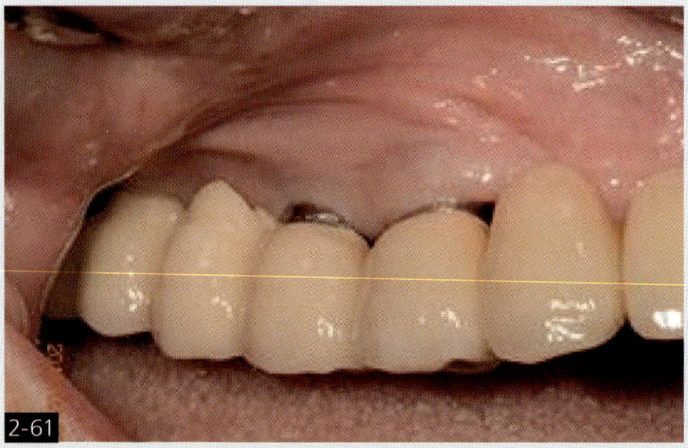

2-61

Eight years post-surgery **(Figure 2-61)**, there is no inflammation in the gingiva, although slight gingival recession is observed. Since the surgery, the patient has not experienced any episodes of inflammation.

The surgical method aimed at reducing the depth of the periodontal pocket has proven to be highly effective. The key to this surgical technique is the degeneration of the epithelial tissue that proliferates into the depth of the alveolar bone. Since it is impossible to completely remove the epithelial tissue during surgical procedures, degeneration is utilized as a means of removal. Therefore, this surgical method is referred to as the Epithelial Isolation Technique by the author and colleagues.

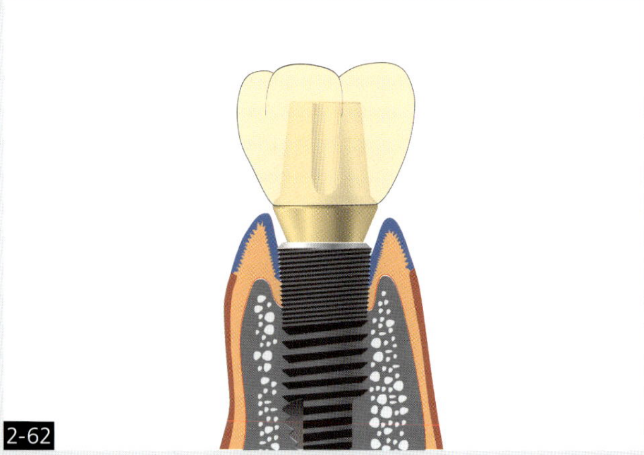

2-62

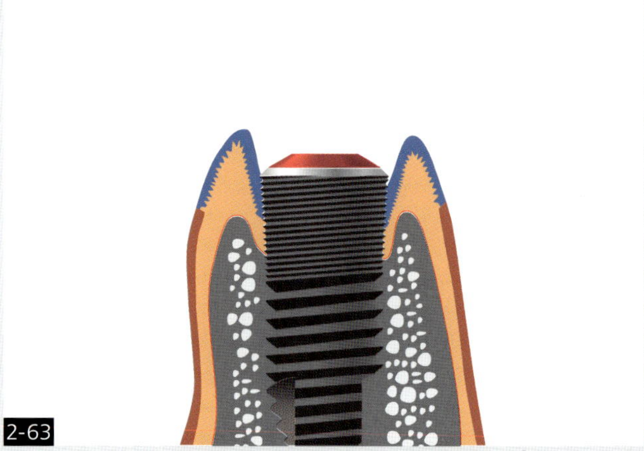

2-63

To facilitate understanding of the clinical procedure and explanations, graphical representations will be provided. In the surgical procedure, when both the abutment and prosthesis are removed and a cover screw is placed, the exposed gingiva will heal normally, allowing the implant to be submerged **(Figures 2-62~64)**.

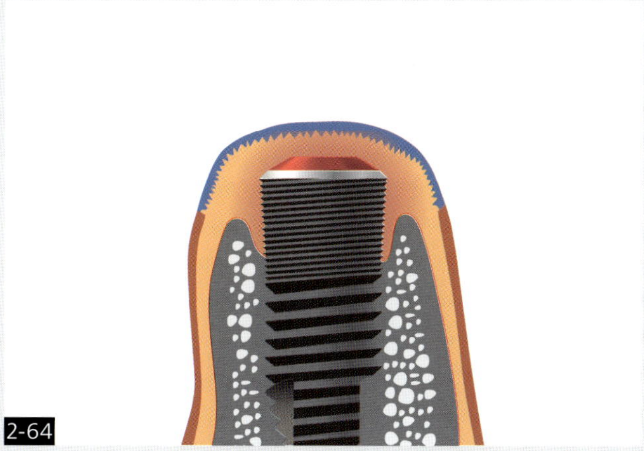
2-64

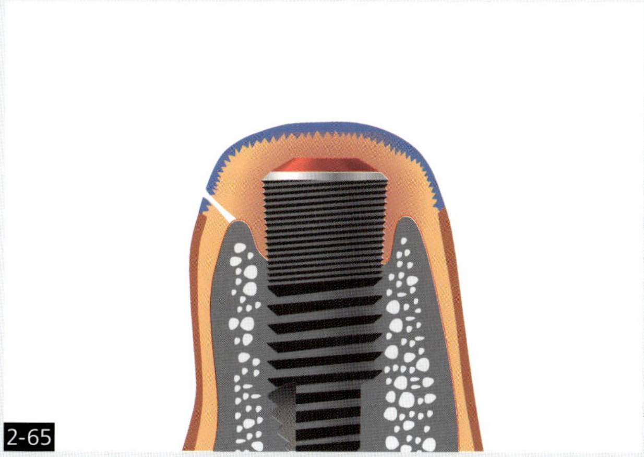
2-65

However, beneath the covered gingiva, infection and inflammation may still persist, necessitating surgical intervention for removal **(Figure 2-64)**. It is also important to note that epithelial tissue contributing to the periodontal pocket may still be present. While inflammatory and epithelial tissues can be surgically excised, it is challenging to guarantee the complete removal of every single epithelial cell **(Figures 2-65~67)**.

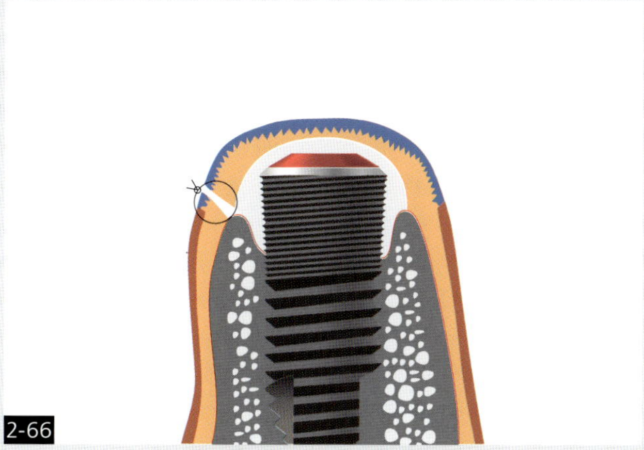
2-66

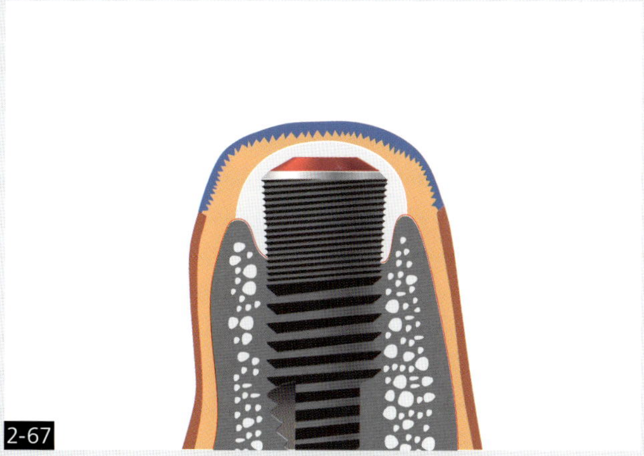
2-67

Along with the removal of inflammatory and epithelial tissues, it is crucial to thoroughly clean the implant surface. The clinical case presented utilizes Astra implants manufactured in Sweden. The Astra implant features a Tioblast surface similar to RBM, which is created by blasting titanium oxide particles.

This surface does not possess the fine honeycomb structure seen in SLA surfaces, making it difficult for bacteria to penetrate deeply into the surface. Therefore, to clean the surface, I opted to use a tetracycline solution without excessive mechanical removal.

The final stage of tissue degeneration is calcification. Over time, contamination on the implant surface can lead to the formation of calcified residues, at which point mechanical removal becomes necessary.

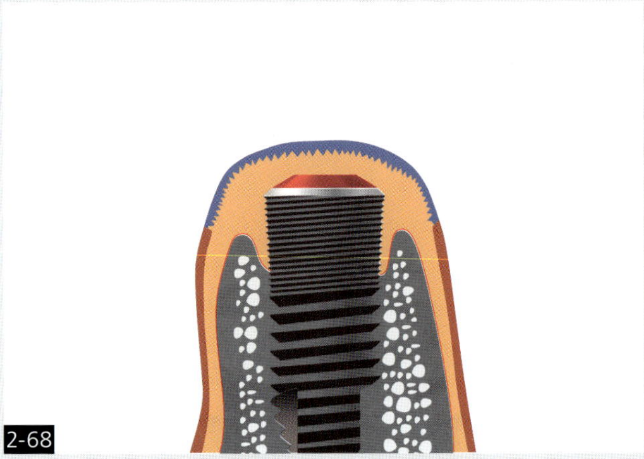

2-68

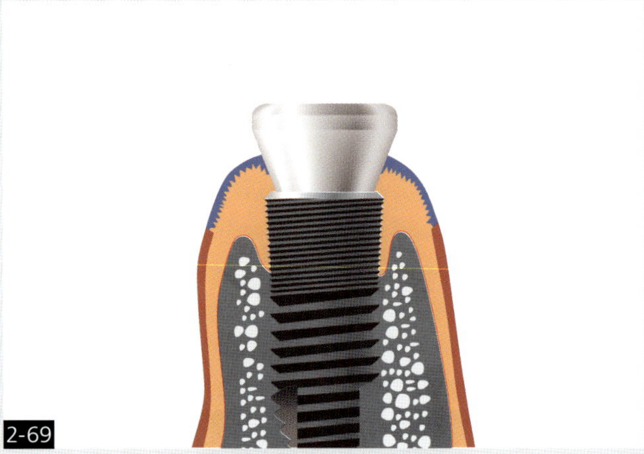

2-69

Once the inflammatory tissue and residual epithelial cells are removed, and the implant surface is cleaned, the voids will be filled with healthy connective tissue devoid of inflammation. If any epithelial cells remain, they will continue to undergo degeneration and eventually disappear. Soft tissue healing typically takes about six weeks, allowing for a secondary surgery to place the healing abutment at the six-week mark **(Figures 2-68, 69)**.

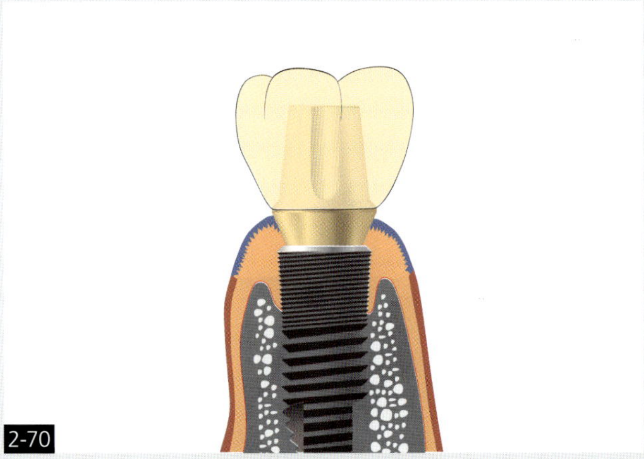

2-70

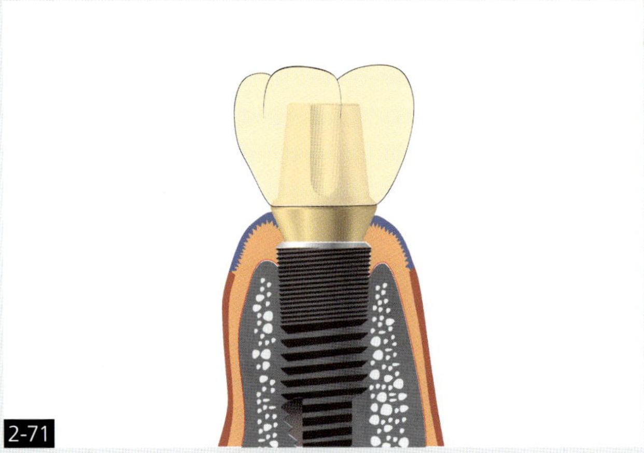

2-71

After the secondary surgery, normal prosthetic procedures can be performed, resulting in epithelial attachment forming on the abutment rather than the implant fixture, transforming deep periodontal pockets into shallow gingival sulci **(Figure 2-70)**. Over time, the intra-bony defects in the alveolar bone will gradually fill with autogenous bone, leading to successful treatment outcomes **(Figure 2-71)**.

I did not perform bone grafting during this procedure. The reason for this decision was to explore how to establish the concept of treating peri-implantitis. I wanted to determine whether bone grafting is a critical element in the treatment of peri-implantitis or if reducing the depth of the periodontal pocket is the key factor. Through multiple surgeries, I have come to believe that reducing the depth of the periodontal pocket is the essential element, while bone grafting serves as a supportive factor that enhances the overall results.

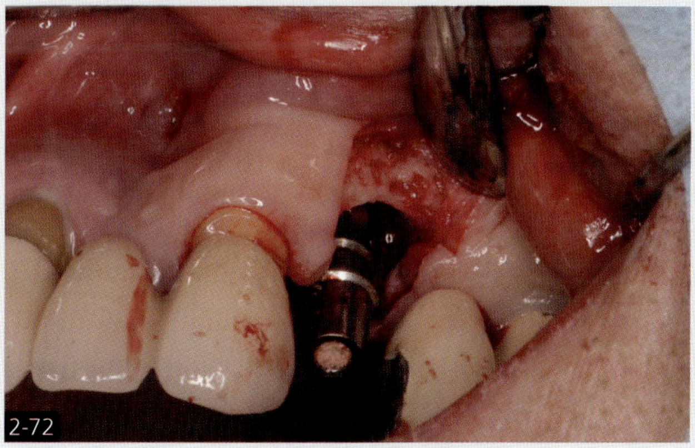

2-72

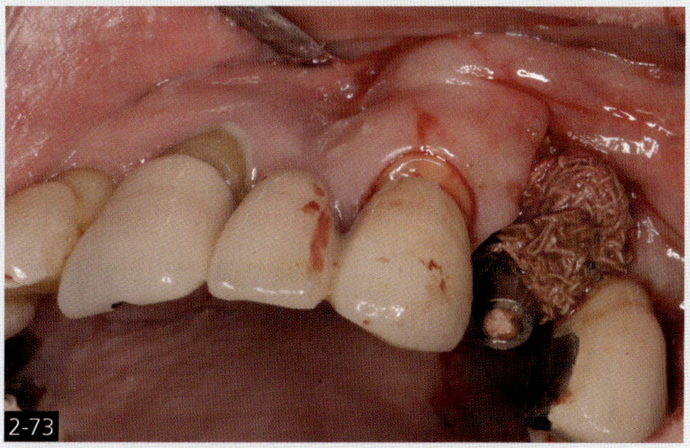

2-73

The development of the Epithelial Isolation Technique stemmed from my experiences with the challenges of reducing the depth of the periodontal pocket. Now, let's examine the outcomes when this surgical method is not employed. As a solo practitioner, I am unable to capture every case photographically. While I would like to document the entire clinical process from initial examination through surgery and prosthetics, it is often impractical. Figures 2-72 and 73 were taken incidentally during the process of performing surgery for peri-implantitis. This approach differs from the previously described method, as it involves a simpler concept of treating peri-implantitis by merely removing the epithelial cells and inflammatory tissue that form the periodontal pocket (Figure 2-72).

The implant surface was cleaned using a tetracycline solution (Figure 2-73). Subsequently, the implant affected by peri-implantitis was allowed to heal without being covered by soft tissue, maintaining the abutment in place (Figure 2-74).

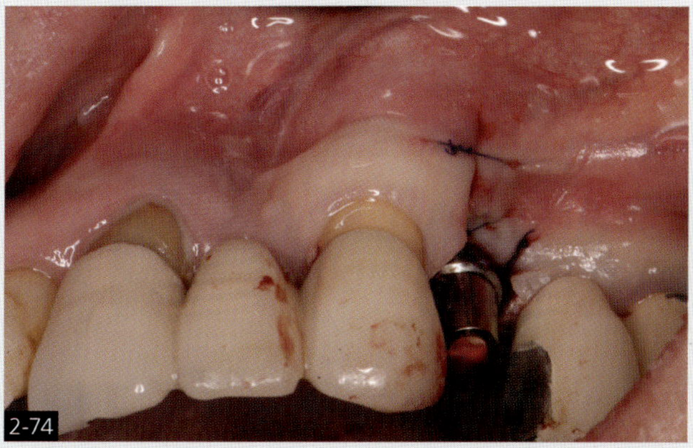

2-74

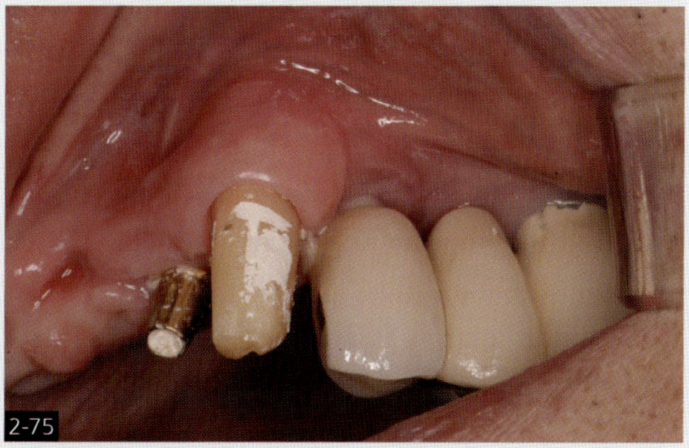

2-75

My intention with this surgery was to shallow the periodontal pocket. After removing the inflammatory tissue and cleaning the implant surface with tetracycline solution, I anticipated that the epithelial cells would attach to the abutment, leading to a shallower periodontal pocket and the filling of the underlying void with normal tissue (Figure 2-74).

Although the initial results appeared promising and the prosthetic work was completed, I observed pus discharge from the buccal side of the 24 implant. Despite the removal of the periodontal pocket and inflammatory tissue, peri-implantitis had recurred, indicating that healing did not occur as intended **(Figure 2-75)**. It seems that the periodontal pocket had reformed.

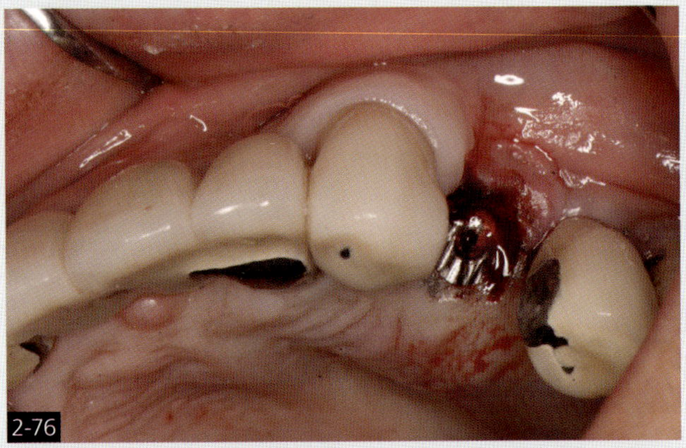
2-76

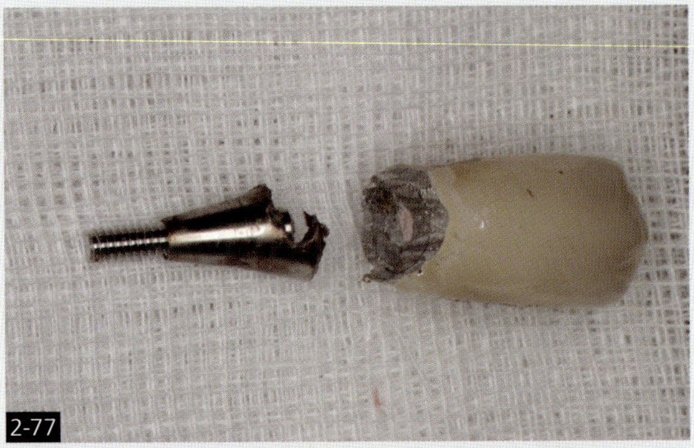
2-77

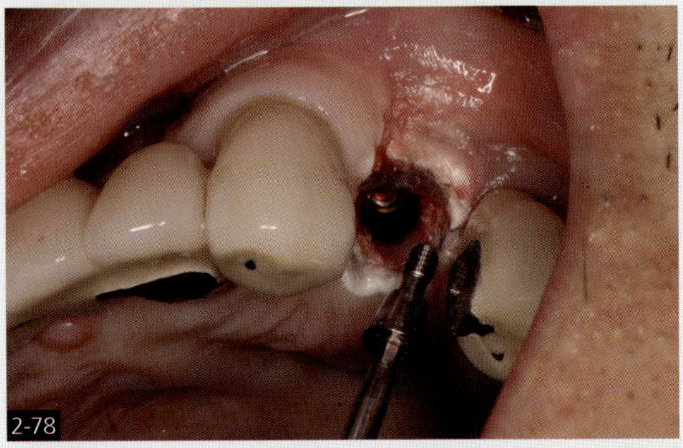
2-78

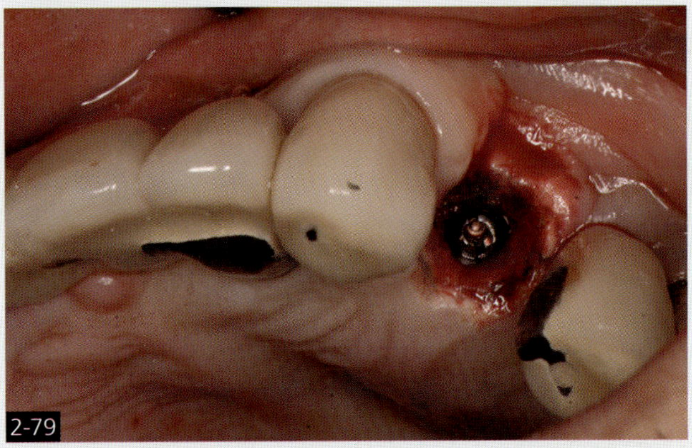
2-79

Reluctantly, I decided to employ the Epithelial Isolation Technique. For this surgical approach, the implant needed to be covered by gingiva, so I cut the abutment, removed the screw, and placed a cover screw **(Figures 2-76~79)**. When removing the implant prosthesis, I prefer this method because cutting the PFM crown takes significantly longer, whereas cutting the abutment with a 330 bur can be done in a much shorter time.

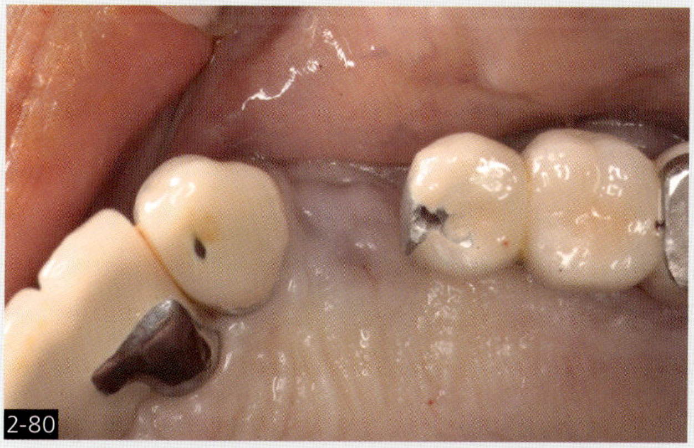
2-80

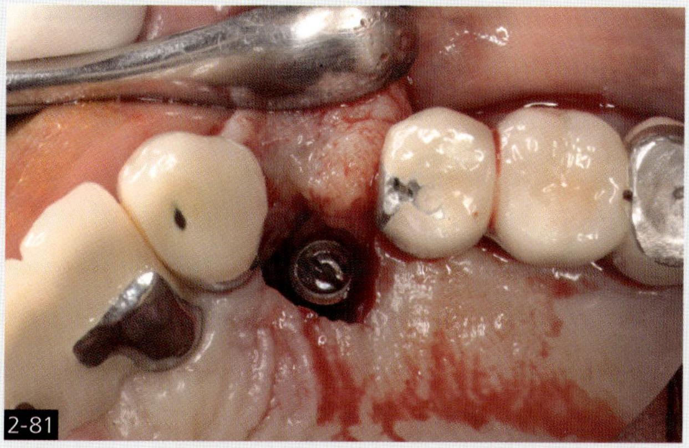
2-81

After placing the cover screw, the soft tissue was closed, but the gingiva still exhibited signs of inflammation **(Figure 2-80)**. Following this, I proceeded with the surgical process similar to the previous case.

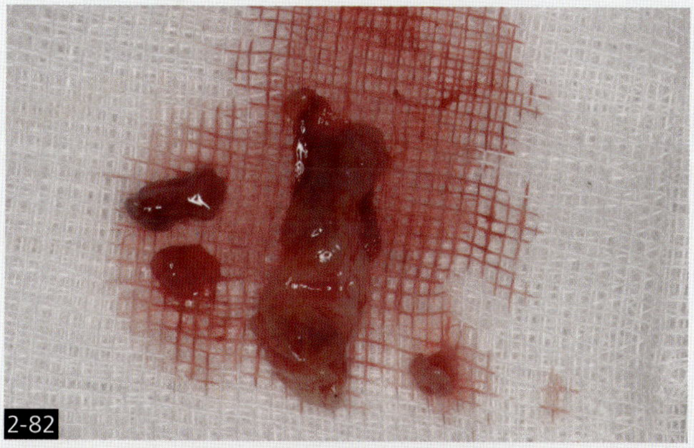
2-82

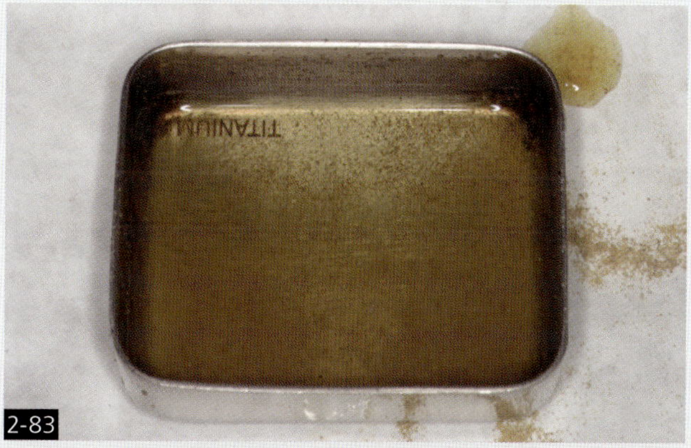
2-83

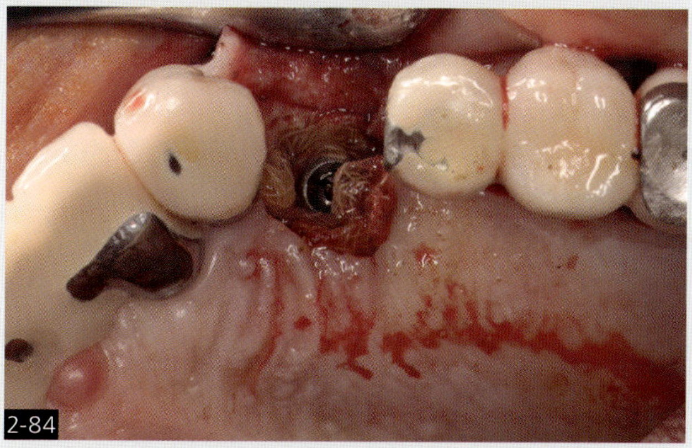
2-84

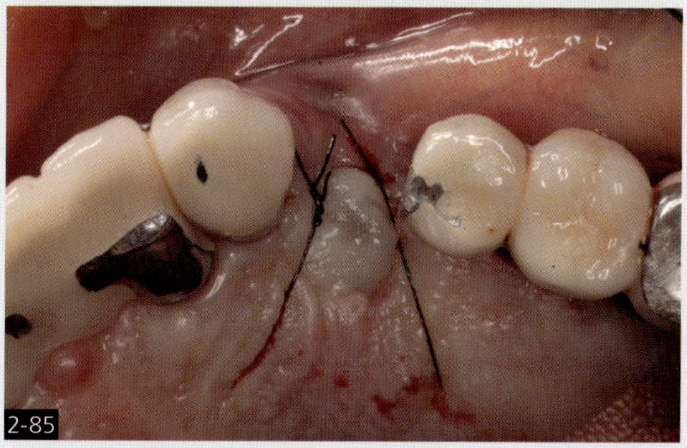
2-85

After elevating the flap, I removed the inflammatory tissue and cleaned the implant surface with tetracycline solution, suturing without bone grafting **(Figures 2-81~85)**.

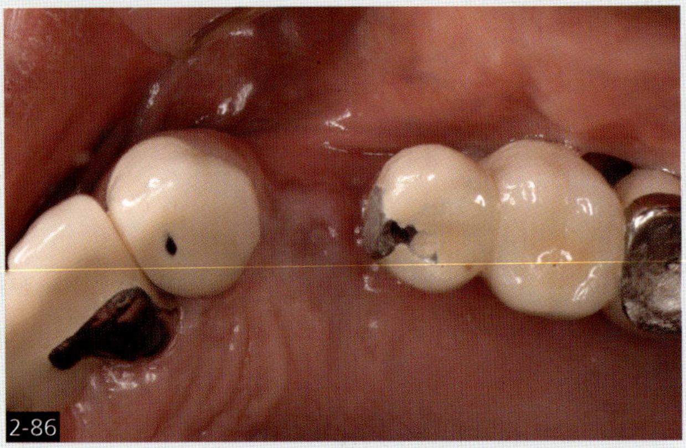
2-86

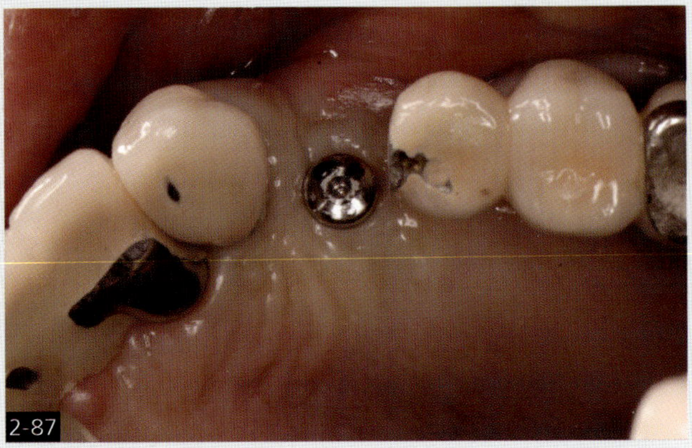
2-87

Six weeks later, I performed the secondary surgery as per protocol and placed the healing abutment (Figures 2-86, 87).

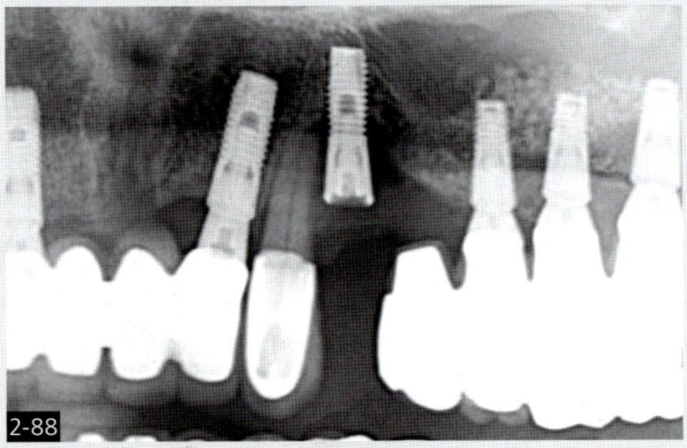
2-88

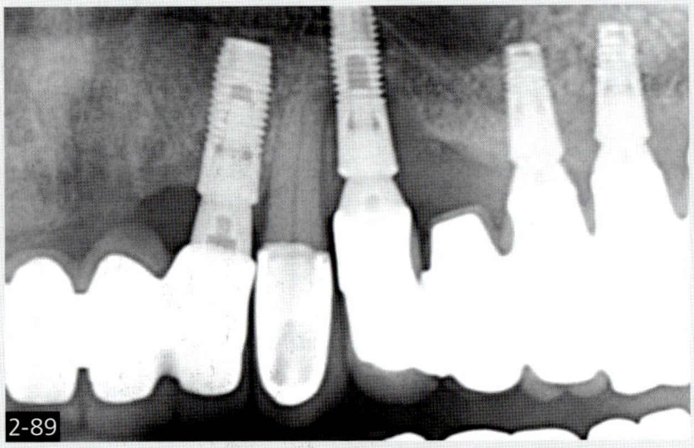
2-89

The case that initially failed with the simple surgical method was successfully resolved using the Epithelial Isolation Technique. After the new prosthesis was placed, I observed progressive healing of the alveolar bone (Figures 2-88, 89).

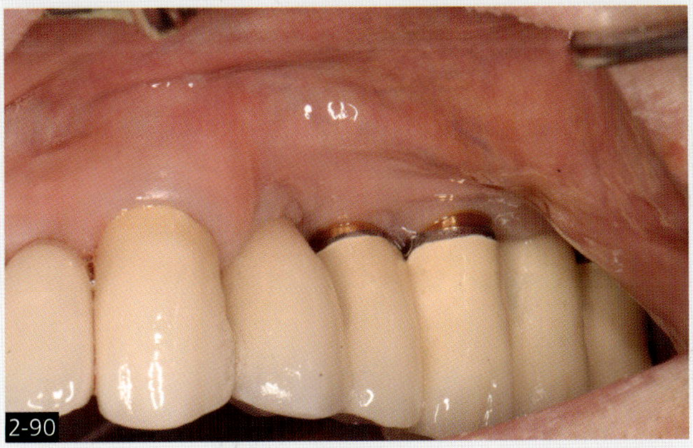

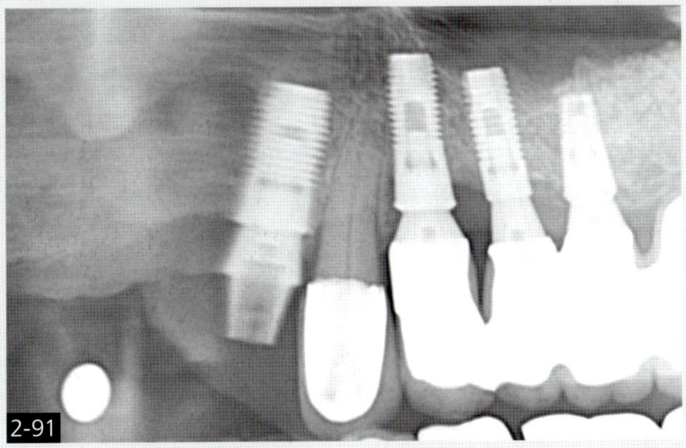

There was no further discharge or inflammation around the 24th implant **(Figure 2-90)**. Approximately four years post-surgery, radiographic images showed significant regeneration of the alveolar bone. This case serves as a meaningful example of the significance of the Epithelial Isolation Technique.

Chapter 3 Another Cause of Peri-implantitis

1. Abutment Mobility (Accompanied by Loose Abutment Screws)

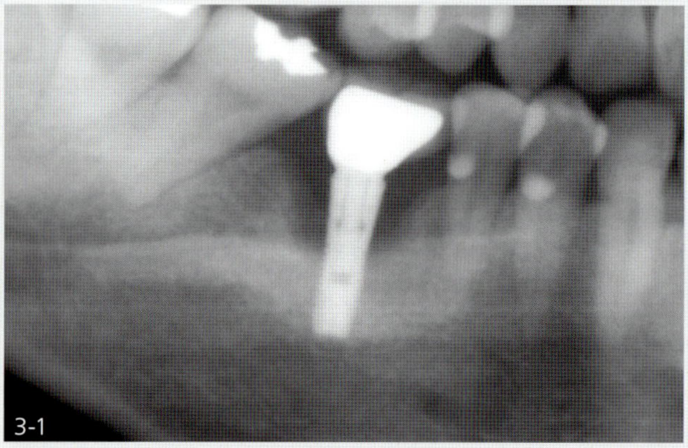
3-1

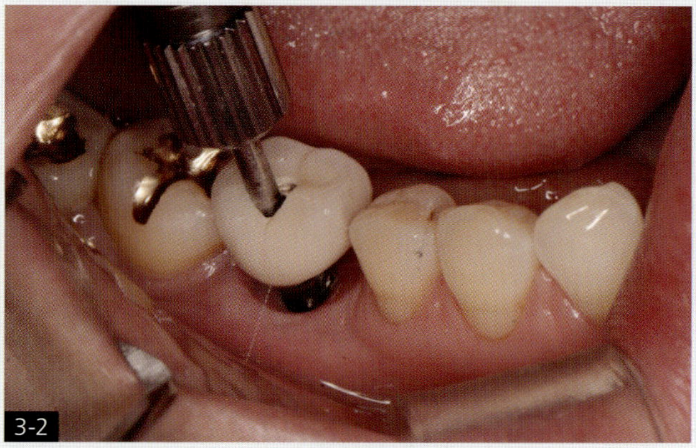
3-2

As seen in the radiographic images, peri-implantitis occurred around implant number 46 **(Figure 3-1)**. To identify the exact cause, a hole was drilled into the occlusal surface to remove the abutment along with the prosthesis; however, no distinct cause was found **(Figure 3-2)**. Consequently, we proceeded with surgery aimed at reducing the depth of the periodontal pocket.

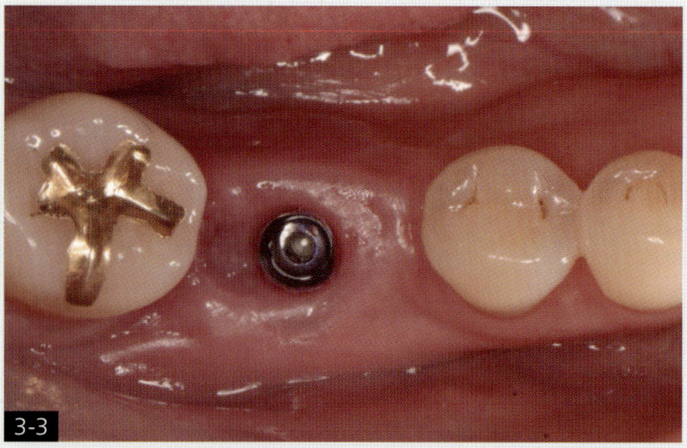
3-3

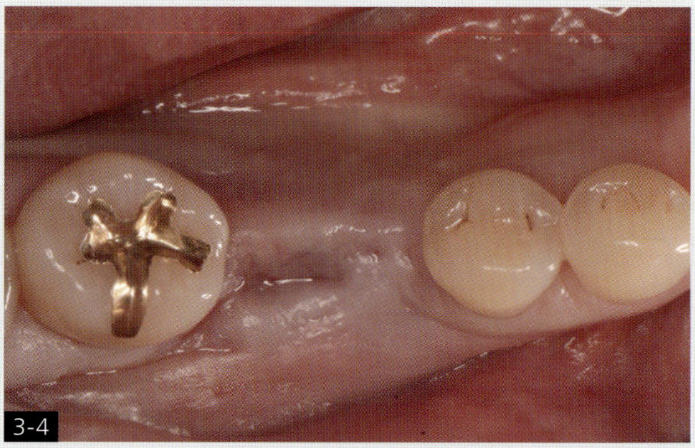
3-4

Although the implant appeared to be deeply placed, it was actually positioned shallowly, and the swollen gingiva made it look deeper than it was **(Figure 3-3)**. After placing the cover screw, we waited for the soft tissue to close, but it did not close as expected **(Figure 3-4)**. Thus, we reluctantly decided to proceed with surgery while the soft tissue remained open.

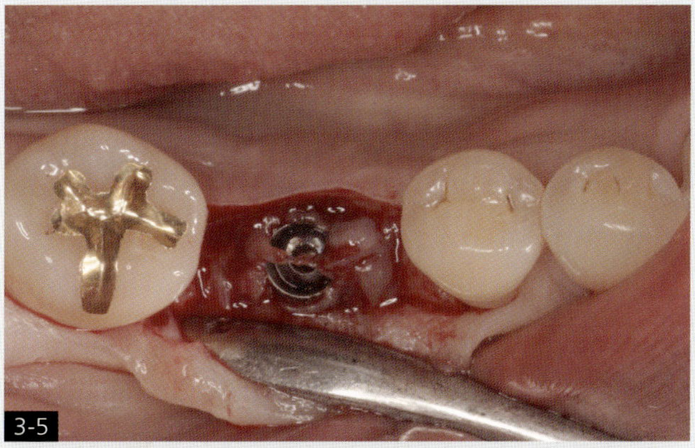
3-5

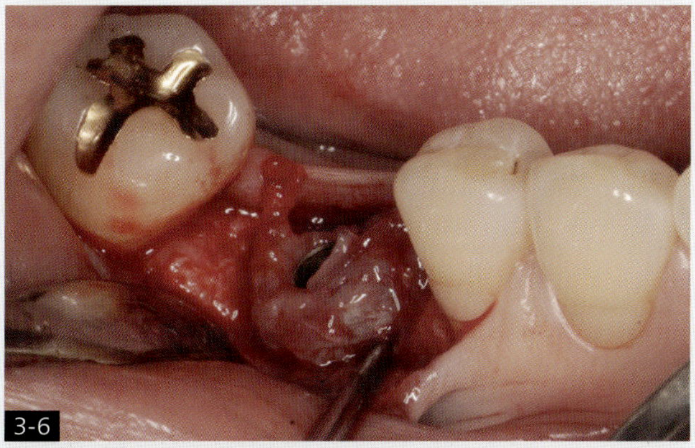
3-6

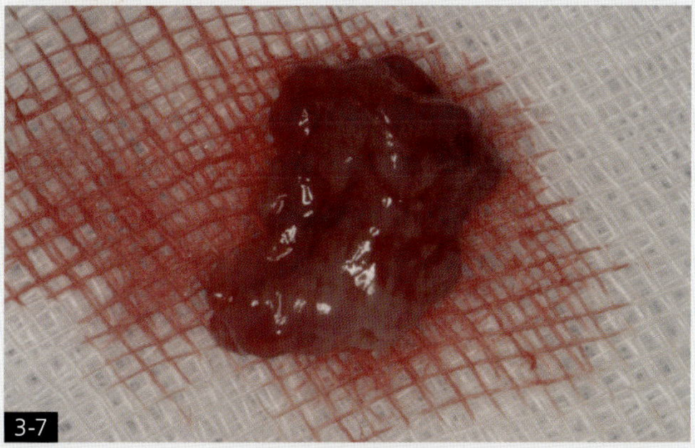
3-7

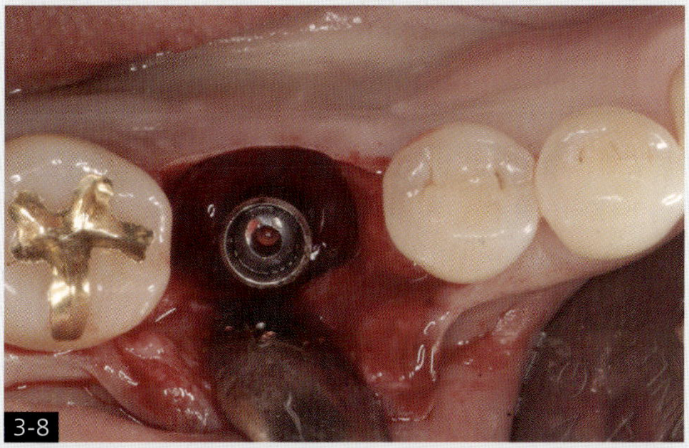
3-8

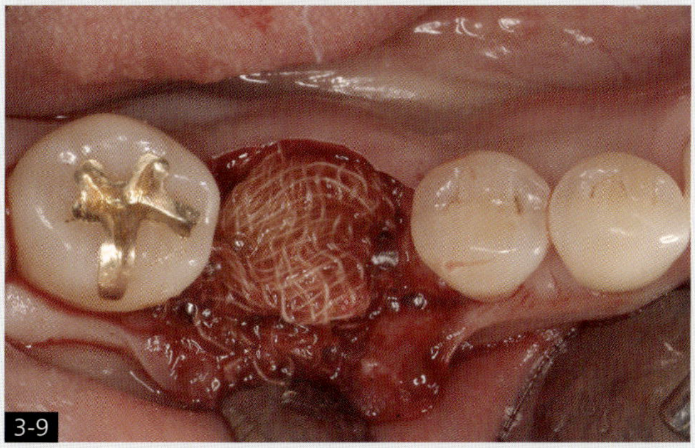
3-9

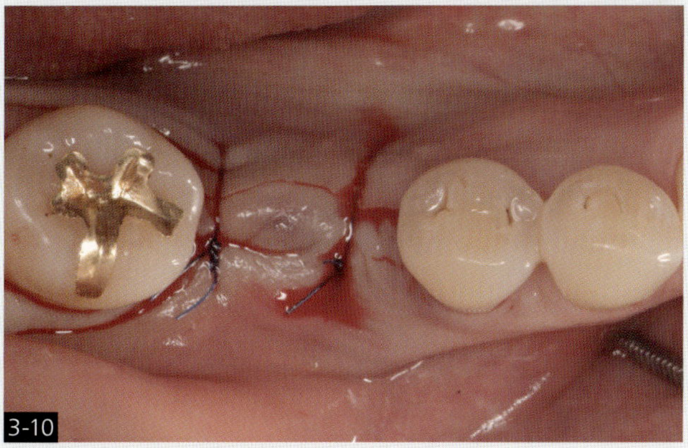
3-10

All surgical procedures were performed in the same manner as in previous cases **(Figures 3-5~10)**. Due to the excessive amount of bone defect, there was a possibility of surgical failure, and if that occurred, the implant would need to be removed; therefore, we opted not to perform bone grafting. We deemed it inappropriate to invest in a surgery with uncertain outcomes. The patient was informed in advance that if the surgical results were unsatisfactory, it would be advisable to remove the implant and place a new one.

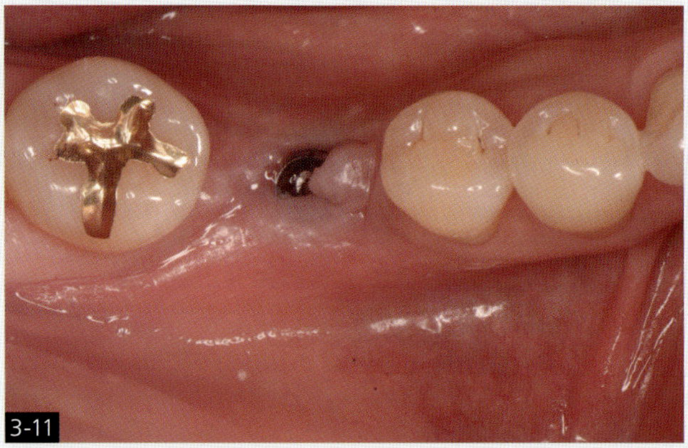
3-11

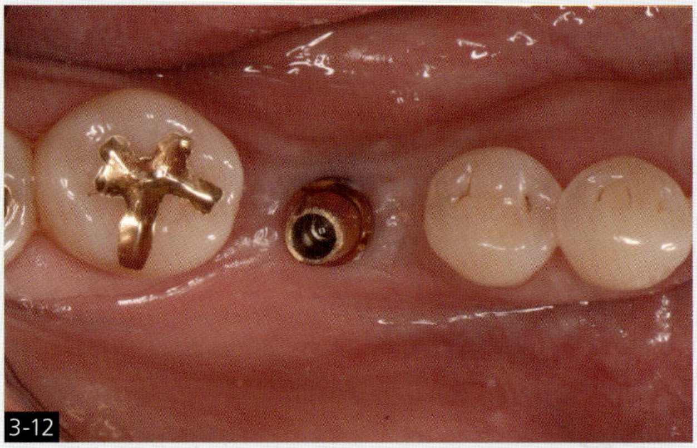
3-12

The inflammation of the soft tissue had resolved **(Figure 3-11)**. Since the implant was initially positioned high, the cover screw and fixture top were exposed above the soft tissue, as shown in the above image. There was concern that the rough surface could harbor bacteria, leading to soft tissue inflammation and a deepening of the periodontal pocket; however, this did not occur, and we proceeded with the prosthetic work as per standard protocol **(Figure 3-12)**. (It was considered fortunate.) The implant used in this clinical case was an Astra implant, which, as previously mentioned, is easy to clean and likely contributed to the success of the treatment.

Peri-implantitis occurring with SLA surface implants would not succeed using the aforementioned method. Currently, there are many seminars in Korea regarding the treatment of peri-implantitis. Various opinions have been expressed regarding surface cleaning methods, and many tools have been developed and sold to facilitate this cleaning. However, since cleaning methods must vary according to the surface treatment, it is recommended that readers first recognize the type of implant surface they are using and respond accordingly.

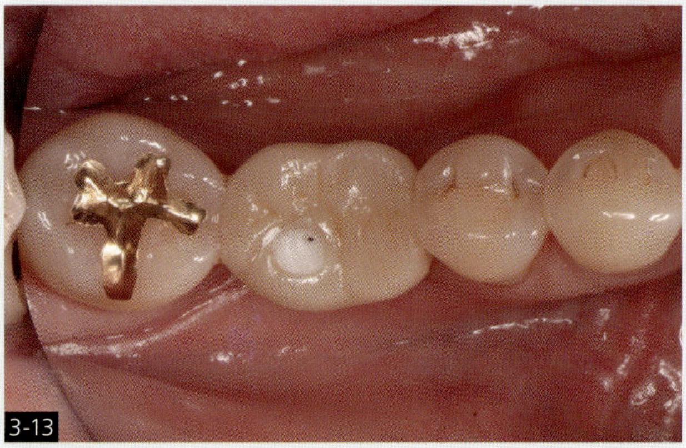
3-13

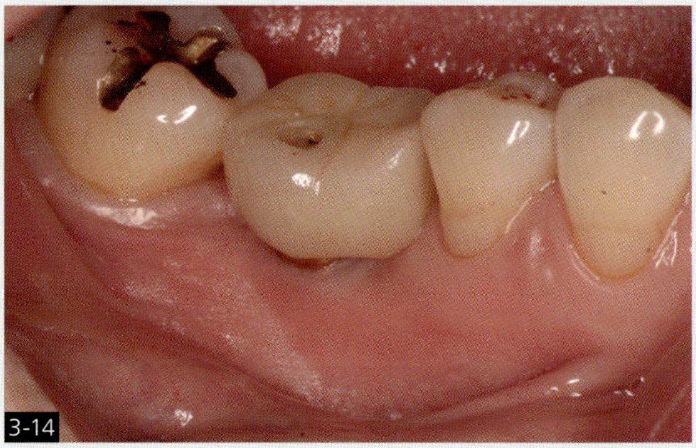
3-14

The case was completed with ceramic prosthetics. Due to the implant being placed on the buccal side, there was a noticeable deficiency of gingiva in that area. However, the vestibule was sufficiently spacious, suggesting that this was not a significant issue **(Figures 3-13, 14)**. Fortunately, all inflammation had resolved, and the periodontal pocket had become shallower.

It is believed that instead of merely removing bacteria, the goal was to shallow the periodontal pocket to a level where only non-pathogenic bacteria could exist in the gingival sulcus.

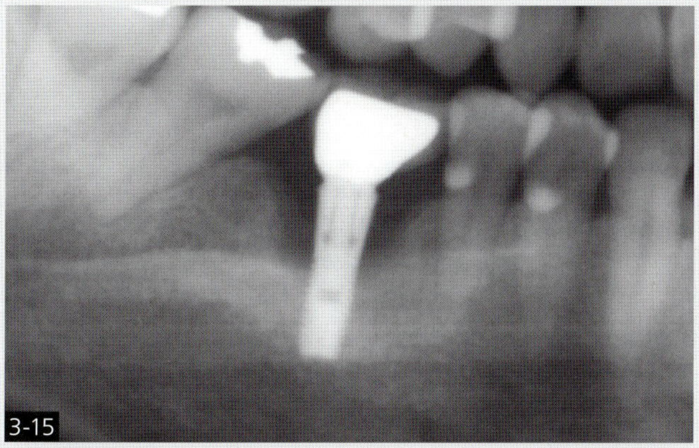
3-15

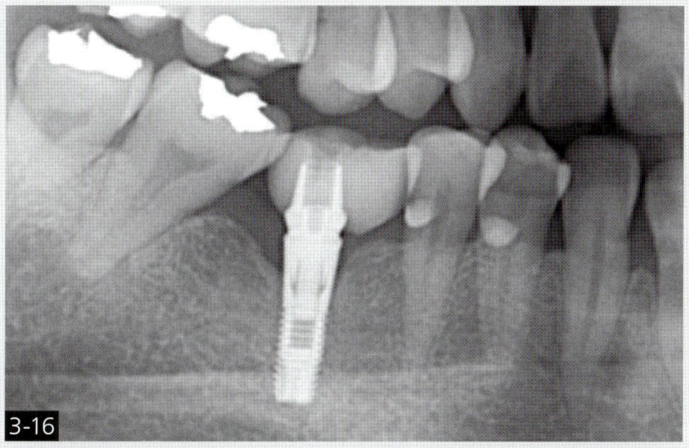
3-16

The initial appearance and the appearance approximately four years later are shown. The alveolar bone had naturally recovered significantly **(Figures 3-15, 16)**. This indicates that bone grafting is not the primary factor in the treatment of peri-implantitis.

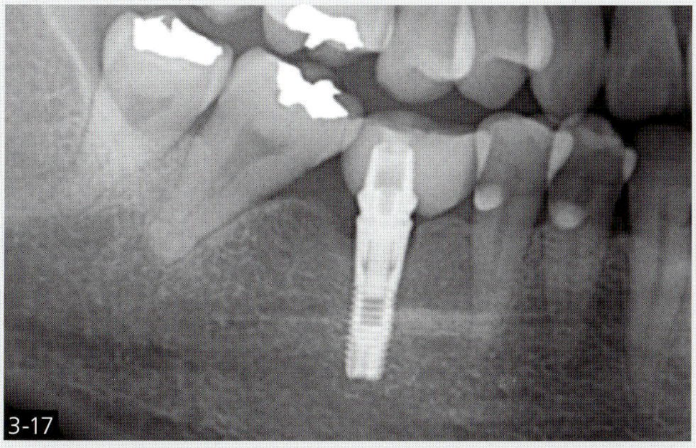
3-17

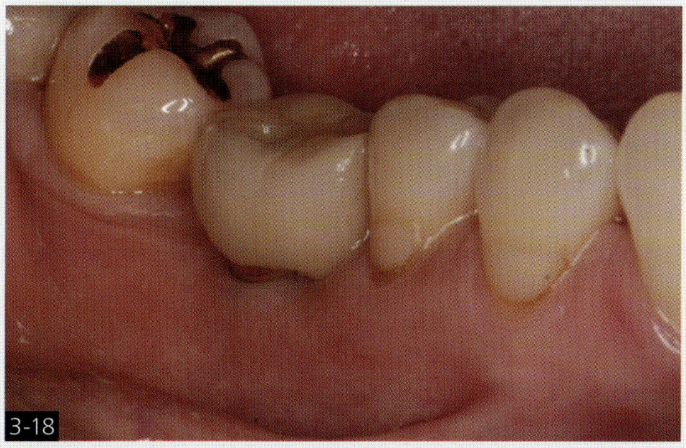
3-18

The appearance after about eight years post-surgery is shown. The alveolar bone continued to proliferate, and clinically, there was still no inflammation **(Figures 3-17, 18)**. Now, I would like to reflect on the causes of peri-implantitis that occurred in this case.

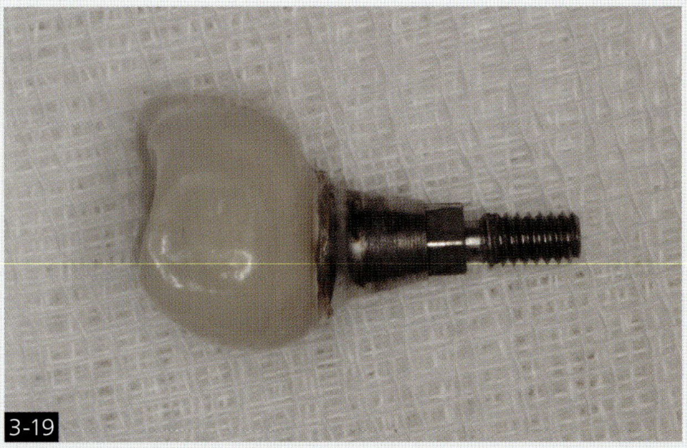

3-19

I observed the above image closely (Figure 3-19). I suspected that there might be some underlying cause for the peri-implantitis. I thought there might be residual adhesive present, but I could not find any. After prolonged observation, I was able to identify the area depicted in the following image.

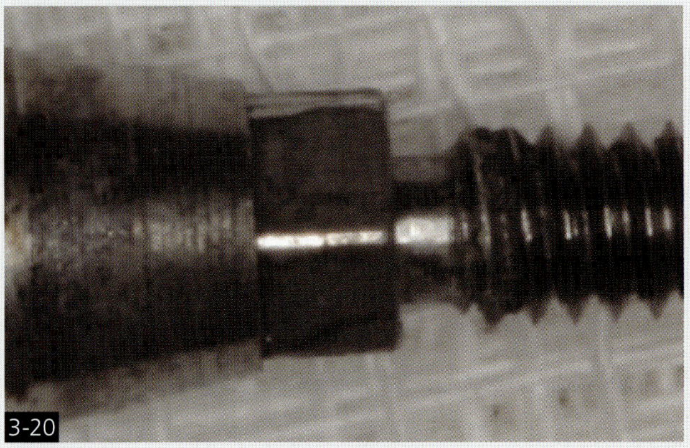

3-20

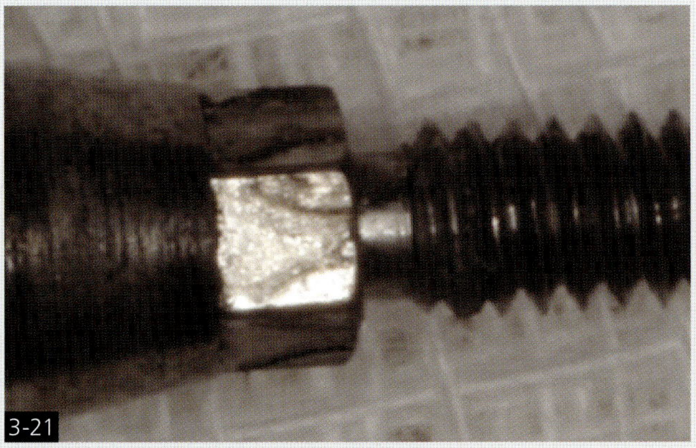

3-21

While examining the hex area of the abutment, I felt a shiver (Figures 3-20, 21). The causes of marginal bone loss around implants can be broadly classified into two categories: micro-gap and micro-mobility. I have long believed that the latter is a significant cause of marginal bone loss. As seen in the images, I suspected that there was continuous micro-movement of the abutment within the fixture, leading to damage in the hex area. The micro-mobility of the abutment destroys the mucosal seal of the soft tissue, allowing bacterial invasion. This invasion by bacteria is what leads to marginal bone loss. It is not merely the presence of bacteria that causes bone loss; rather, it is the absence or destruction of the mucosal seal that permits bacterial invasion.

Once peri-implantitis occurs, the periodontal pocket deepens, and this deepened pocket becomes a breeding ground for pathogenic bacteria, making spontaneous healing impossible. Therefore, it is essential to reduce the depth of the periodontal pocket through surgery and eliminate the micro-mobility that contributes to the problem. The methods for eliminating micro-mobility at the fixture-abutment connection will be discussed in the next chapter.

Let's examine more clinical cases to see if abutment mobility can indeed lead to peri-implantitis. (Presenting just one clinical case could be seen as coincidental, but if there are many similar cases, it is difficult to dismiss them as mere coincidence.)

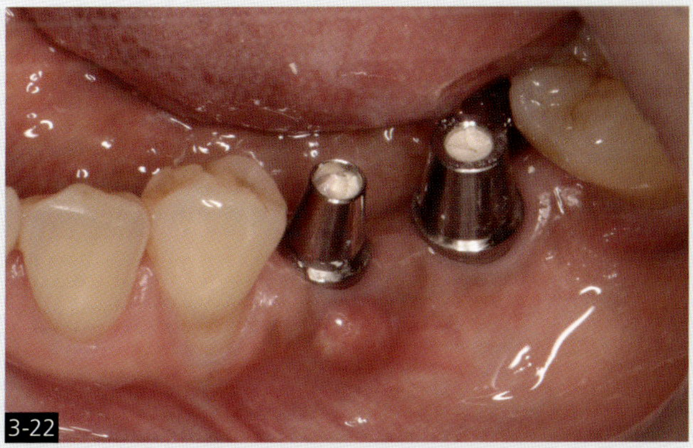

3-22

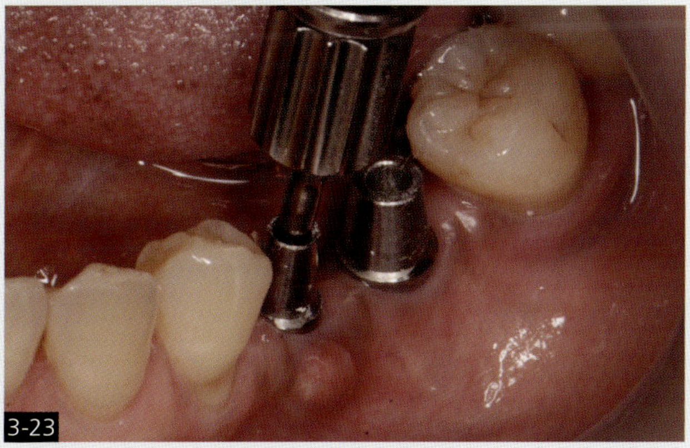

3-23

Inflammation of the gingiva was observed around implant number 35 **(Figure 3-22)**. Bacterial invasion was suspected. The mere presence of bacteria in the oral cavity cannot be considered the sole cause of infection; there must be some underlying reason.

I believed that the mobility of the abutment led to the destruction of the mucosal seal, allowing for bacterial invasion. Without any disinfection or antibiotic treatment, I simply tightened the loose abutment screw using a hex driver (the abutment screw was loose, and the abutment was in a state of mobility) **(Figure 3-23)**.

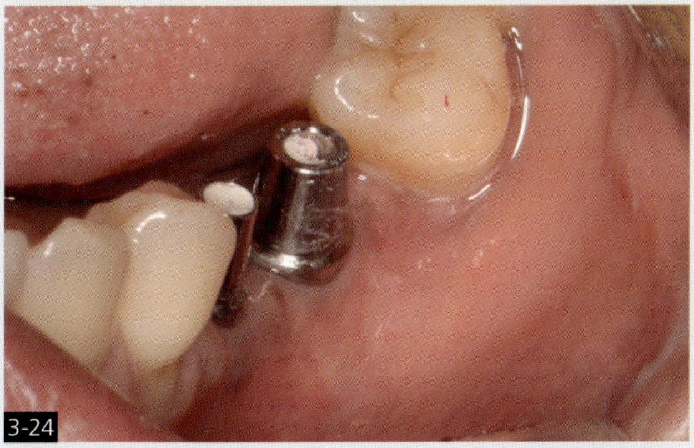

3-24

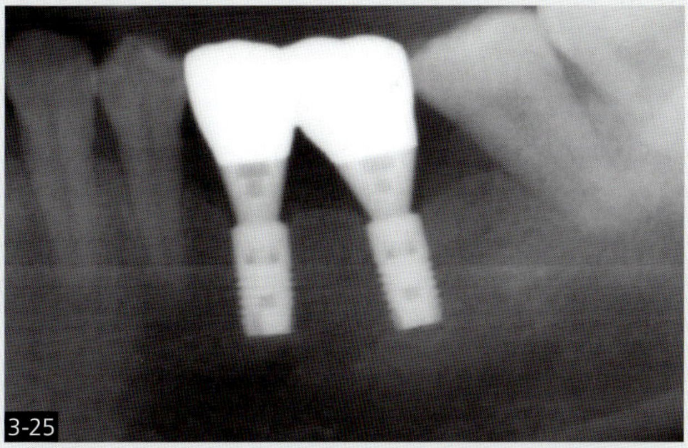

3-25

A week later, miraculously, the gingival inflammation had disappeared **(Figure 3-24)**. It was confirmed that the loosening of the abutment screw was the cause. Fortunately, no bone loss was detected in the radiographic images **(Figure 3-25)**.

Had the abutment screw remained loose for an extended period, I believe that marginal bone loss would have occurred, leading to peri-implantitis. Therefore, the loosening of the abutment screw is a matter that clinicians must carefully monitor.

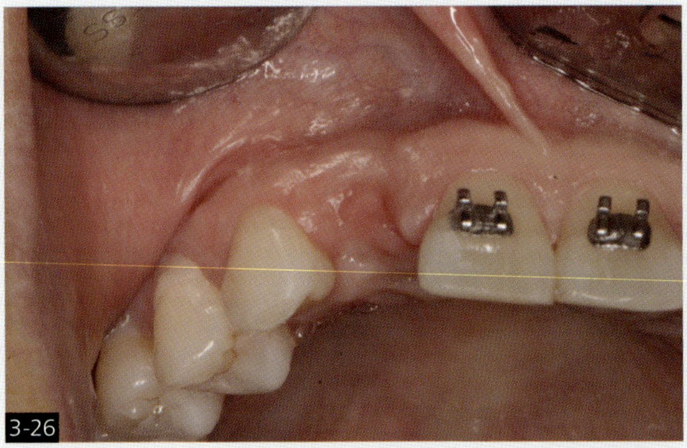

3-26

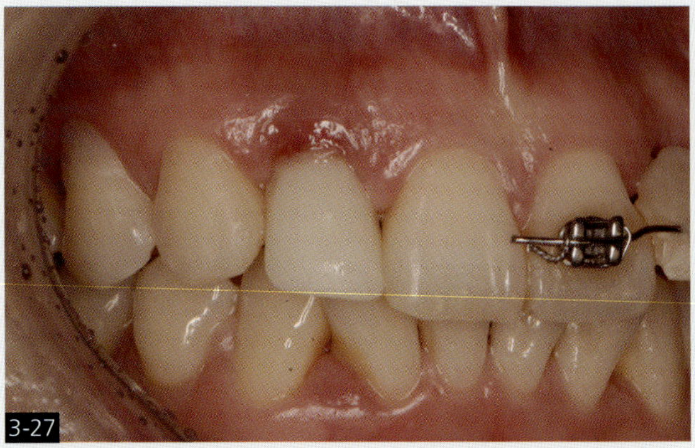

3-27

Let's look at another clinical case. The patient had a temporary restoration on implant number 12, and inflammation with swelling was observed in the gingiva **(Figure 3-27)**.

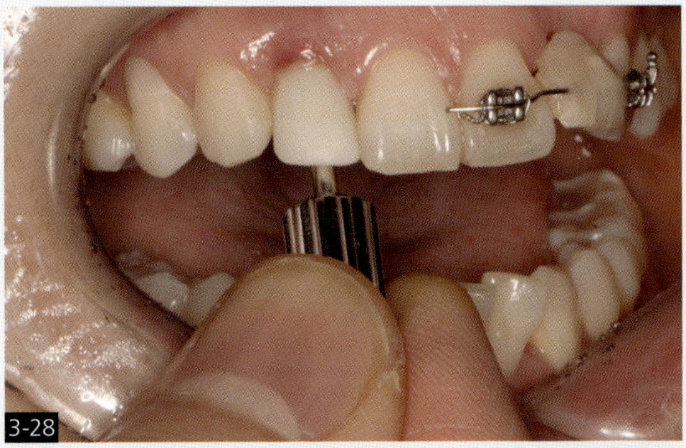

3-28

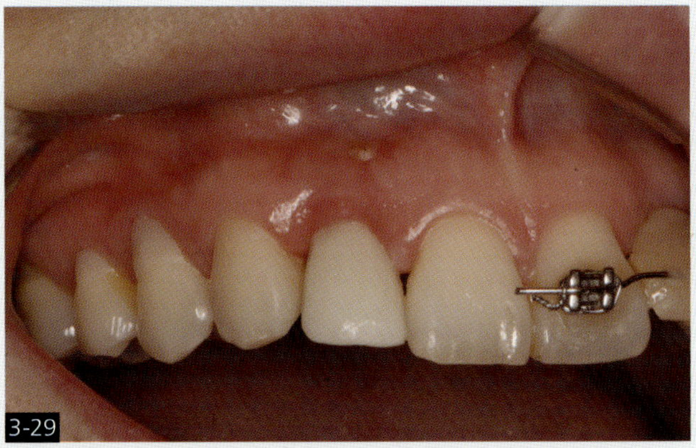

3-29

I did nothing other than tighten the screw **(Figure 3-28)**.

A week later, most of the inflammation had subsided **(Figure 3-29)**. This indicates a clear correlation between screw loosening and gingival inflammation. A mechanical issue caused a biological problem. Loosening of the screw is not merely a mechanical issue; it is closely related to biological problems.

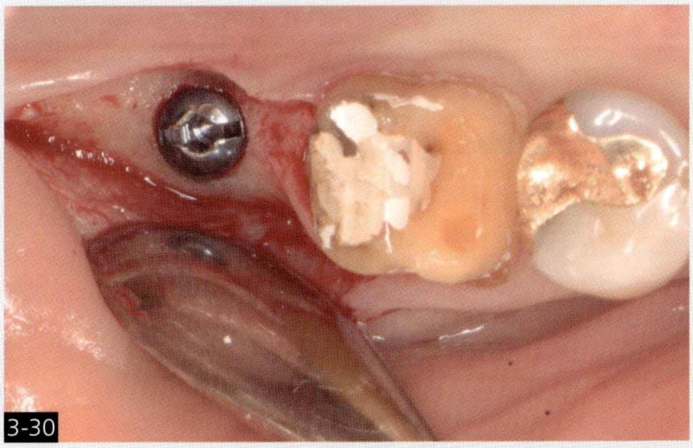
3-30

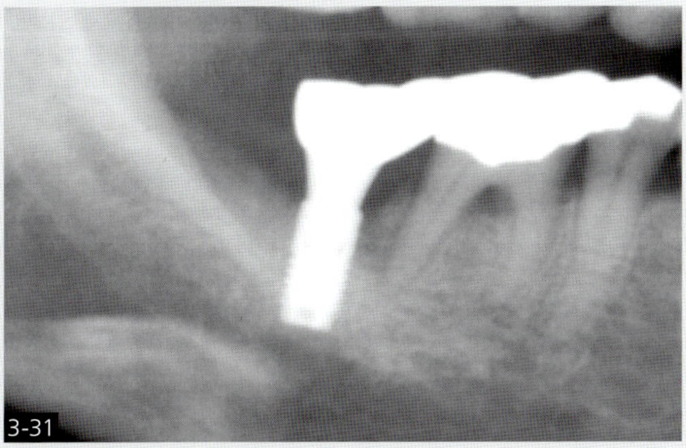
3-31

The surgical and radiographic images of implant number 47 show no bone loss and excellent bone response (Figures 3-30, 31).

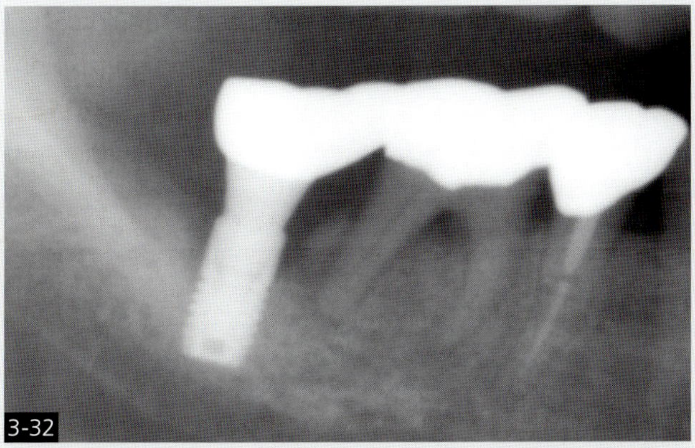
3-32

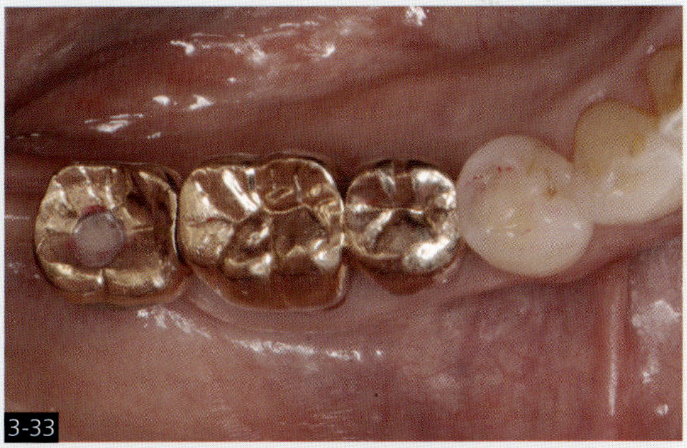
3-33

However, after about eight years, marginal bone loss was observed, and peri-implantitis developed (Figure 3-32). The abutment screw was already loose, the periodontal pocket had deepened, and bone loss was observed, making it too late to intervene.

Ultimately, this implant had to be extracted (Figure 3-33). Preventing screw loosening is crucial, and if it cannot be prevented, immediate action must be taken upon discovery. Failing to do so could lead to the necessity of implant removal. Loosening of screws and abutment mobility should never be treated as trivial issues.

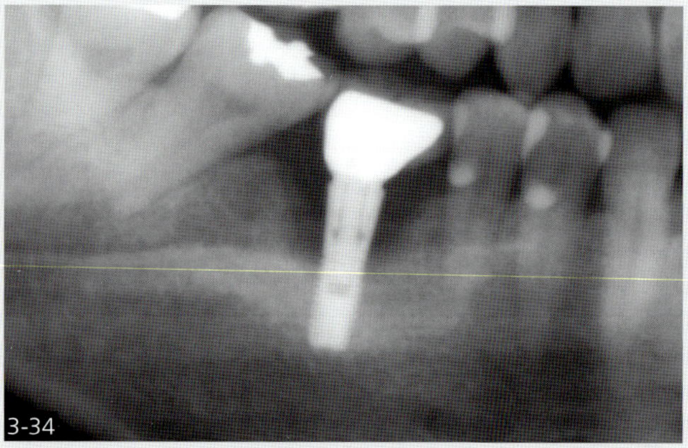

3-34

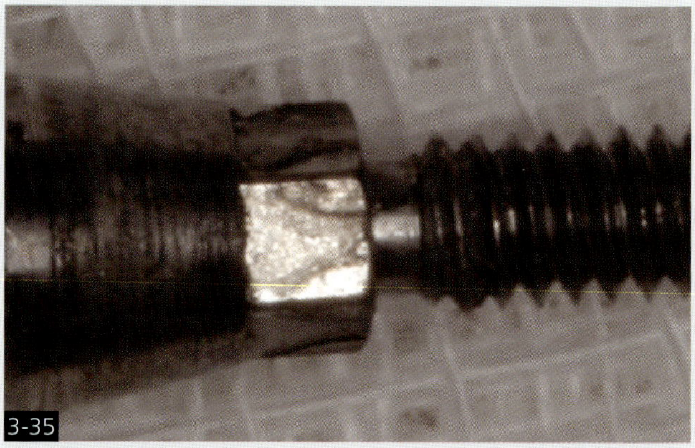

3-35

I prefer to use non-hex abutments unless there are special circumstances. There are various opinions regarding whether to use hex type or non-hex type abutments. Personally, I do not think it is crucial which type is used, nor do I believe that one type is superior to the other. However, the reason I favor and frequently use non-hex abutments is quite simple.

When using hex type abutments, as shown in the images, it is often difficult to detect screw loosening and abutment mobility until peri-implantitis occurs **(Figures 3-34, 35)**. In contrast, with non-hex abutments, both the prosthesis and the abutment move together, prompting the patient to visit the clinic due to discomfort.

In other words, my preference for non-hex abutments is to easily identify screw loosening after the prosthesis is placed. In many cases where hex type abutments are used, the abutment screws may actually be loose, but this often goes unnoticed clinically. (In cases where more than three months have passed since the prosthesis was placed, one can easily find that the screw turns significantly when tightened through the occlusal access hole.)

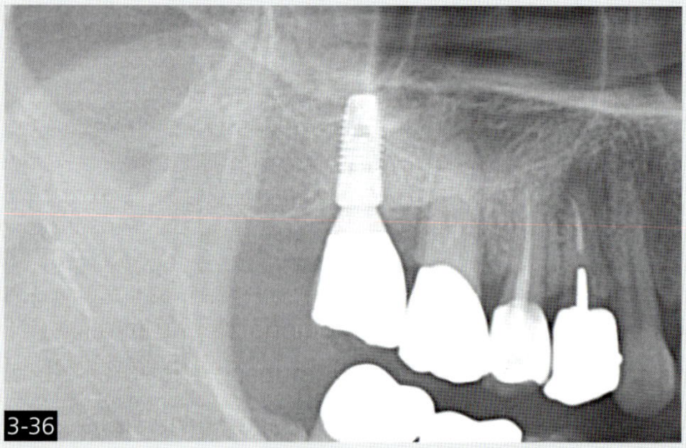

3-36

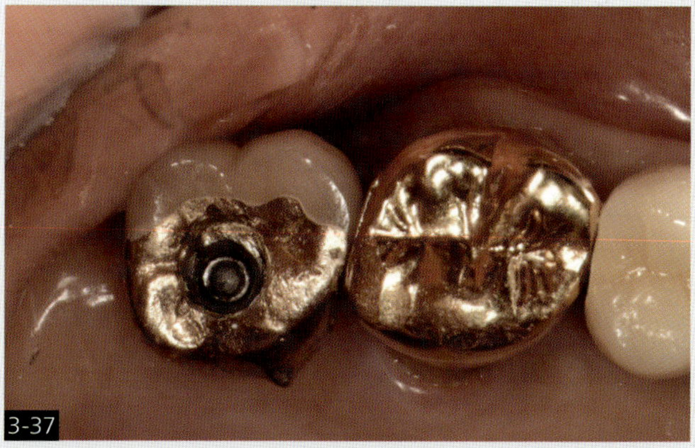

3-37

A patient presented with a complaint that the prosthesis on implant number 17 was loose. Suspecting that the abutment screw was loose, I created an access hole in the occlusal surface of the prosthesis and removed both the prosthesis and the abutment simultaneously **(Figures 3-36, 37)**.

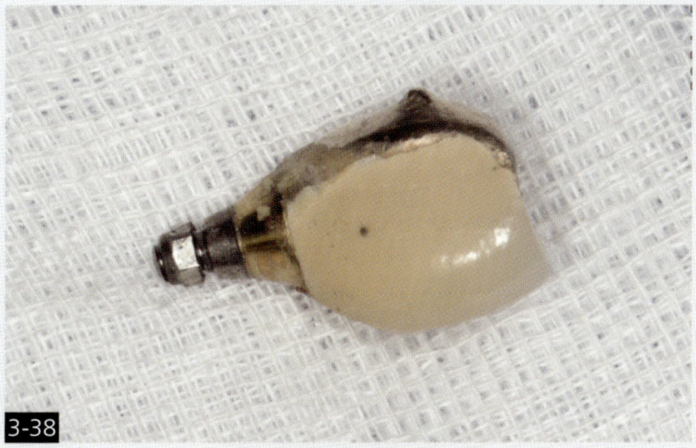
3-38

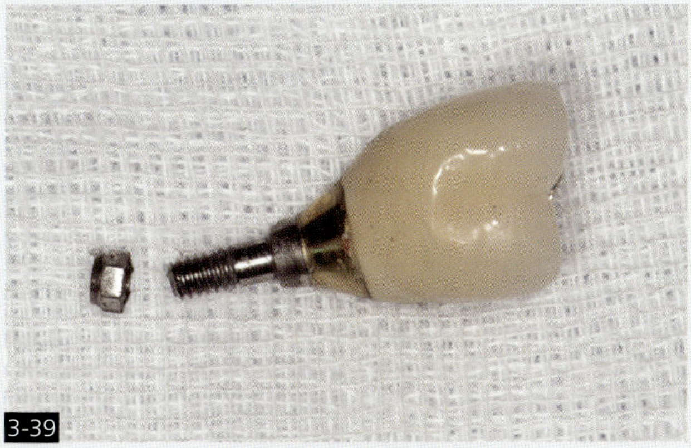
3-39

To my surprise, I found that the hex portion of the removed abutment was broken **(Figures 3-38, 39)**. The patient reported that it had been ten years since the prosthesis was placed. The original purpose of the hex was to aid in the proper placement of the implant into the alveolar bone, but it is now being used as a prosthetic tool. Observing such damage raises doubts about whether we clinicians can rely on hex as a prosthetic means.

I believe that for stable connections, we should not depend on hex. The hex is a complementary tool for prosthetics, not an absolute one. The concepts and clinical techniques necessary for achieving stable connections will be discussed in the next chapter, as noted by Professor Yeoinseong.

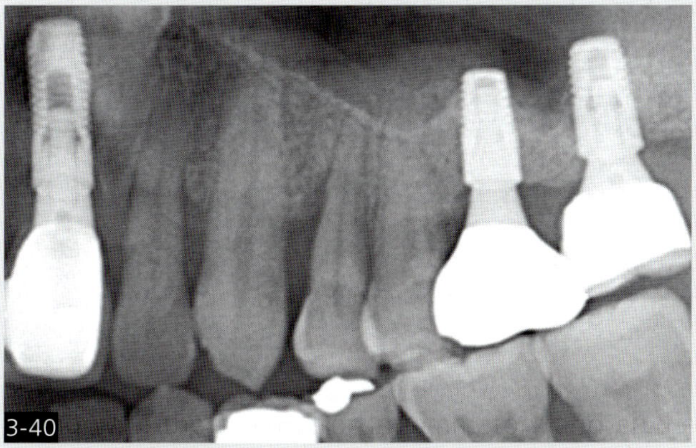
3-40

The periodontal condition of tooth number 24 is significantly poor **(Figure 3-40)**.

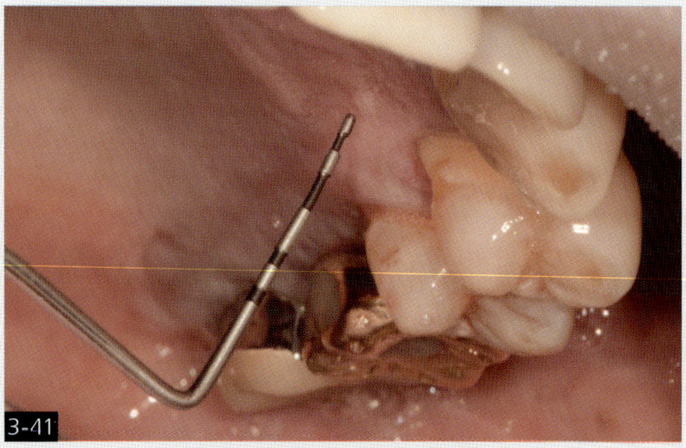

3-41

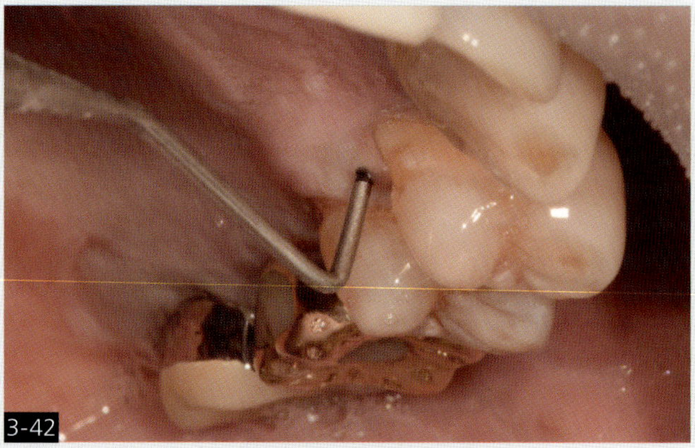

3-42

We clinicians often witness deep periodontal pockets on the palatal side of maxillary premolars. There can be various causes for this, but I focus on the buccal cusp's palatal surface of tooth number 24. There is no cusp tip phenomenon on tooth number 25, but it is present on tooth number 24. During mastication, excessive lateral forces were applied to the buccal cusp's palatal surface of tooth number 24.

I believe that these forces caused movement towards the buccal side, leading to the formation of a palatal periodontal pocket. Since such movement did not occur on tooth number 25, the depth of the palatal periodontal pocket did not increase **(Figures 3-41, 42)**.

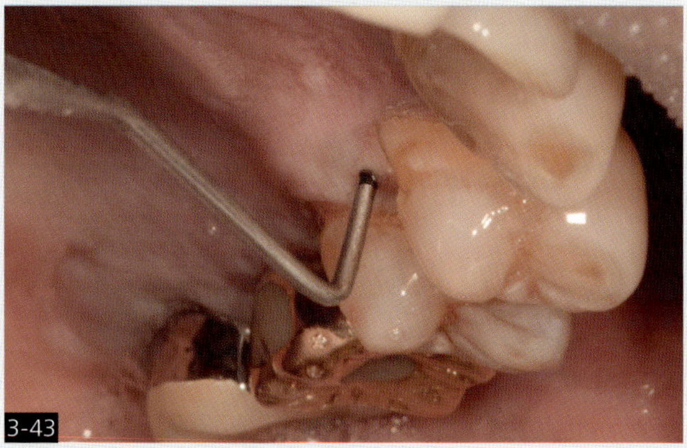

3-43

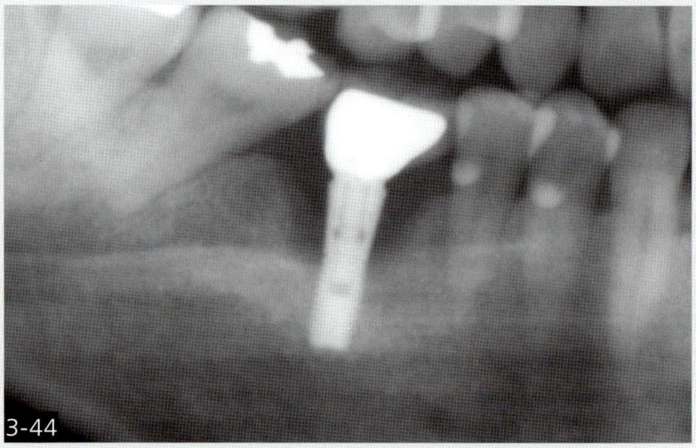

3-44

Just as the buccal movement of the maxillary premolar destroyed the palatal mucosal seal and formed a periodontal pocket **(Figure 3-43)**, the movement of the implant abutment also appears to have destroyed the mucosal seal, leading to the formation of a periodontal pocket **(Figure 3-44)**. This phenomenon applies the same principles to both natural teeth and implants.

2. Frenum

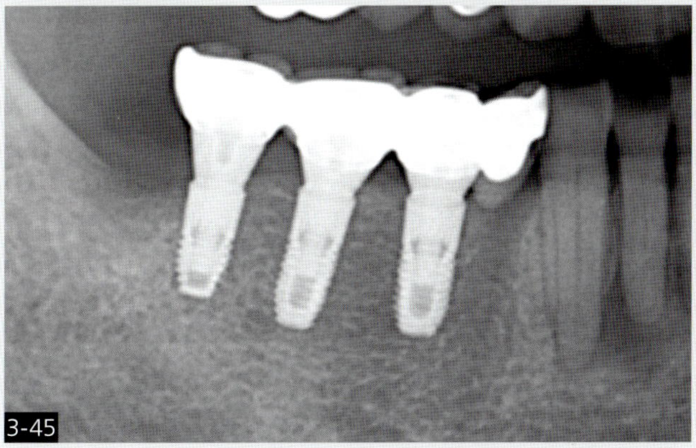
3-45

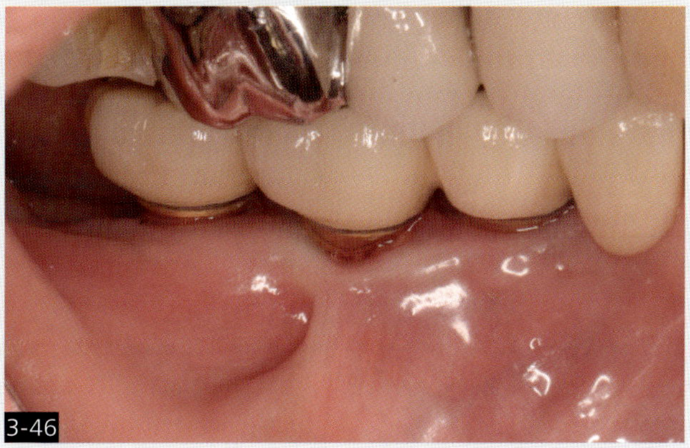
3-46

Implants were placed in the areas of teeth 45, 46, and 47, and prosthetic treatment was completed **(Figure 3-45)**.

As seen in the image, the frenum is attached high on the buccal surface of implant number 46. This frenum pulls on the gingiva, destroying the mucosal seal on the buccal surface of the abutment **(Figure 3-46)**. The destruction of this mucosal seal allows for bacterial invasion, so it should be addressed immediately upon observation.

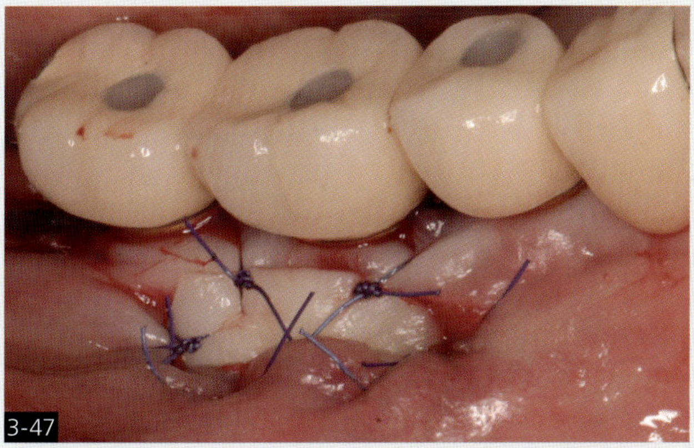
3-47

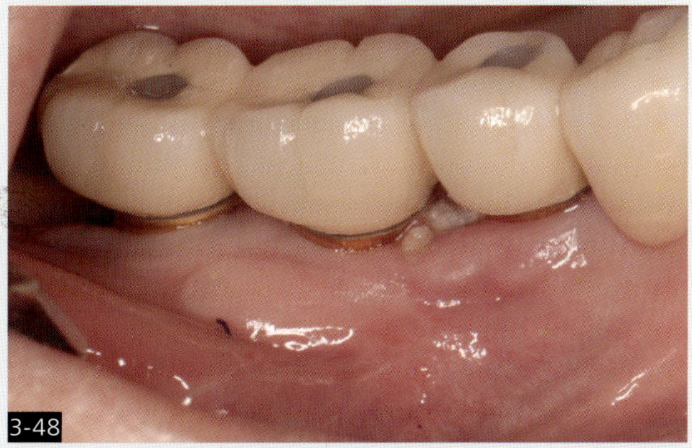
3-48

A gingival graft was harvested from the palatal side and transplanted to the buccal side **(Figure 3-47)**. To eliminate the buccal frenum, it is necessary to release the frenum towards the root apex, and the exposed area must undergo gingival grafting. Simply incising the frenum will not be effective, as it will likely reattach soon after, rendering the surgery ineffective. In **Figure 3-48**, we can observe a small piece of bone forming on the mesial buccal side of tooth number 46.

This indicates that bacterial invasion occurred rapidly, leading to necrosis before the alveolar bone could undergo resorption.

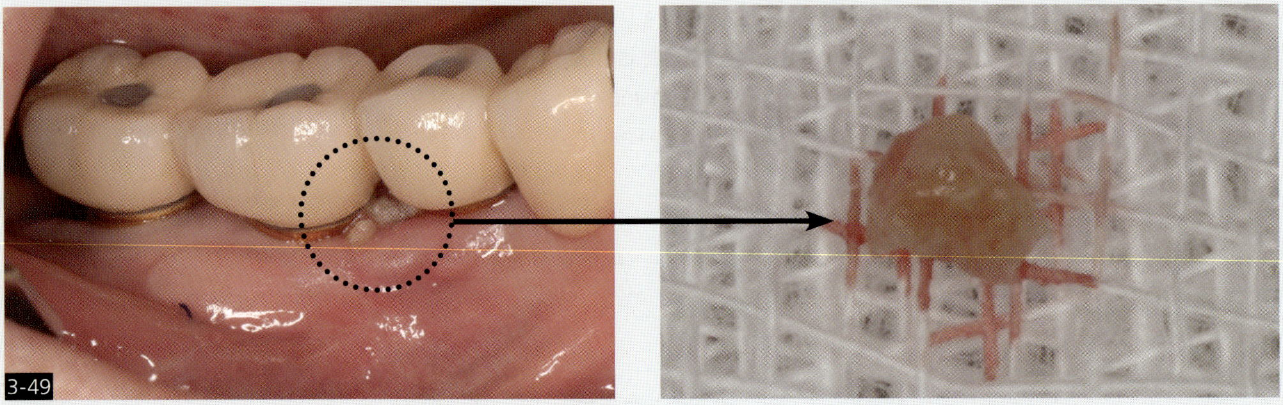

3-49

The appearance of the removed bone is shown in **Figure 3-49**. As seen in this clinical case, just like the movement of the abutment in implants, the movement of the gingiva caused by the frenum can also destroy the mucosal seal, potentially leading to peri-implantitis.

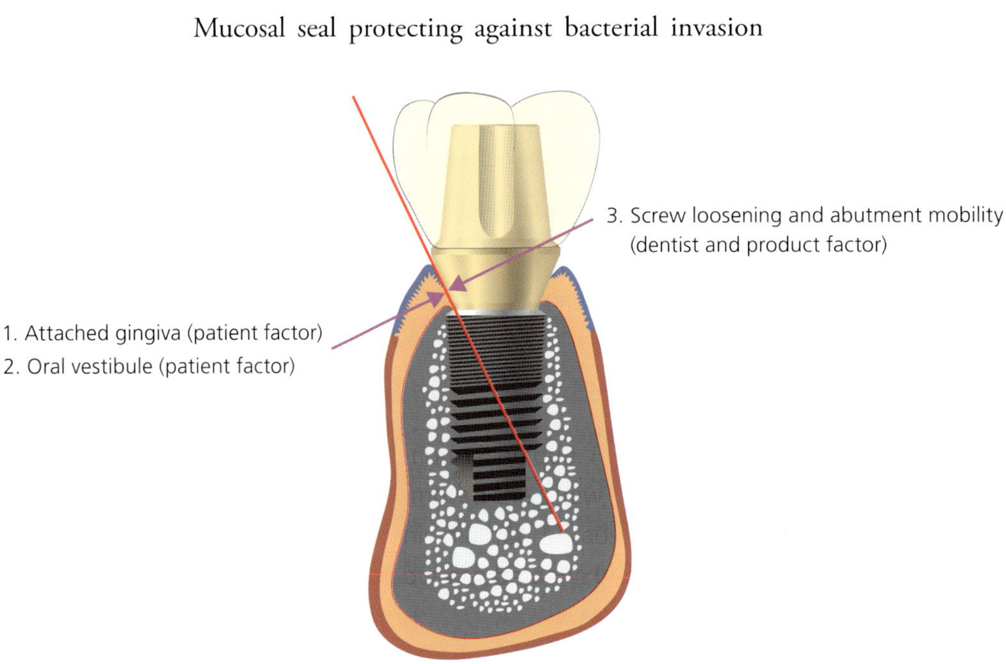

3-50

When illustrating this concept **(Figure 3-50)**, it becomes evident that most issues with implants arise at the connection site. Peri-implantitis also occurs at this location. Bacteria can invade the gingiva and alveolar bone through the gingival sulcus, leading to bone resorption and the downward proliferation of the periodontal pocket epithelium, which deepens the periodontal pocket. To fundamentally prevent these issues, a perfect mucosal seal must form around the abutment to protect the alveolar bone from bacteria. The abutment should not move at the top of the implant, and the movements of the buccal and lingual soft tissues should not be transmitted to the marginal gingiva. To prevent movement of the marginal gingiva, the implant and abutment should be surrounded by attached gingiva rather than mucosa. It is effective for the gingiva to be attached gingiva rather than free gingiva. For the gingiva to be attached, the alveolar bone beneath it must not be lost. Clinically, if there is insufficient or inadequate attached gingiva, a deeper vestibule may help to some extent.

To prevent peri-implantitis and ensure long-term stability, the following conditions must be met:

1. Product Requirements: Use of implant products that minimize screw loosening (the implant should also be free from fractures).
2. Dentist Responsibilities: The dentist should place the implant in the center of the gingiva and perform tightening to prevent screw loosening.
3. Patient Conditions: The patient should maintain sufficient gingival width, have a deep vestibule, and practice thorough oral hygiene.

If these three conditions are perfectly fulfilled, I believe that implants can be maintained in the patient's mouth for a semi-permanent duration.

Through the cases discussed, readers should now understand the concept of the mucosal seal. The mucosal seal refers to the histological attachment of epithelial cells and the circular gingival fibers that tightly bind the gingiva to the abutment. This seal acts both biologically and mechanically to prevent bacterial invasion.

Chapter 4

Surgical Techniques for Preventing Peri-implantitis

1. Case of Periodontitis Affected Natural Tooth (Maxillary Anterior Region)

In the treatment of peri-implantitis, the author has argued that the formation of a mucosal seal around the abutment can lead to the spontaneous regeneration of lost alveolar bone. Based on this concept, this section introduces surgical techniques aimed at preventing peri-implantitis and facilitating the natural recovery of alveolar bone when extracting periodontally affected teeth and immediately placing implants.

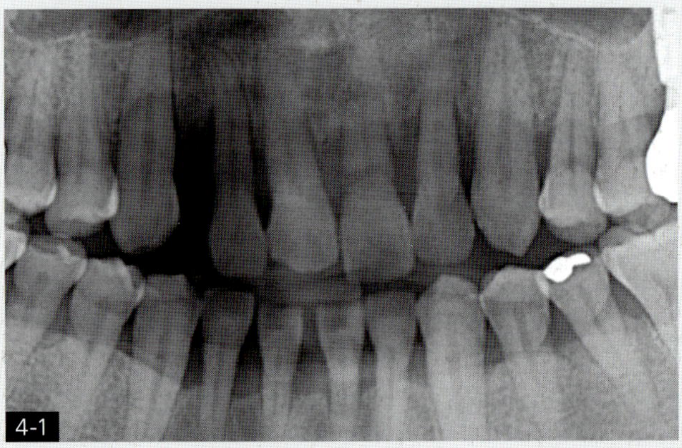

4-1

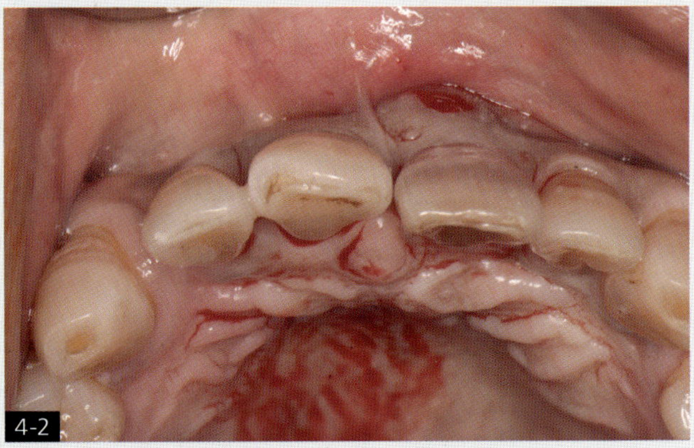

4-2

Figure 4-1 and 4-2 illustrate the presence of a periodontal abscess on tooth #21 after anesthesia. Typically, in cases where an active abscess is present, implant placement is not recommended.

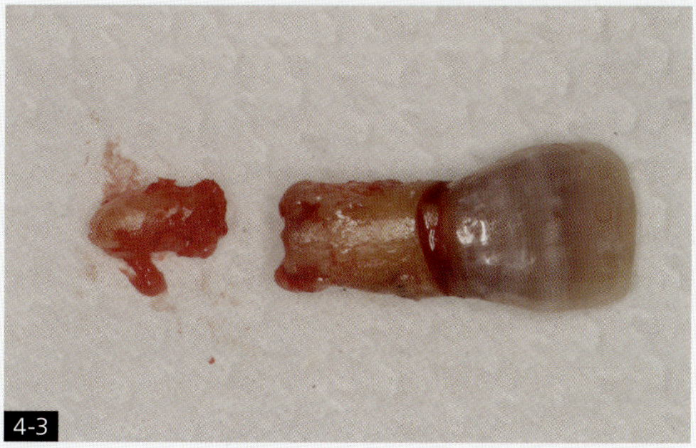

4-3

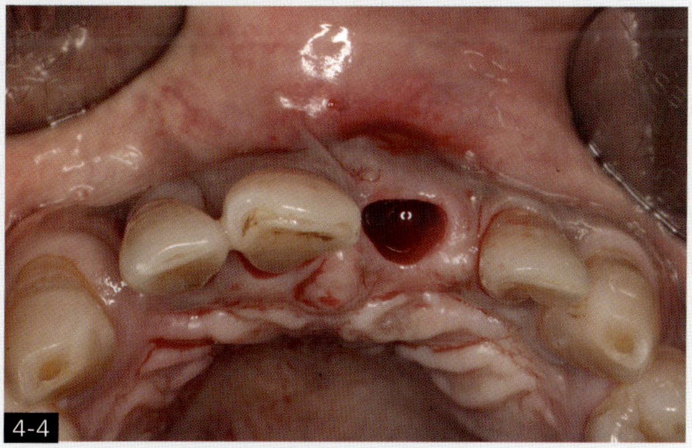

4-4

Figures 4-3 and 4-4 show the extracted tooth and the post-extraction site. Tooth #21 was fractured, and such fractures can lead to tooth mobility. Tooth mobility disrupts the mucosal seal, allowing bacterial invasion and resulting in periodontitis. (This principle applies equally to both implants and natural teeth.)

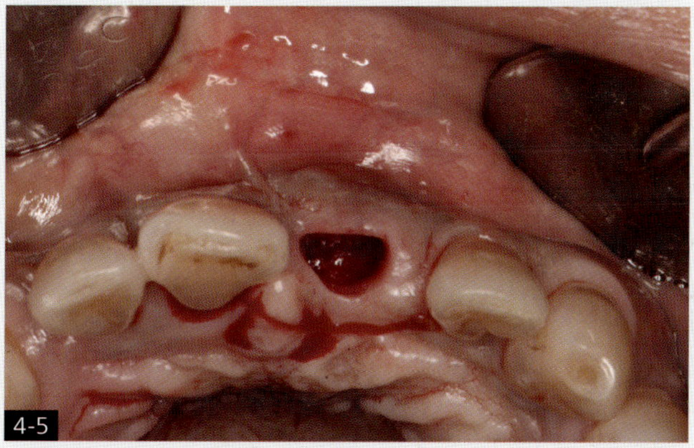

4-5

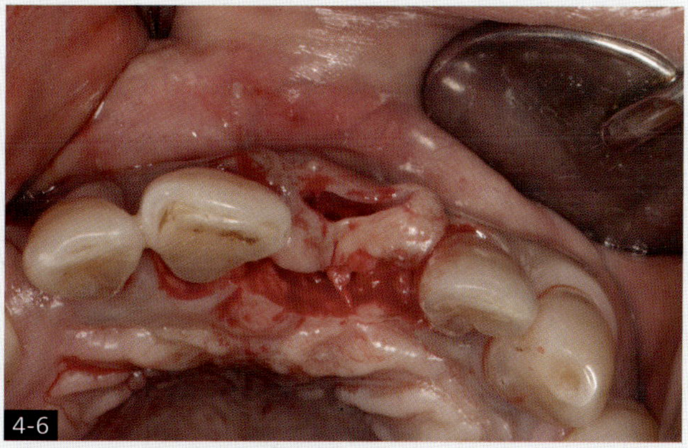

4-6

Among the various methods to restore the extracted tooth (such as bridges or implants), it was decided to place an implant with the patient's consent. When extracting a periodontally affected tooth and placing an implant, I perform a palatal incision to ensure that the extraction site is not directly included in the incision **(Figures 4-5, 6)**.

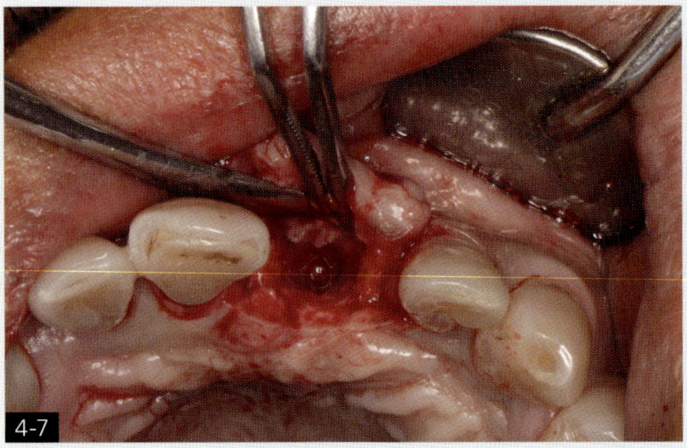

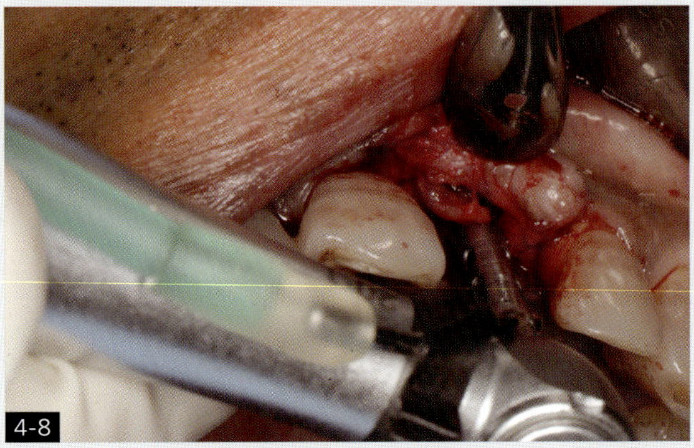

Soft tissue dissection should include the soft tissue and epithelial hyperplasia formed around the periodontally affected tooth. It is crucial to perform this dissection cleanly and in one piece without tearing. To achieve this, the soft tissue should not be scraped with a surgical curette; instead, the alveolar bone should be scraped **(Figure 4-7)**.

As is well known, when placing an implant in the maxillary anterior region, drilling should not be done at the center of the extraction site but rather more palatally, which can be challenging. I frequently use a trephine drill for this purpose **(Figure 4-8)**.

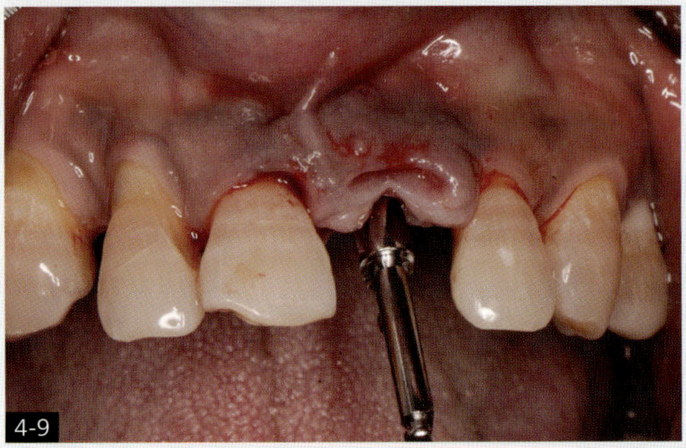

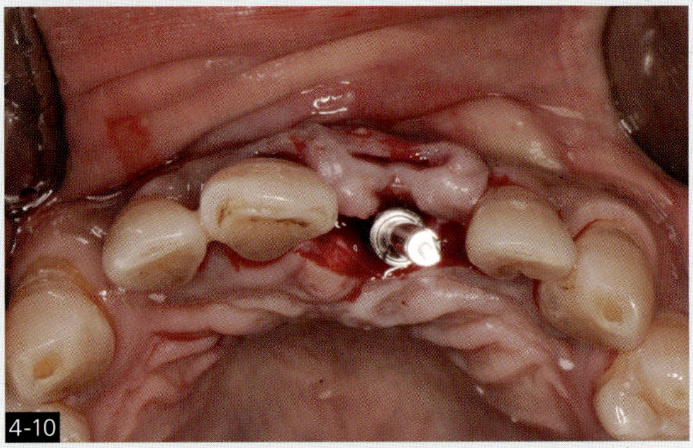

After implant placement, I believe it is more accurate to state that the implant is placed for prosthetic restoration. It is essential to predict whether the prosthetic restoration will be aesthetically pleasing during the surgery. The position and direction of the drilling can be easily verified using the final drill employed. If the drilling is performed satisfactorily, an aesthetically pleasing prosthetic restoration can be anticipated **(Figures 4-9, 10)**.

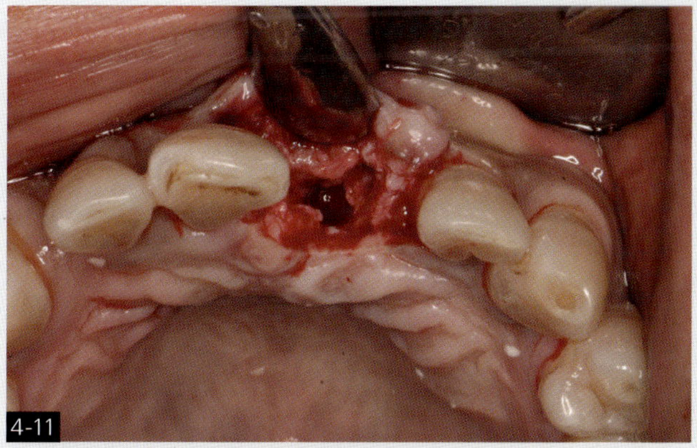

4-11

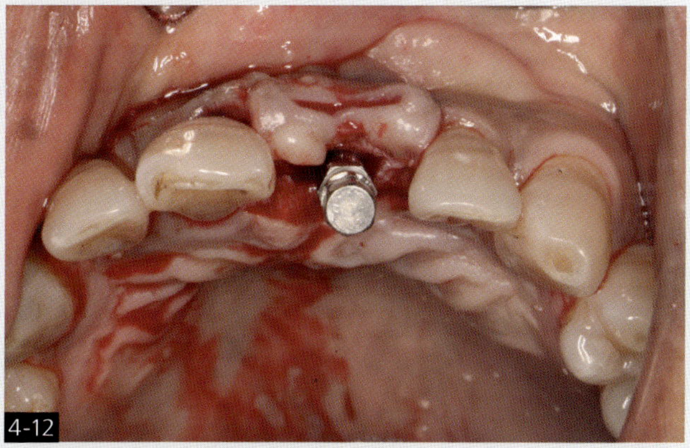

4-12

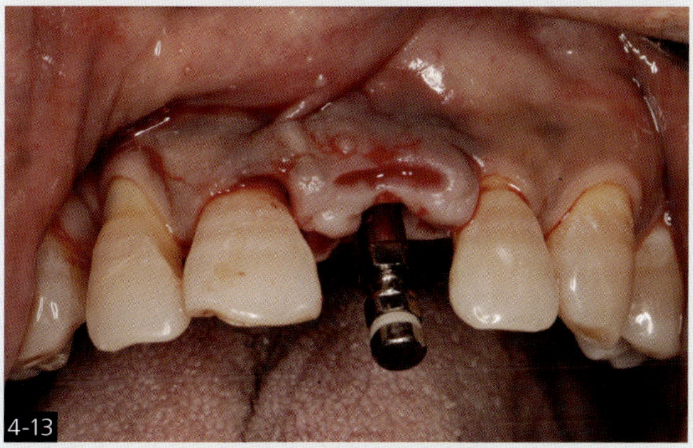

4-13

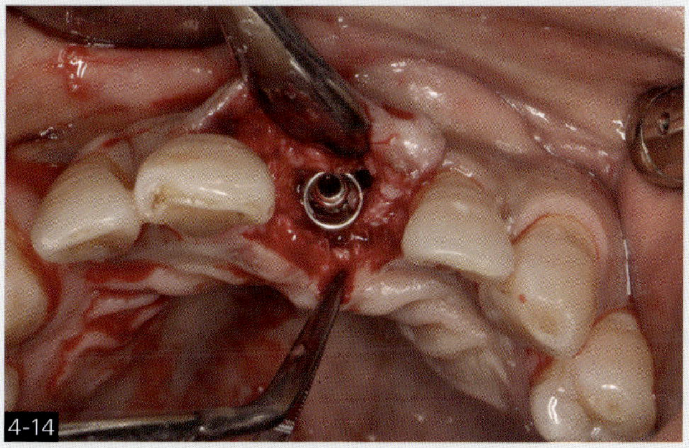

4-14

After drilling, the implant is in place. I always use a mount during implant placement, as it is very useful for confirming the position and direction of the implant after placement. Additionally, it allows for the prediction of the final prosthetic state **(Figures 4-11~14)**.

During anterior implant surgery, I do not position the screw hole of the restoration to emerge from the cingulum of the tooth. To achieve this, the upper part of the implant would need to be tilted significantly palatally, which can be risky as the apex of the implant fixture may penetrate the buccal alveolar bone. Furthermore, during prosthetic restoration, a shorter palatal length of the abutment can reduce the retention of the prosthesis, leading to its dislodgement.

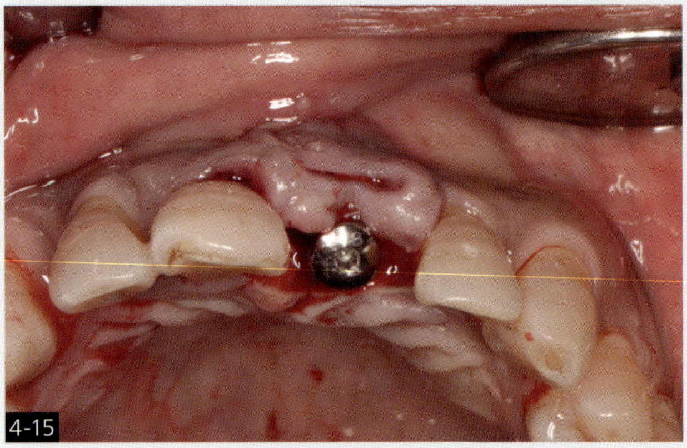
4-15

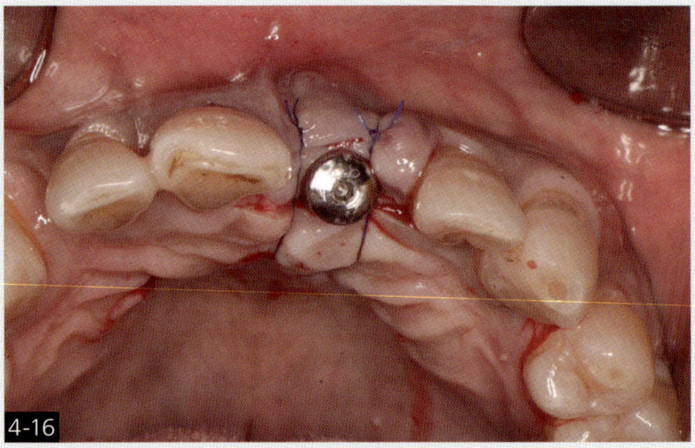
4-16

Soft tissue management is crucial. The soft tissue was entirely positioned buccally before suturing **(Figures 4-15, 16)**. This holds significant importance, and the concept will be graphically explained below. While it may seem that the volume of buccal soft tissue was increased to prevent buccal tissue collapse, this was not my intention. Regardless of how much soft tissue is positioned buccally, if the alveolar bone is resorbed, the volume will decrease, and creating volume solely with soft tissue is not easily achievable.

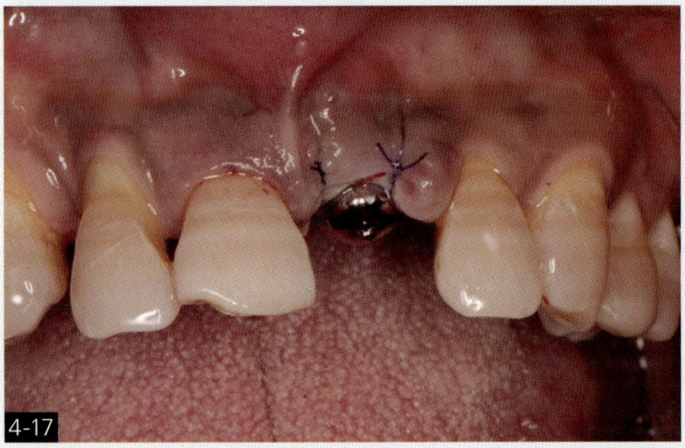
4-17

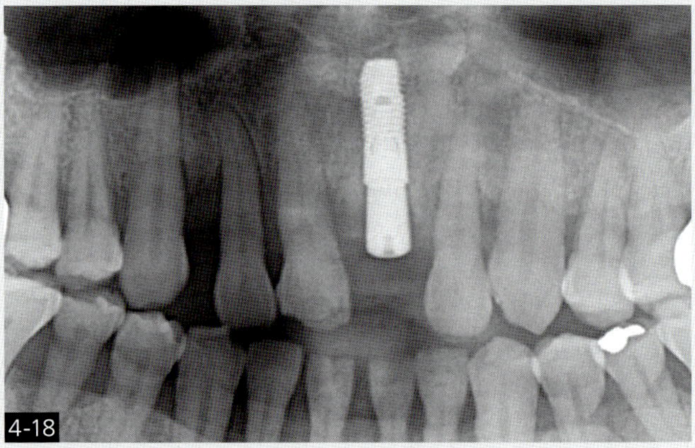
4-18

The inflammatory tissue and epithelial tissue that had hyperplastic growth due to periodontitis were all positioned buccally **(Figure 4-17)**. An X-ray image shows that the surgery was performed successfully **(Figure 4-18)**.

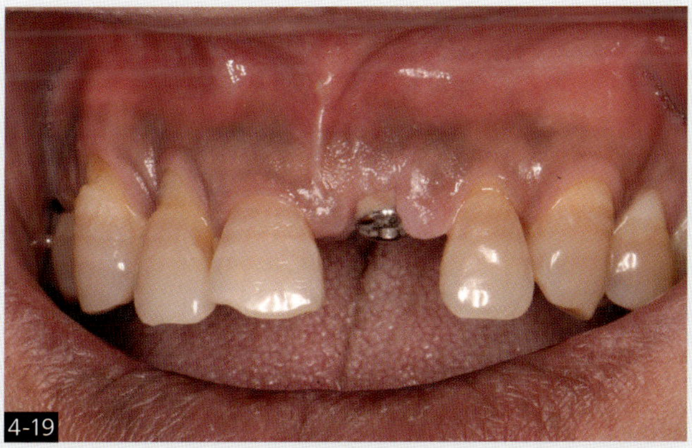
4-19

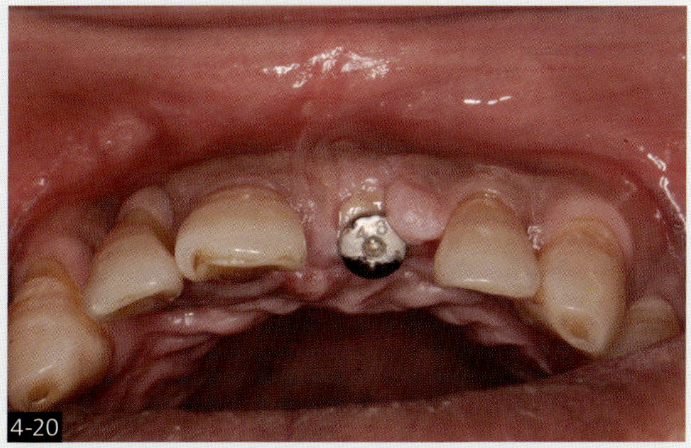
4-20

One week after suture removal, the soft tissue surrounding the buccal extraction site has healed well, with no visible holes remaining (Figures 4-19, 20).

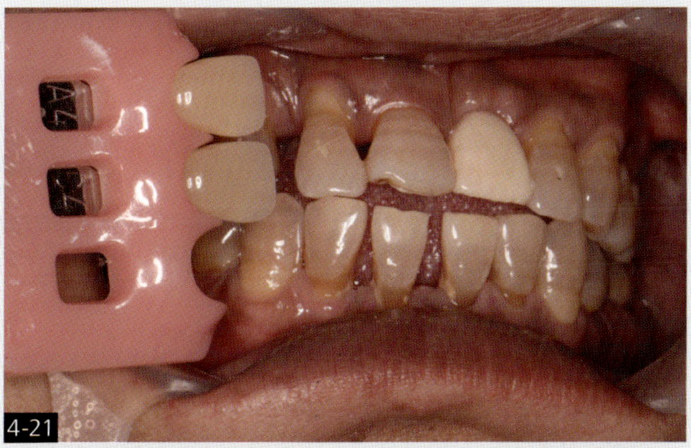
4-21

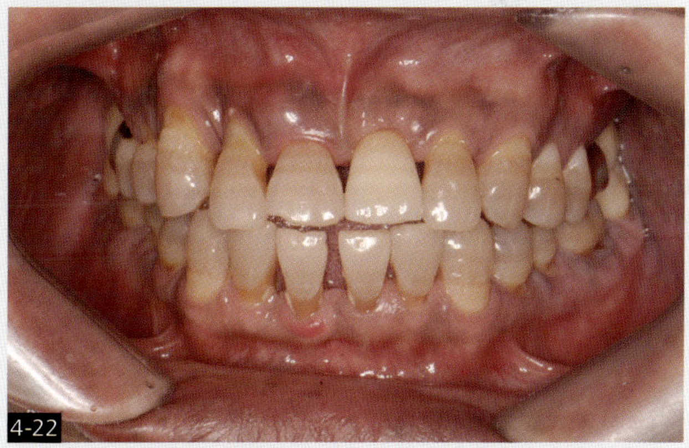
4-22

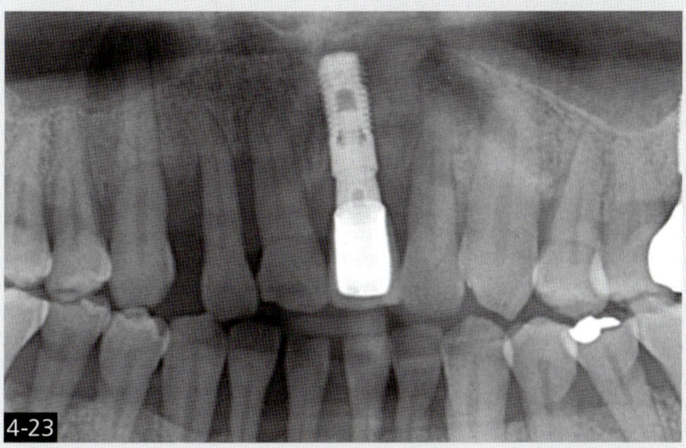
4-23

After fitting a temporary crown, the patient reported no discomfort, allowing for the completion of the final prosthetic restoration (Figures 4-21, 22). Although the color of the final prosthesis was not perfect, the patient was satisfied with the treatment. The gingiva has completely healed, with no recurrence of abscesses or unresolved periodontitis. Radiographic images also show no issues (Figure 4-23).

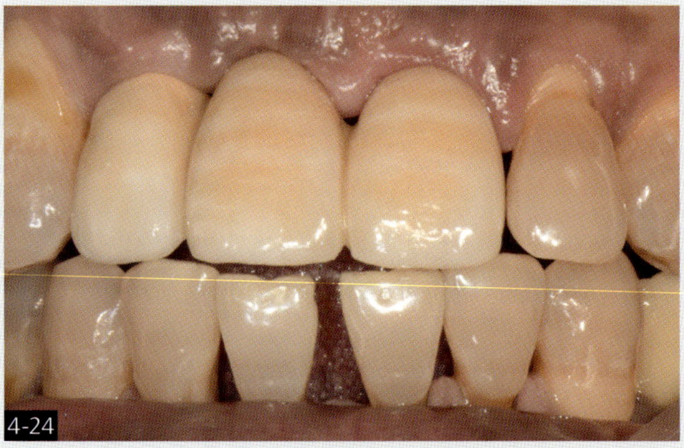
4-24

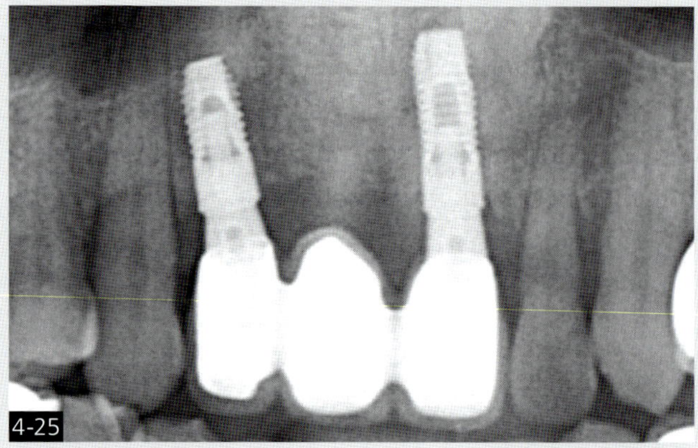
4-25

The patient's right central and lateral incisors also exhibited poor periodontal conditions, leading to extraction and subsequent implant placement, followed by bridge restoration. Six years after the placement of the implant for tooth #21, there have been no clinical issues **(Figures 4-24, 25)**.

Both natural teeth affected by periodontitis and implants can develop deep periodontal pockets. If these pockets persist after implant placement, peri-implantitis may occur. This section examines how to manage soft tissue to prevent peri-implantitis. To facilitate understanding, the following graphics will illustrate these concepts.

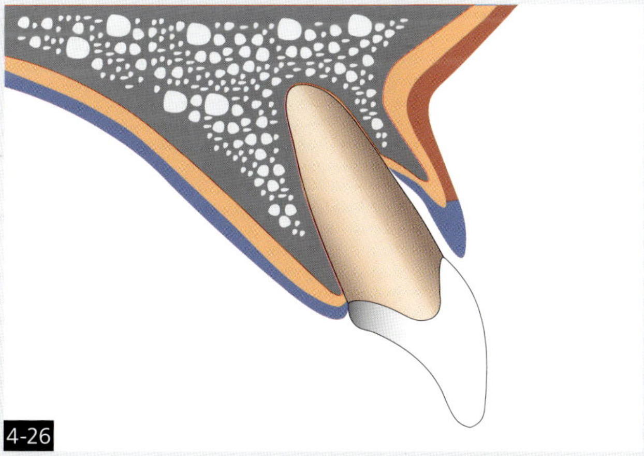
4-26

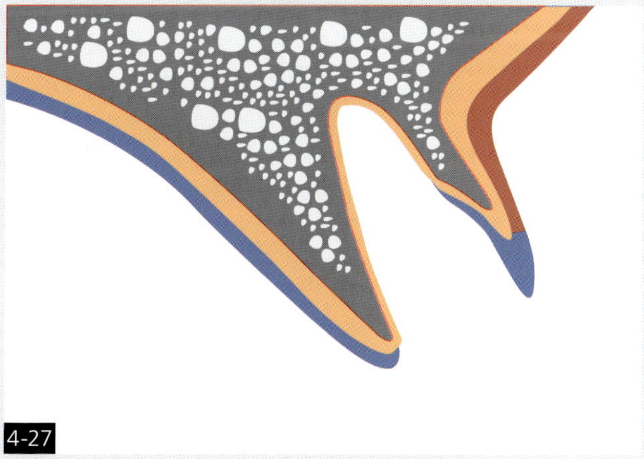
4-27

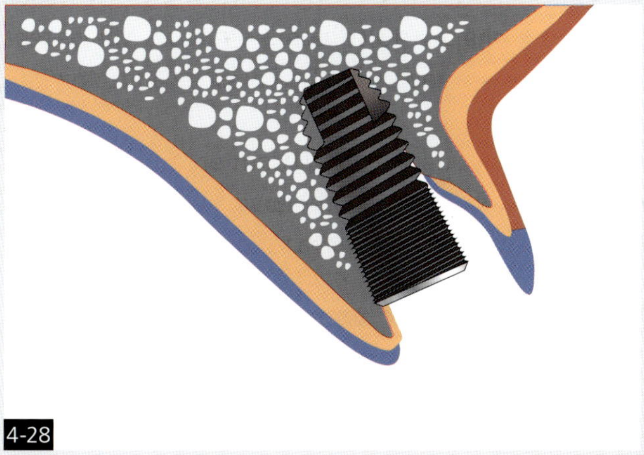
4-28

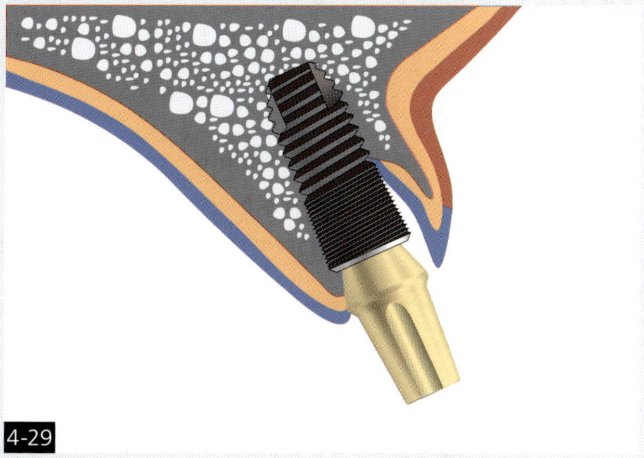
4-29

These figures depict a scenario where an implant is placed directly into an extraction site without soft tissue management after periodontal disease **(Figures 4-26~29)**.

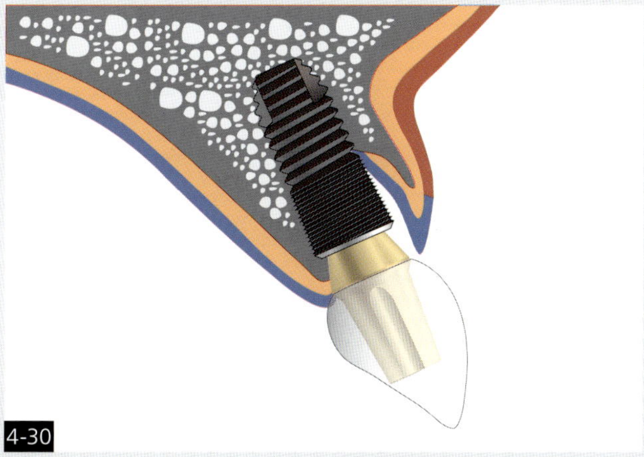
4-30

The buccal periodontal pocket present in the natural tooth remains after the implant procedure **(Figure 4-30)**. The periodontitis from the natural tooth can directly progress to peri-implantitis.

To prevent this, implants can be placed after the soft tissue around the extraction site has healed. However, for patient convenience, immediate implant placement is often performed. To prevent peri-implantitis, it is crucial to eliminate the periodontal pocket, and the surgical techniques for this will be discussed.

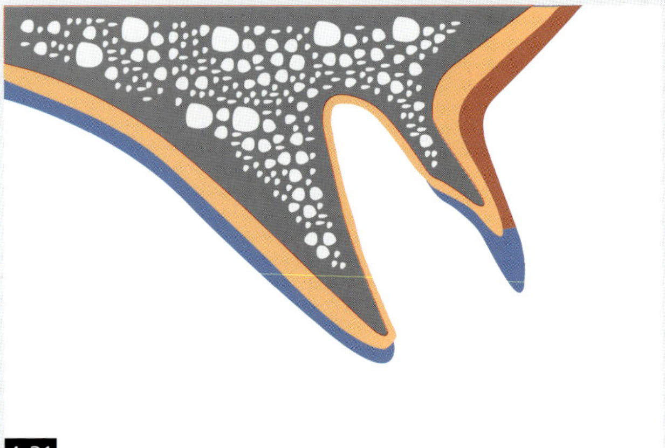

4-31

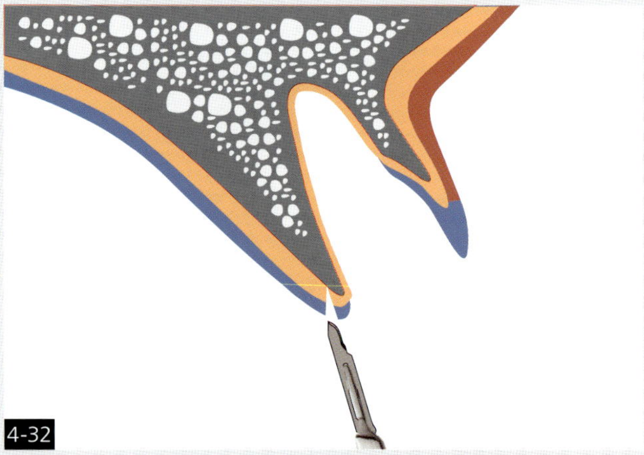

4-32

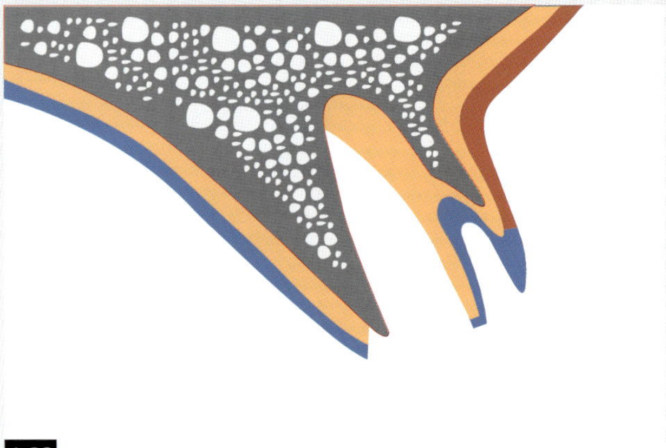

4-33

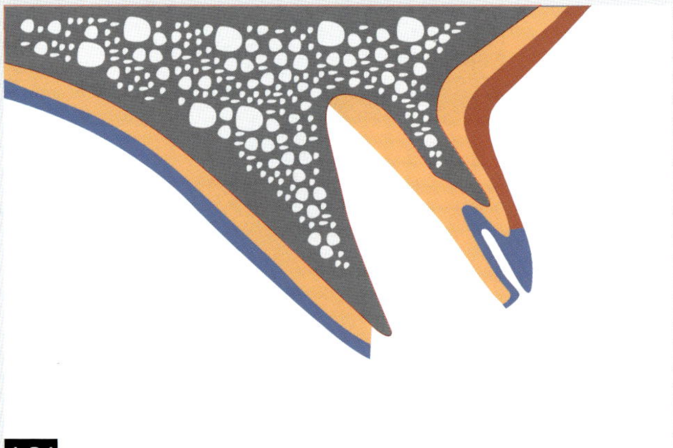

4-34

An incision is made on the buccal side after extracting the periodontally affected tooth **(Figure 4-32)**. As seen in the clinical photos, the alveolar bone at the extraction site is scraped to gradually push the inflammatory and epithelial tissues buccally **(Figures 4-33, 34)**.

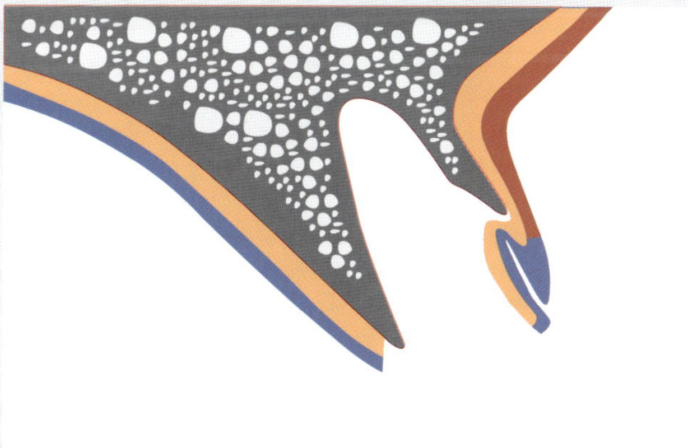
4-35

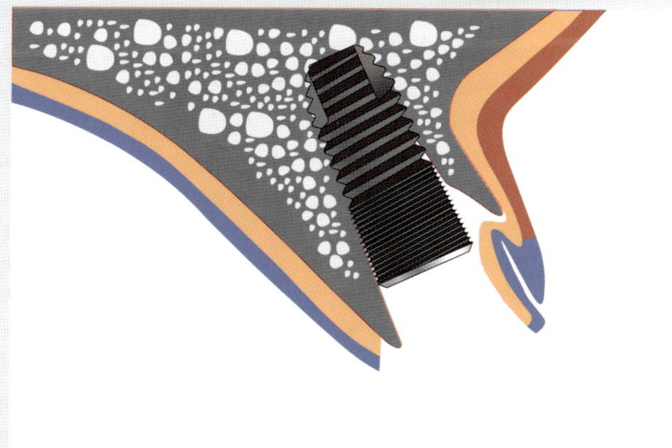
4-36

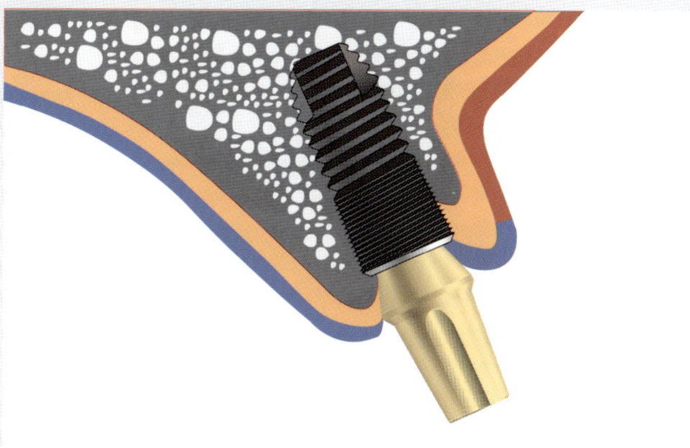
4-37

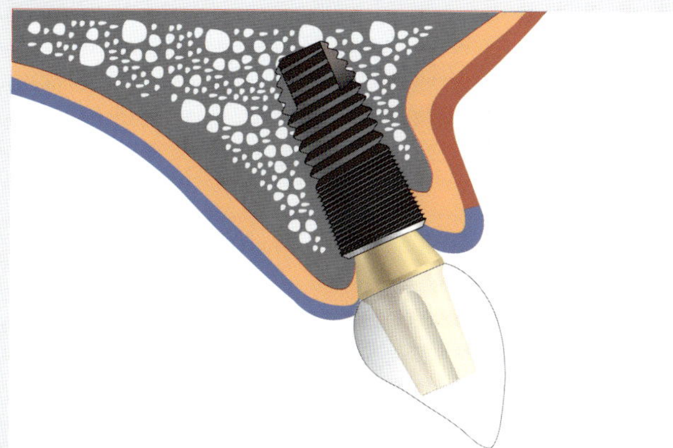
4-38

To promote alveolar bone regeneration, it is advisable to expose all the bone covered by inflammatory tissue. The soft tissue should be pushed buccally until the buccal bone's edge is visible. If the buccal surface of the bone is exposed, it is expected that bone loss will occur, so dissection should not extend beyond that point.

Once the soft tissue is completely pushed buccally, the implant can be placed. Following this, the prosthetic restoration will ensure that the epithelial cells do not contact the abutment but rather that connective tissue does. The epithelial cells from the periodontal pocket that existed at the extraction site will be trapped between the connective tissue and will eventually degenerate and disappear. This means that a periodontal pocket will not form buccally; instead, a gingival sulcus will develop. Since the gingival sulcus cannot harbor pathogenic bacteria, periodontitis will heal, and peri-implantitis will not occur **(Figures 4-35~38)**.

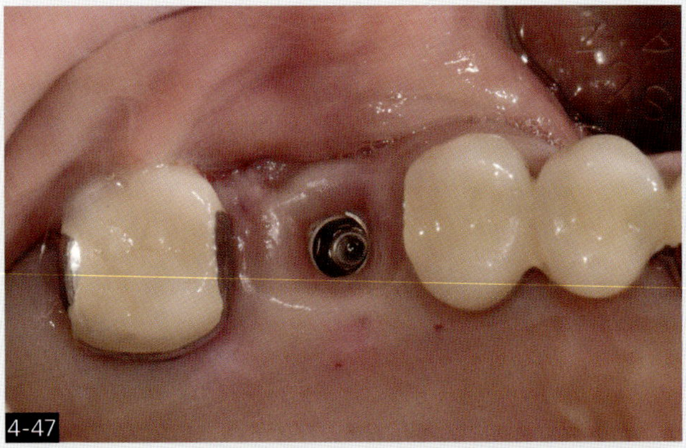
4-47

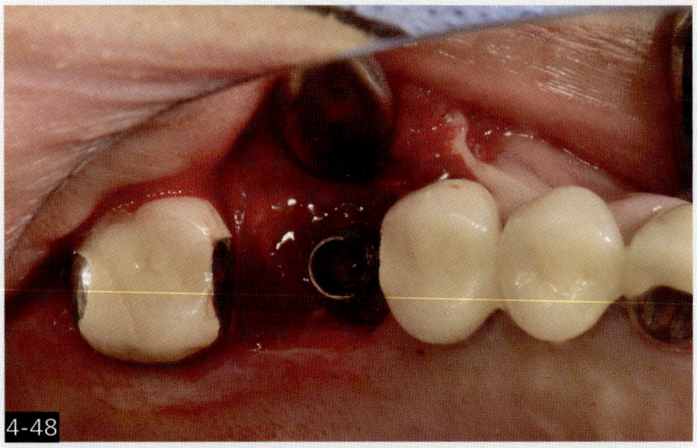
4-48

The prosthesis has been removed **(Figure 4-47)**. It is crucial to consider not only the alveolar bone loss but also the inflammatory tissue and epithelial cells that have migrated deeper. Ignoring this and placing an implant in the same location could lead to recurrent peri-implantitis. The same principles used in the maxillary central incisor implant surgery should be applied here as well.

A palatal incision that does not include the soft tissue surrounding the implant and abutment is necessary **(Figure 4-48)**. After the incision, the inflammatory tissue and surrounding tissues are scraped and pushed buccally.

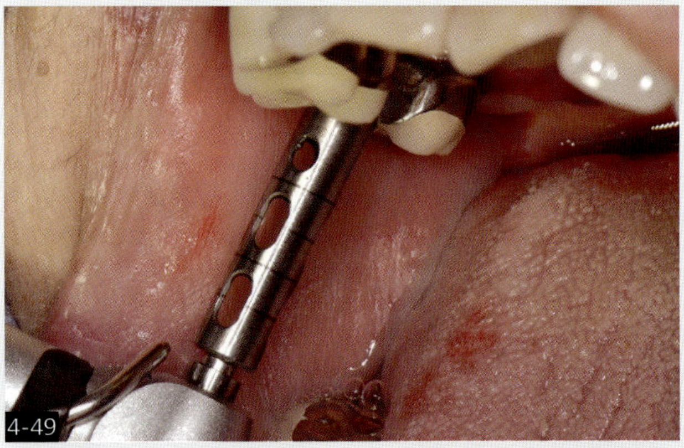
4-49

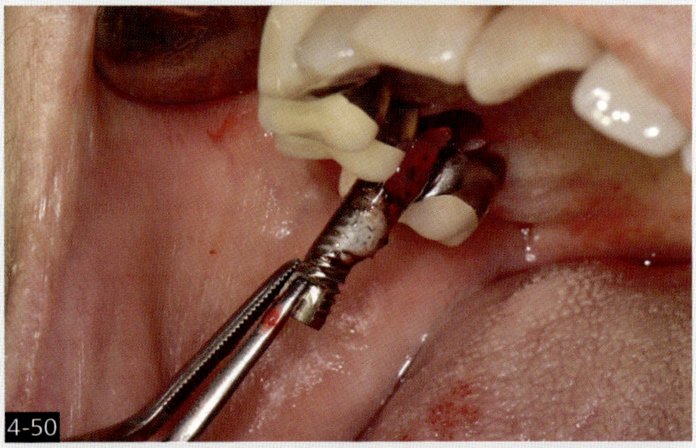
4-50

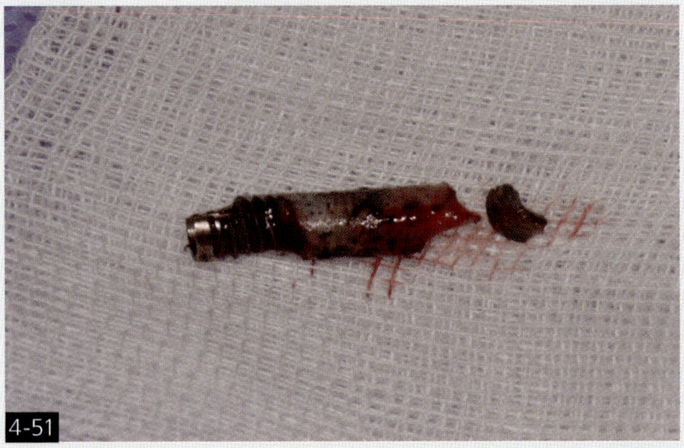
4-51

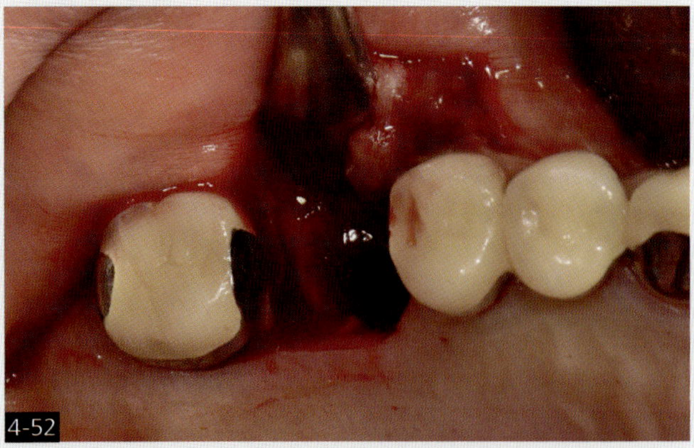
4-52

The removal of the implant is performed according to standard methods. While there are various techniques, I prefer using a trephine drill **(Figures 4-49~52)**. The removed implant shows a fracture at the top **(Figure 4-51)**. Readers should choose products that are less prone to fracture. It is important to note that simply using a thicker implant does not guarantee that fractures will not occur.

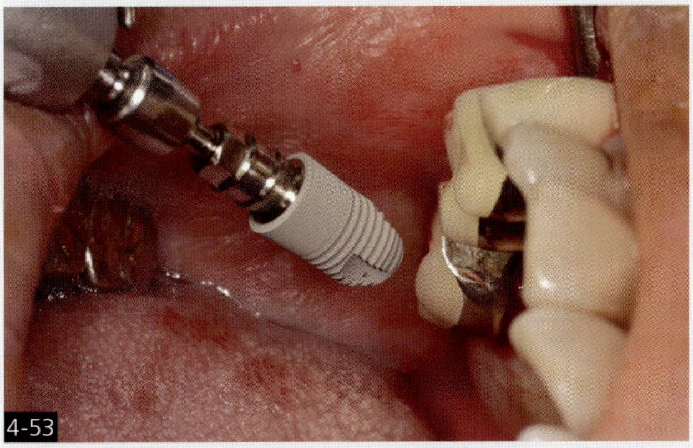
4-53

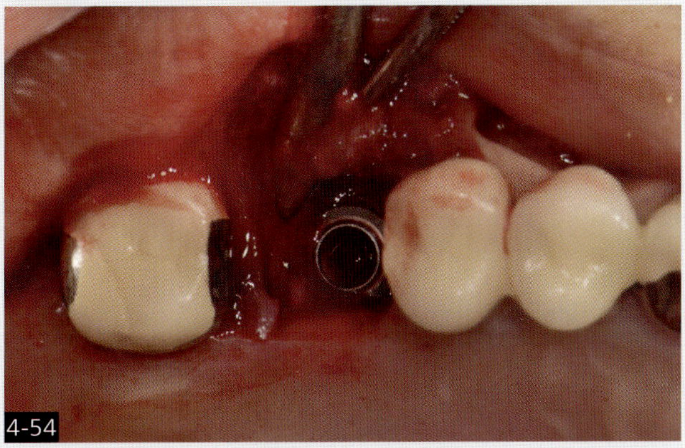
4-54

When placing an implant immediately after removal, several considerations must be made. First, achieving stability is crucial. There are various methods to obtain stability; if the width of the alveolar bone and the gingiva is sufficient, simply placing a thicker implant may suffice. The inner diameter of the trephine drill used for removal is 4mm, and the outer diameter is 5mm. Therefore, the diameter of the hole formed in the alveolar bone is at least 5mm. While a 5.5mm implant could be placed, a 6.0mm diameter implant was used for assured stability **(Figures 4-53, 54)**.

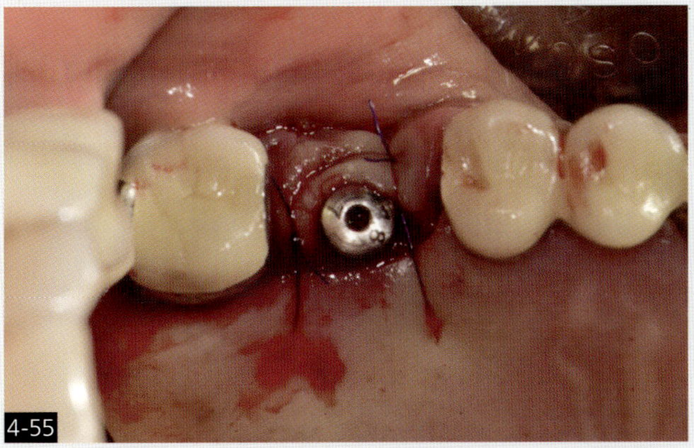
4-55

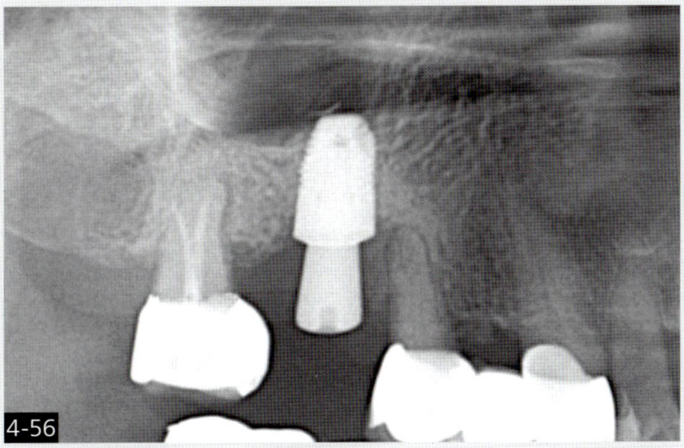
4-56

After achieving sufficient stability, all granulation tissue and the downward-proliferated epithelial tissue caused by peri-implantitis were pushed buccally **(Figure 4-55)**. As previously explained, this soft tissue management is intended to prevent the formation of periodontal pockets around the abutment and to create a shallow gingival sulcus. Radiographic images confirm that the surgery was successfully performed **(Figure 4-56)**.

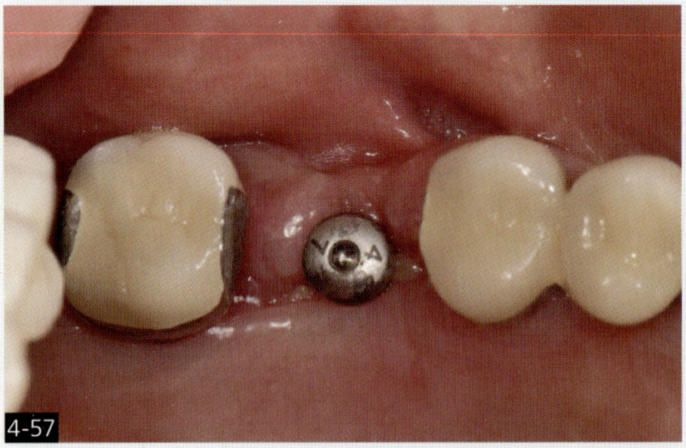

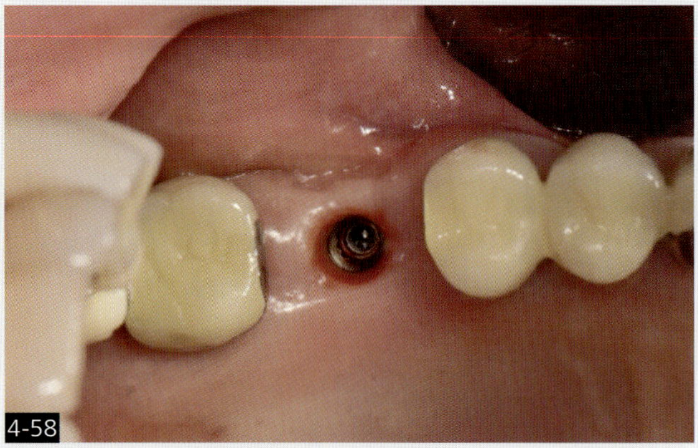

One week and six weeks post-surgery, the healing process appears normal **(Figures 4-57, 58)**.

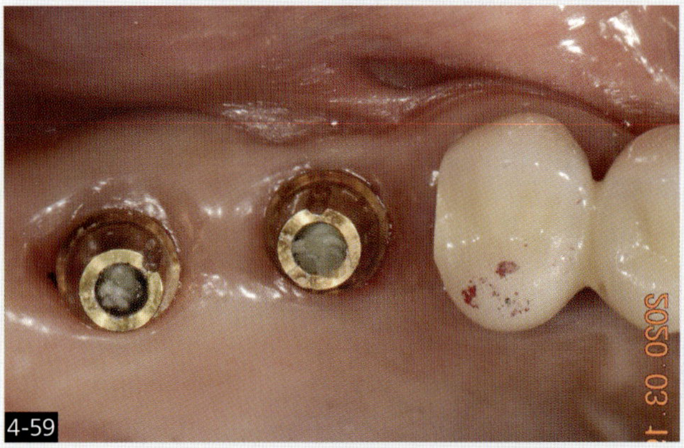

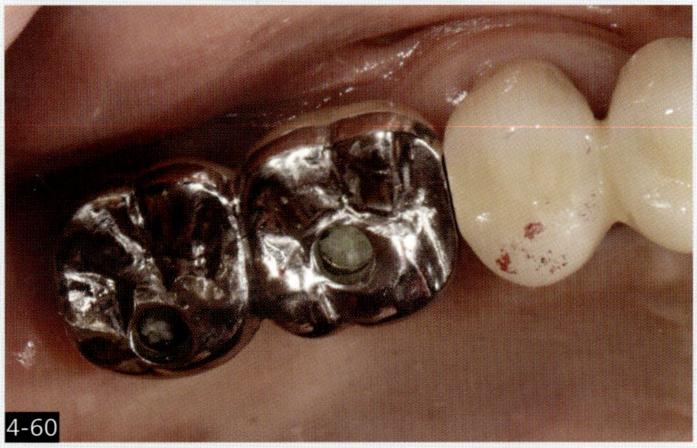

Tooth #17 also exhibited poor condition, leading to immediate implant placement after extraction, with both implants being connected for prosthetic completion **(Figures 4-59, 60)**.

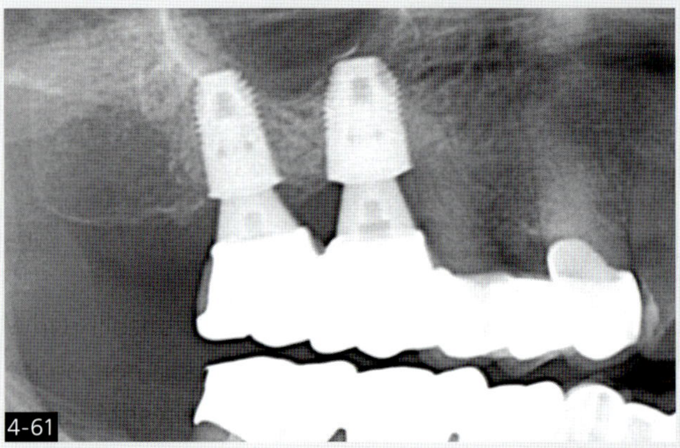

Approximately 1.5 years post-procedure, the condition is excellent, with complete recovery of the lost alveolar bone **(Figure 4-61)**.

To aid in understanding this case, graphics will be utilized for further explanation.

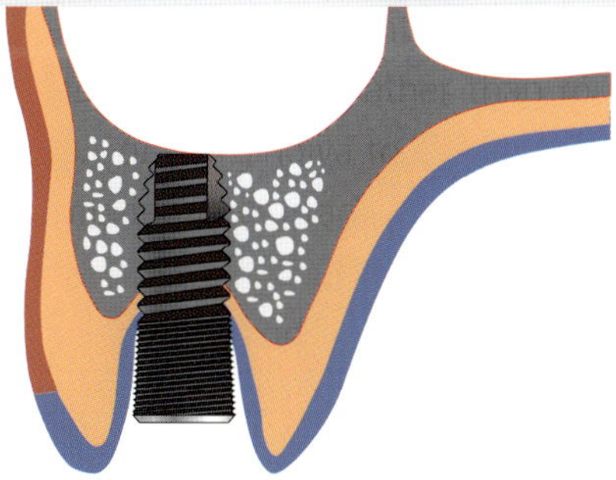
4-62

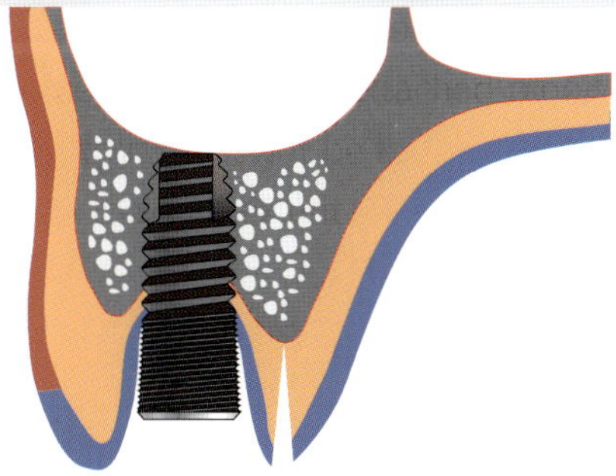
4-63

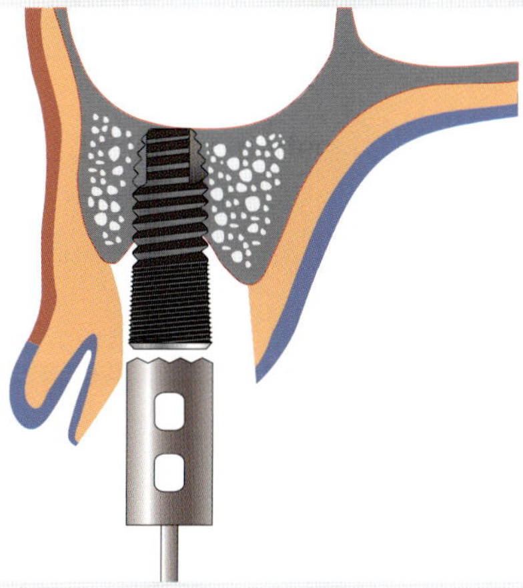
4-64

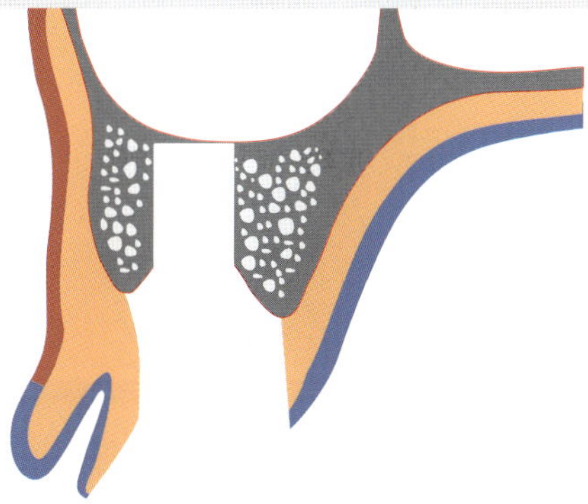
4-65

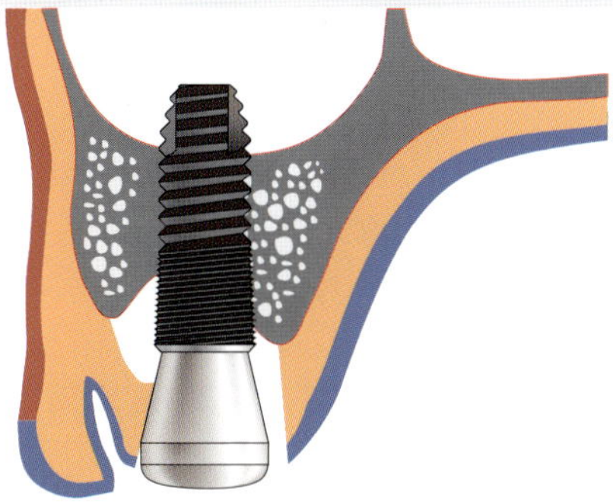
4-66

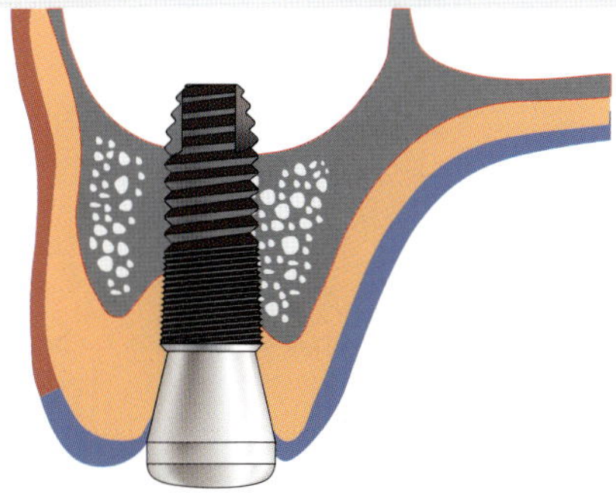
4-67

When complications such as peri-implantitis arise due to implant fractures and associated alveolar bone loss, it is crucial to understand that re-implanting without addressing the underlying issues can lead to the persistence of deep periodontal pockets and the recurrence of peri-implantitis.

Therefore, a palatal incision should be made to displace normal connective tissue and epithelial cells from the periodontal pocket buccally, ensuring that the healing abutment comes into contact with healthy connective tissue, thereby forming a gingival sulcus instead of a periodontal pocket **(Figures 4-62~67)**.

The epithelial cells that contribute to the formation of periodontal pockets do not proliferate downward unless there is inflammation in the connective tissue. In the case described above, since the new implant does not induce inflammation in the connective tissue, the epithelium remains attached at the top, preventing the formation of a periodontal pocket and instead allowing only a gingival sulcus to form.

There are two methods to eliminate the periodontal pocket during peri-implantitis surgery: one involves pushing out the inflammatory tissue and epithelial cells, while the other method focuses on different techniques to remove the pocket entirely.

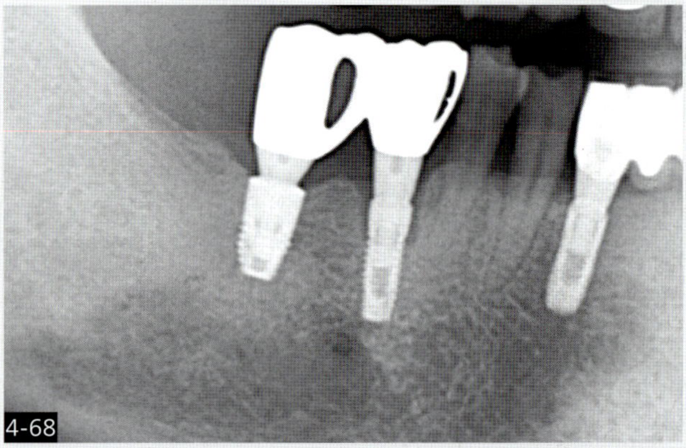
4-68

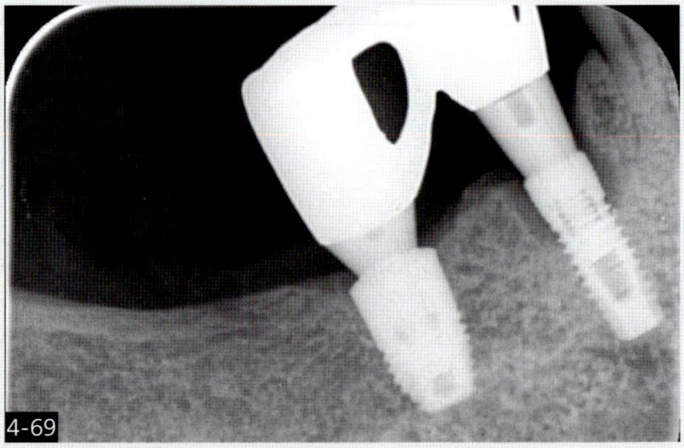
4-69

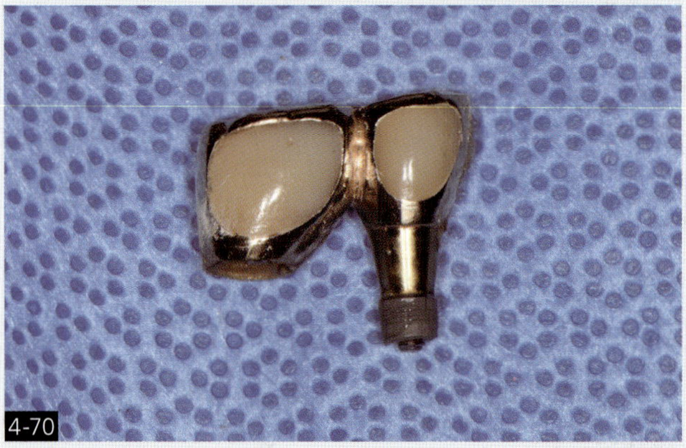
4-70

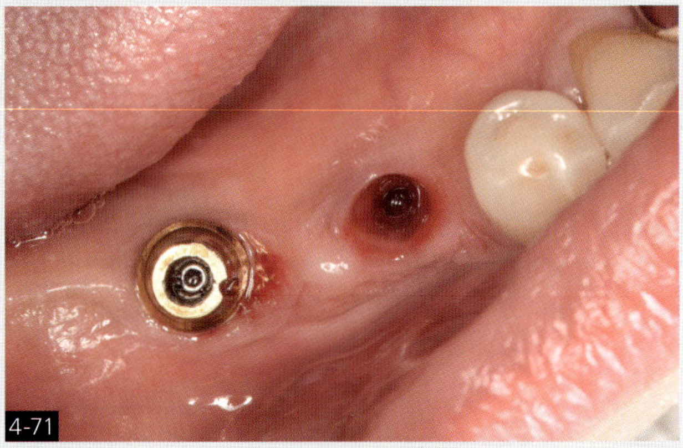
4-71

Figures 4-68 and **4-69** show the broken state of implant #45 and the associated alveolar bone loss. Clinical photographs of the removed implant reveal that it is not just the alveolar bone loss that is present; inflammatory tissue has formed within, and there is also downward proliferation of epithelial cells **(Figures 4-70, 71)**. If an implant is placed immediately in this condition, it is anticipated that the periodontal pocket will reform, necessitating an unconventional surgical approach.

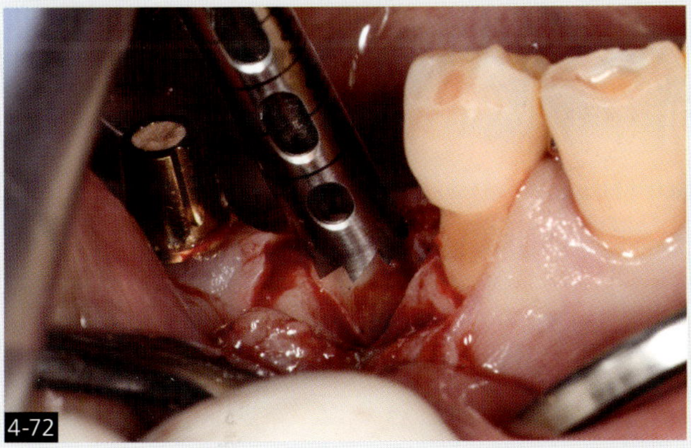
4-72

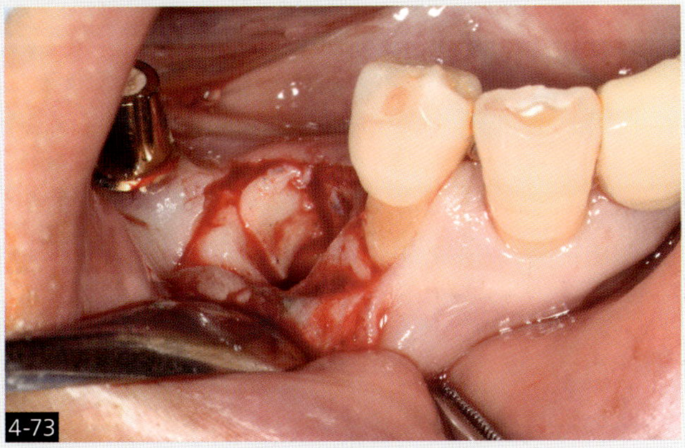
4-73

The surgery was performed one week later, at which point the soft tissue openings were nearly closed. Unfortunately, I did not capture this photograph. The implant removal utilized a trephine drill with an inner diameter of 4 mm and an outer diameter of 5 mm, resulting in a minimum 5mm diameter hole in the alveolar bone. To achieve stability in this enlarged hole, an implant with a diameter of 5.5 mm or 6mm should be placed; however, this would significantly thin the remaining alveolar bone and lead to considerable marginal bone loss.

The implant was positioned slightly buccally rather than centrally in the alveolar ridge, resulting in particularly thin buccal bone and some degree of bone resorption. In this situation, placing a thicker implant would lead to severe bone loss, potentially leaving the buccal side of implant #45 without attached gingiva or only with non-attached mucosa. Therefore, a crescent-shaped autogenous bone graft was harvested using a trephine drill from the posterior aspect of the implant removal site **(Figures 4-72, 73)**.

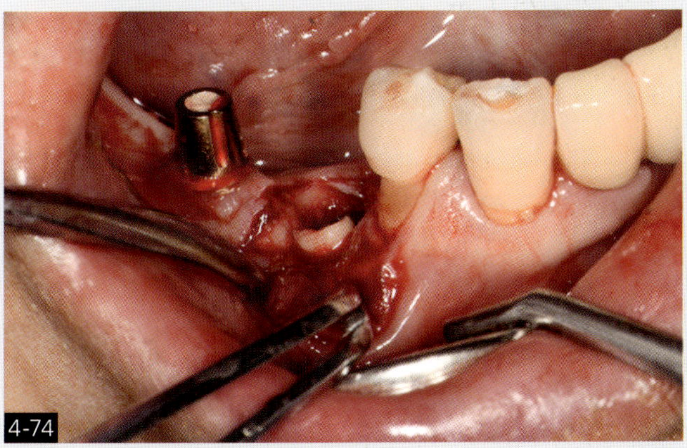
4-74

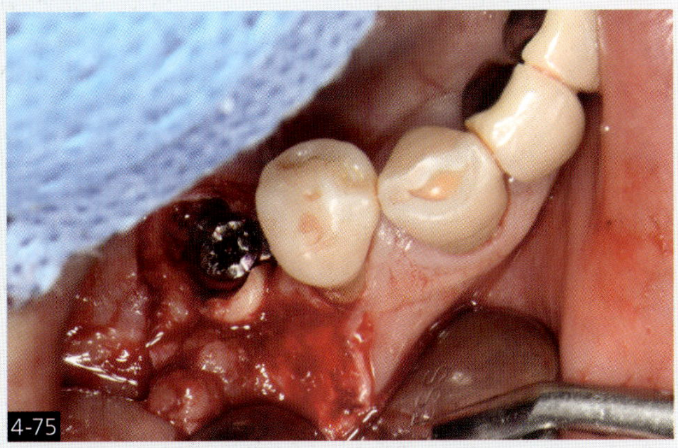
4-75

The crescent-shaped alveolar bone graft harvested from the buccal side was inserted, and a 5.0mm diameter implant was placed to achieve initial stability (the stability was not strong enough, necessitating a three-month wait until the second surgery). The graft placed on the buccal side compensates for the buccal bone resorption, and the implant can achieve stability using the graft **(Figures 4-74, 75)**. Achieving initial stability using the lingual alveolar bone and the buccal graft increases the complexity of the surgery and requires meticulous handling.

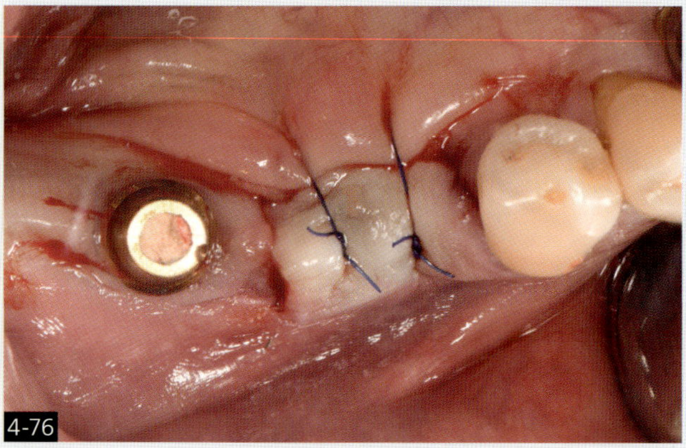
4-76

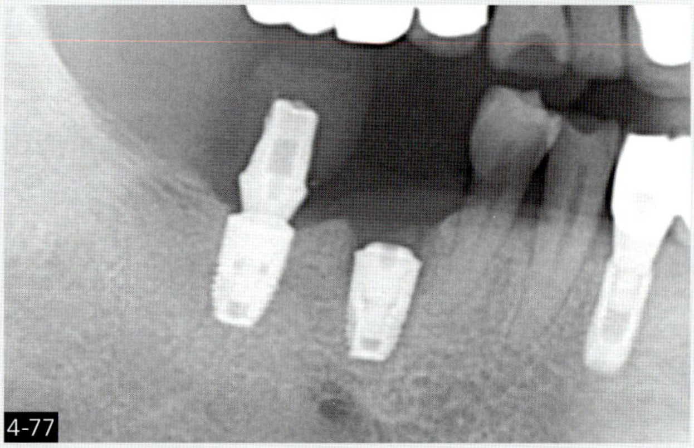
4-77

The surgery was performed one week after the removal of the fractured implant, and the soft tissue opening from the implant removal is nearly closed **(Figures 4-76, 77)**. As seen in the images, the top of the implant is positioned significantly lower than the alveolar ridge. This positioning is intentional to ensure that the implant and the graft are adequately covered by soft tissue, reducing the risk of exposure (if the implant is positioned too high, the risk of exposure increases).

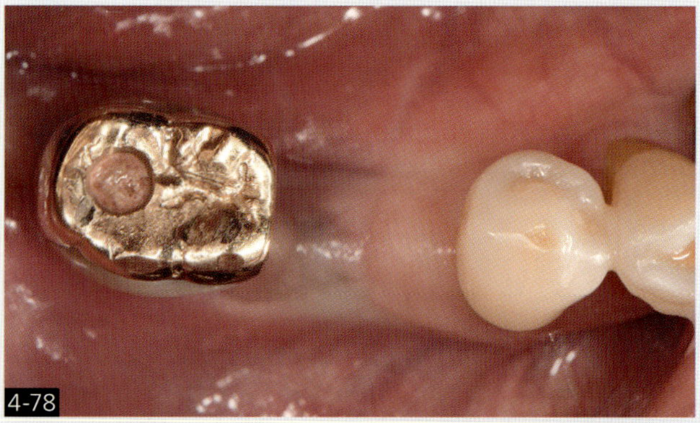
4-78

Four weeks post-surgery, the implant and the graft are well covered by soft tissue **(Figure 4-78)**, indicating that the surgery was highly successful. When soft tissue completely covers the surgical site, it effectively prevents epithelial cells from forming periodontal pockets. Even if epithelial cells remain after the gingival incision and flap elevation, they will eventually degenerate. This concept aligns with the Epithelial Isolation Technique.

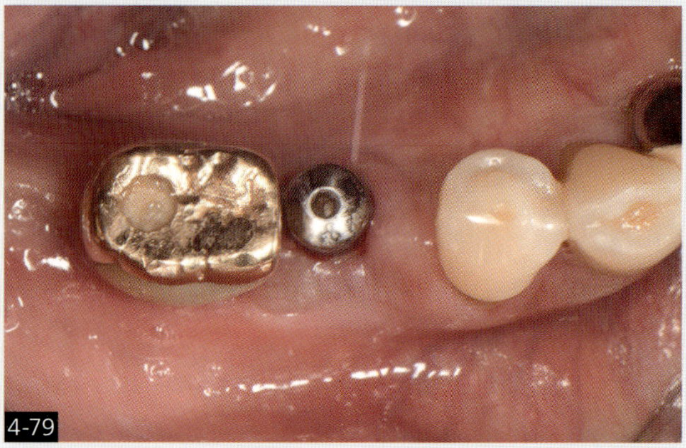
4-79

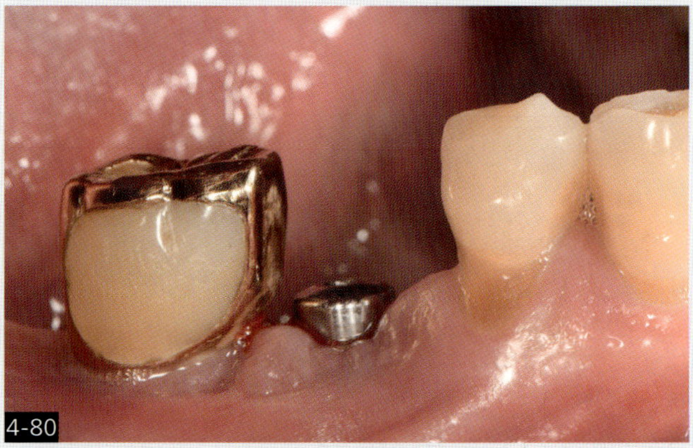
4-80

The secondary surgery was performed three months later, and all procedures went smoothly. The implant (fixture) showed good osseointegration, and the autogenous bone graft also integrated well with the buccal bone **(Figures 4-79, 80)**.

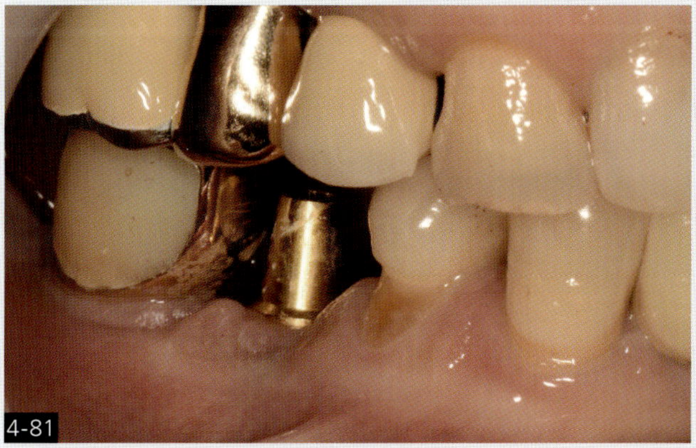

4-81

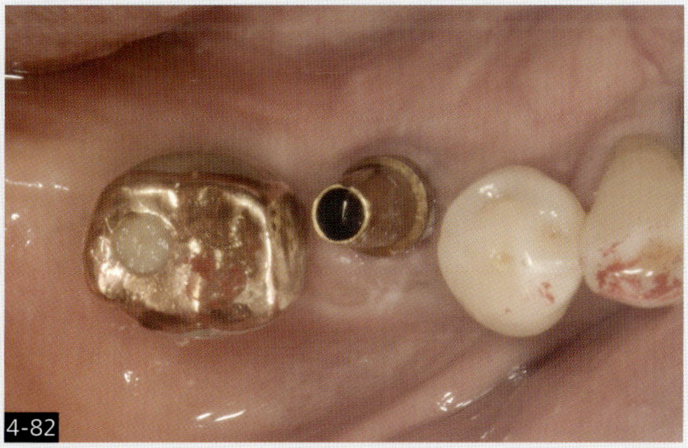

4-82

Due to the placement of the crescent-shaped autogenous bone graft on the buccal side to secure the initial stability, the implant was positioned significantly lingually **(Figures 4-81, 82)**.

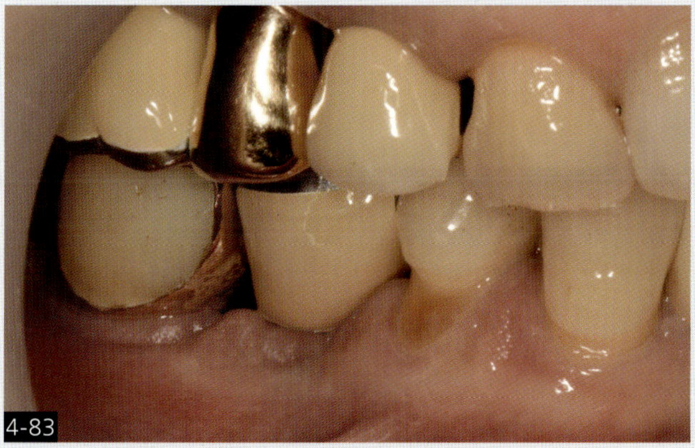

4-83

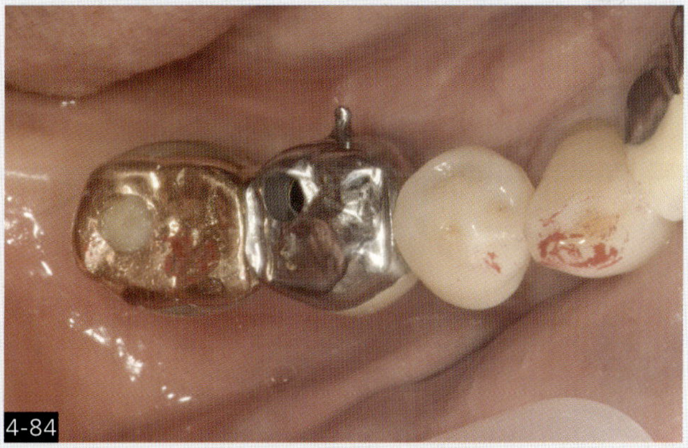

4-84

The lingual positioning of the implant resulted in a thicker restoration on the lingual side; however, no further mechanical or biological issues are anticipated **(Figures 4-83, 84)**.

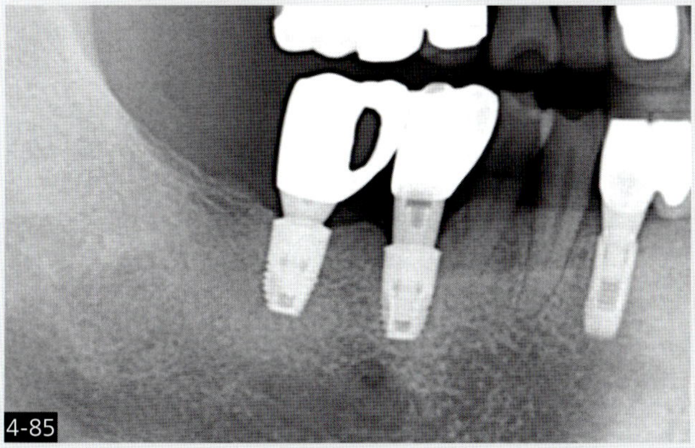

4-85

Radiographic images show that the alveolar bone has healed cleanly **(Figure 4-85)**.

To aid understanding, this case will also be examined graphically.

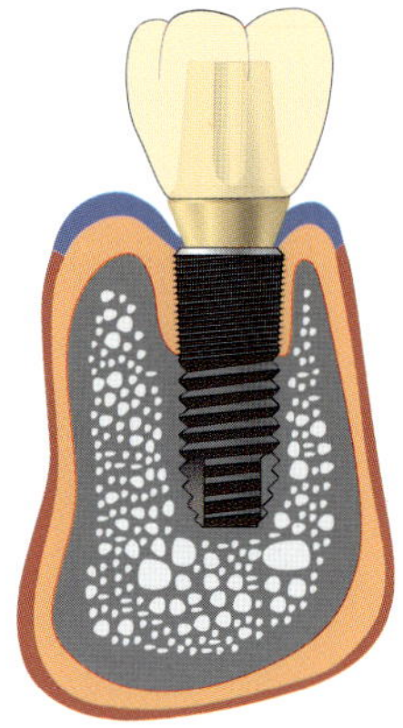

4-86

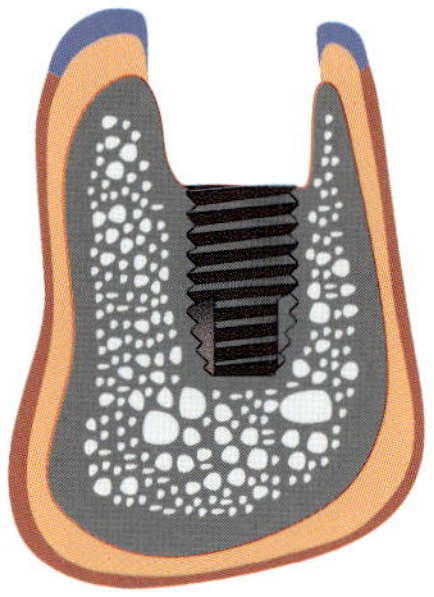

4-87

Due to the fracture of the implant, some degree of periodontal pocket formation was present, necessitating treatment **(Figures 4-86, 87)**.

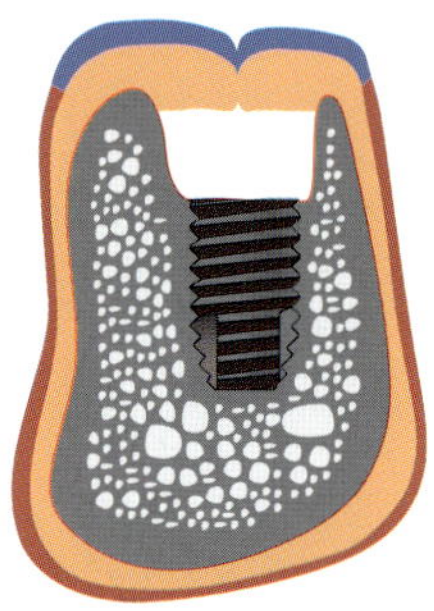

4-88

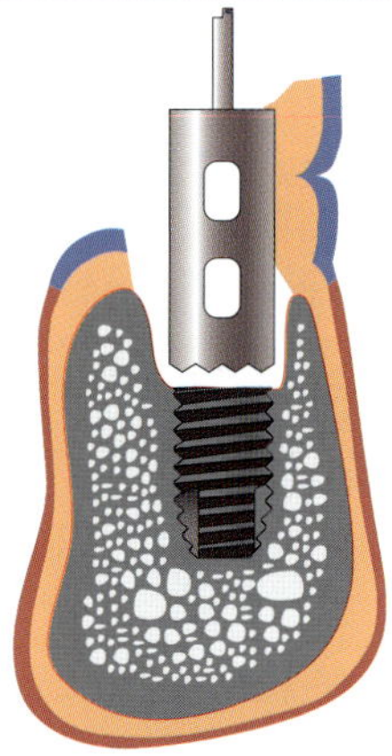

4-89

One week later, the soft tissue opening had significantly reduced, and a lingual incision was made to elevate both the inflammatory tissue and epithelial tissue simultaneously **(Figures 4-88, 89)**.

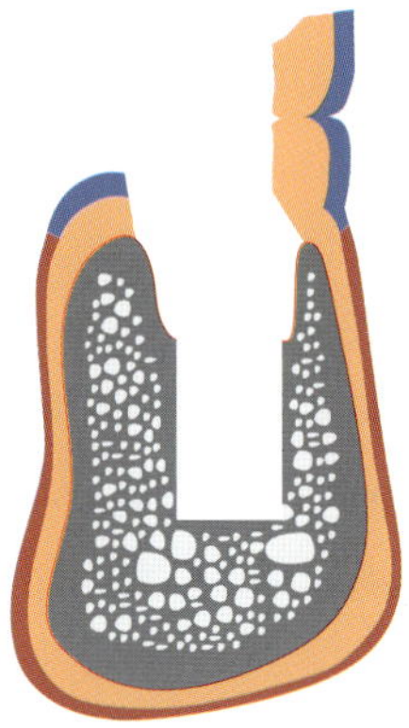

4-90

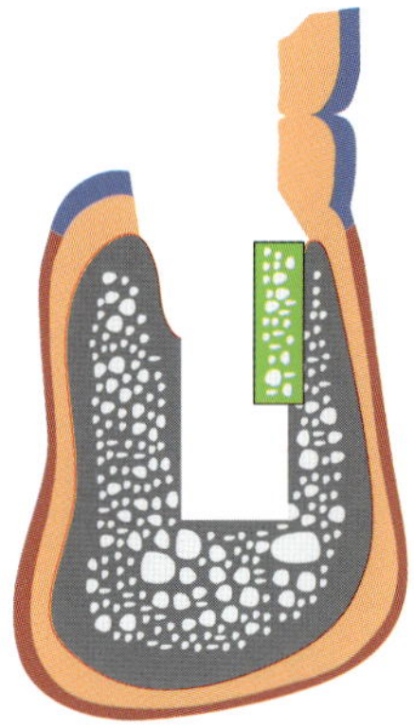

4-91

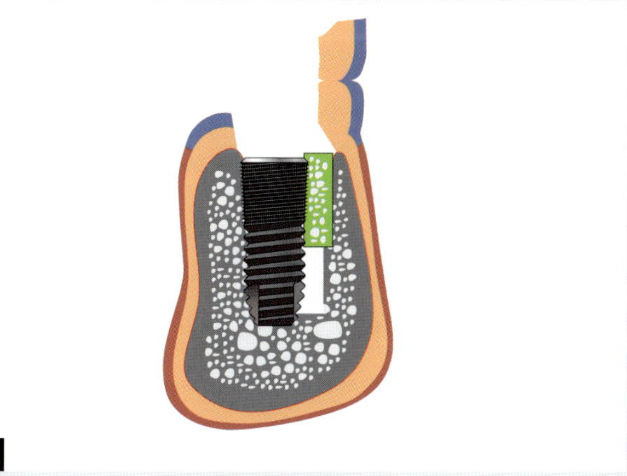

4-92

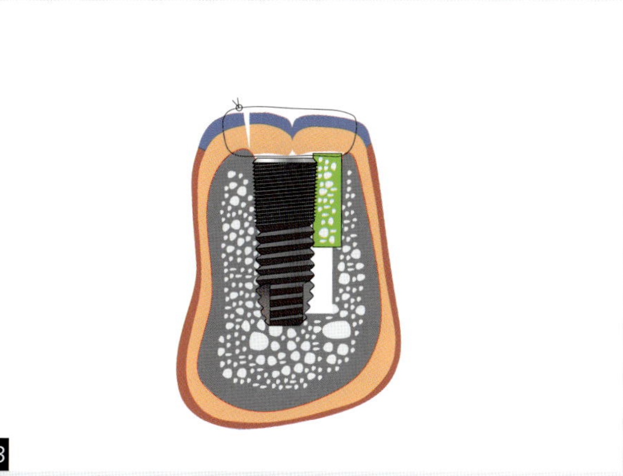

4-93

Bone was harvested from the centrifugal area of the implant removal site and placed on the buccal side to secure the implant **(Figures 4-90~93)**.

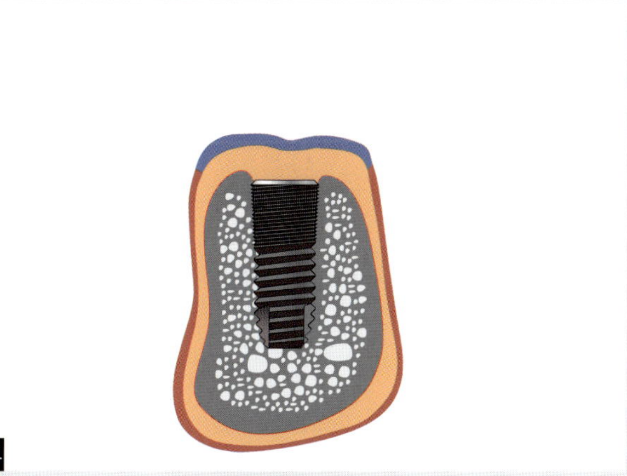

4-94

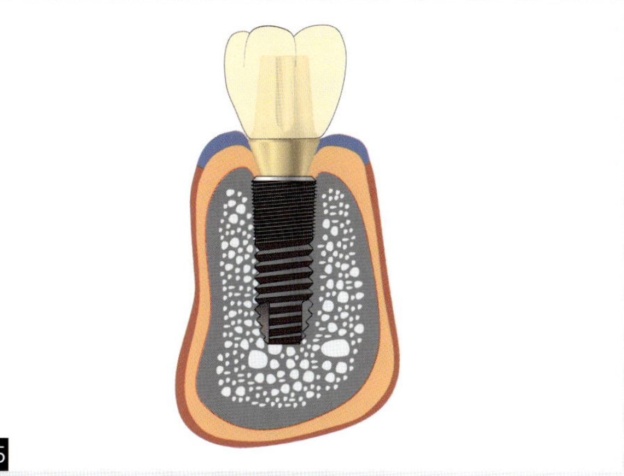

4-95

The grafted bone fused with the buccal bone, resulting in normal alveolar bone, and the implant achieved osseointegration with the surrounding bone, leading to excellent clinical outcomes. No periodontal pockets formed, preventing peri-implantitis **(Figures 4-94, 95)**.

Simultaneously performing bone grafting and placing a new implant immediately after removing a fractured implant while managing soft tissue is quite challenging. However, allowing sufficient healing time can simplify the surgical process.

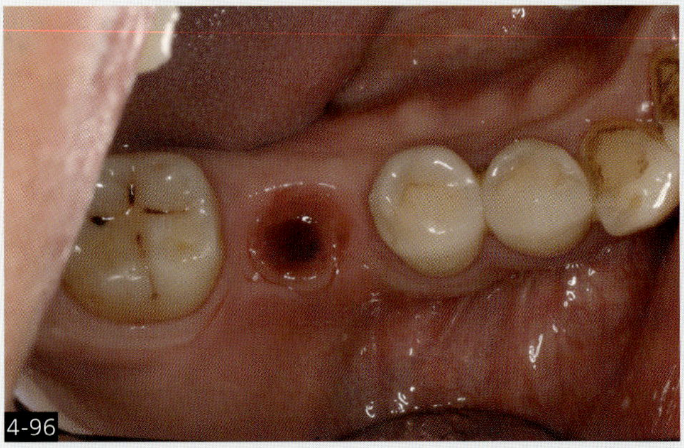

4-96

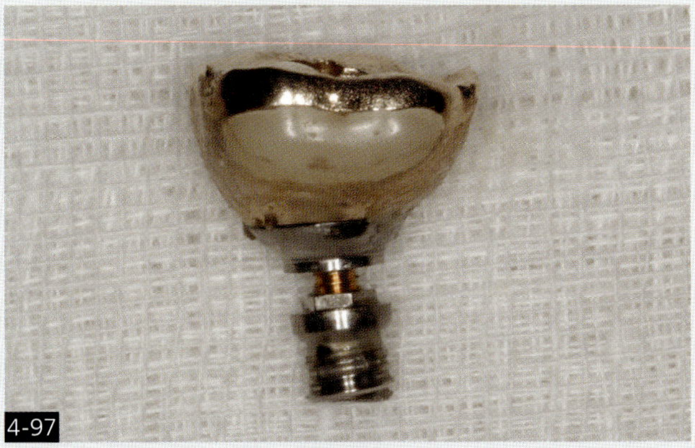

4-97

The implant was fractured, and the intraoral view after removing the fractured pieces is shown **(Figures 4-96, 97)**. Various methods can be employed to cover the surgical site with soft tissue, and waiting approximately two months can be an effective strategy.

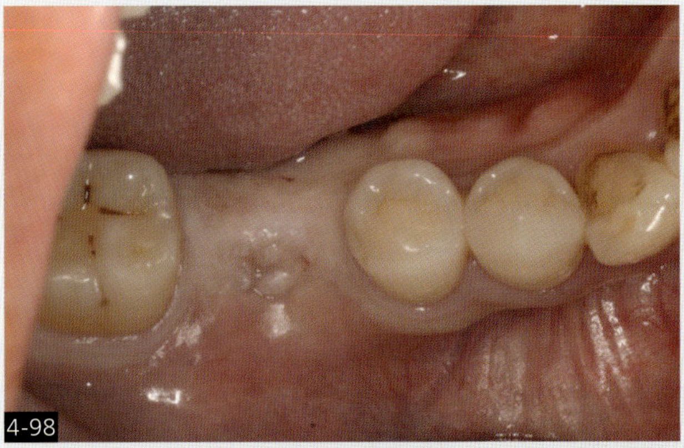

4-98

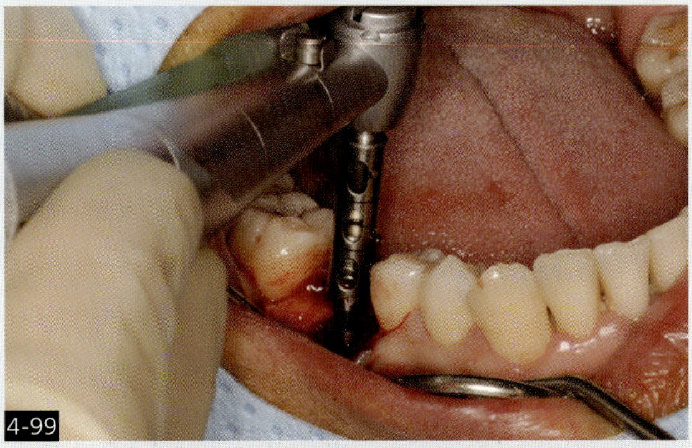

4-99

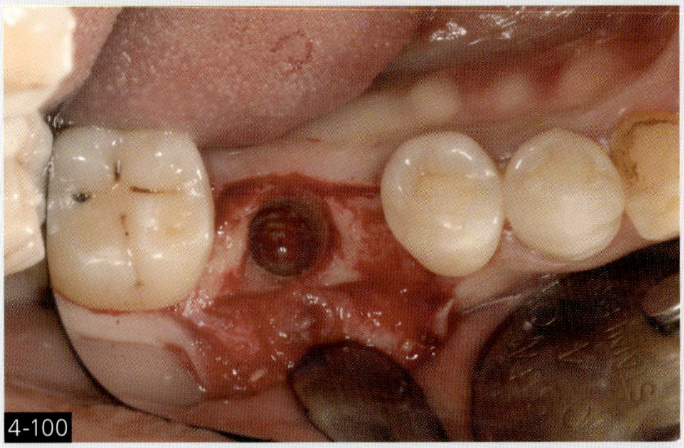

4-100

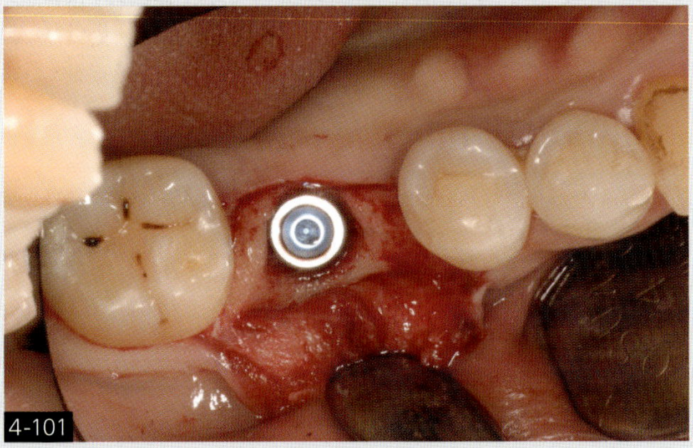

4-101

After two months following the removal of the upper fractured implant pieces, the soft tissue defect was completely covered **(Figure 4-98)**.

If the remaining fractured pieces are positioned shallowly rather than deeply, the soft tissue may not cover well. Once the soft tissue has healed, removing the fractured implant and re-implanting a new one after flap elevation will prevent the formation of periodontal pockets, making the surgery significantly easier **(Figures 4-99~101)**.

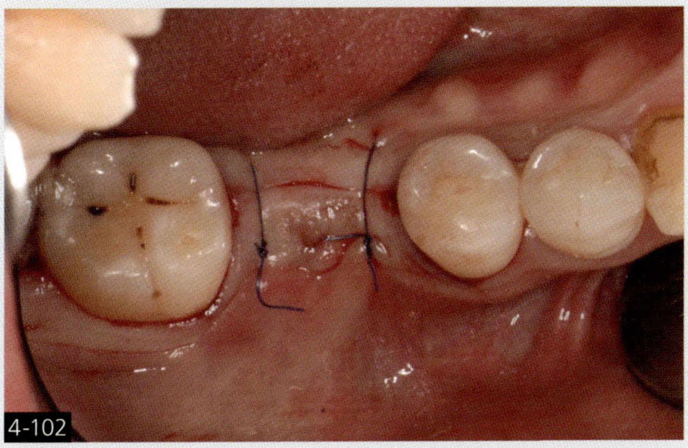
4-102

The completed suturing is shown **(Figure 4-102)**. The downward proliferation of epithelial cells due to peri-implantitis will not occur, effectively eliminating the possibility of peri-implantitis. However, this approach may extend the overall treatment duration for the patient.

Sometimes, implants may fail to withstand occlusal forces and become mobile. In such cases, a thin gap may exist between the implant and the alveolar bone, disrupting osseointegration. Surgical techniques that involve covering the flap can be beneficial in preventing the formation of periodontal pockets in these clinical scenarios.

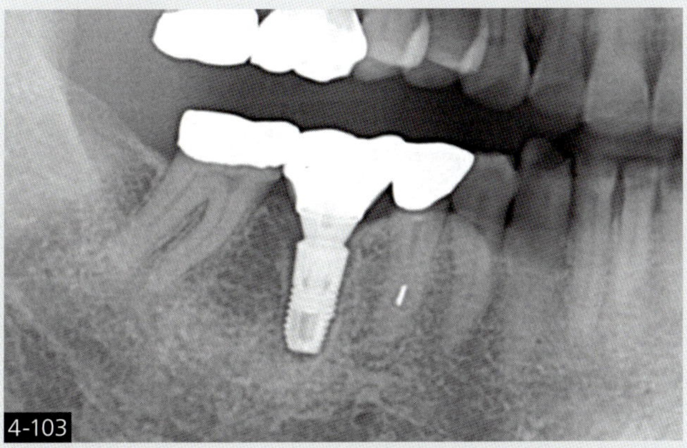
4-103

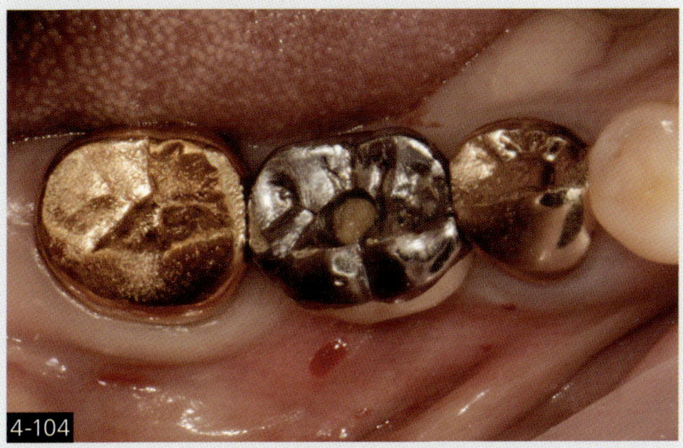
4-104

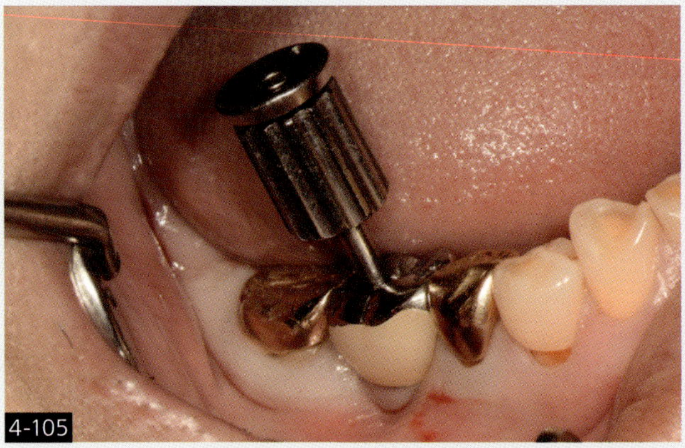

4-105

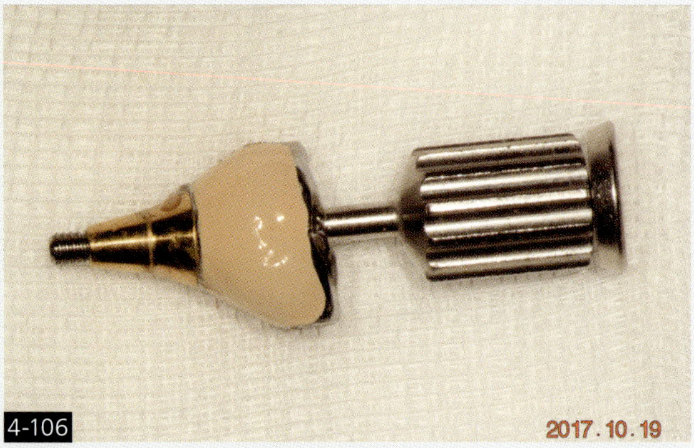

4-106

Implant #46 exhibited poor bone quality, leading to mobility due to inadequate resistance to occlusal forces **(Figure 4-103)**. It was decided to remove the implant and place a new one. To remove the implant, the prosthesis must first be taken off **(Figures 4-104~106)**.

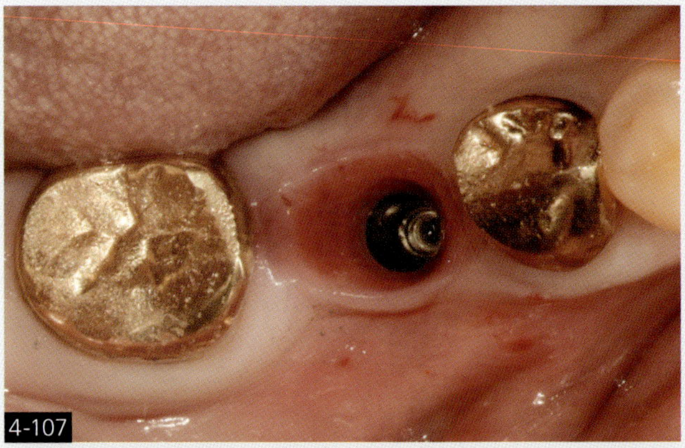

4-107

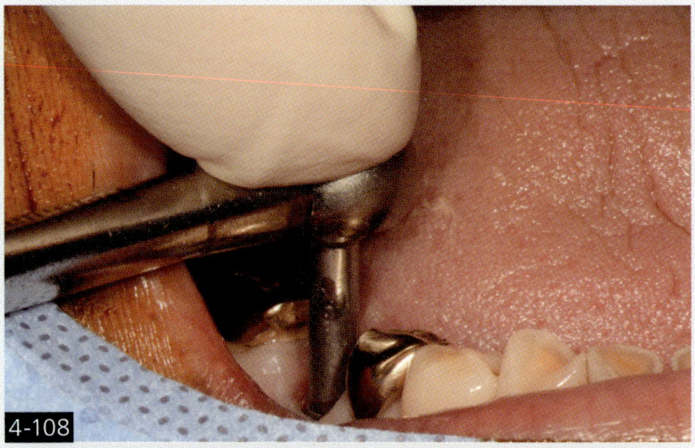

4-108

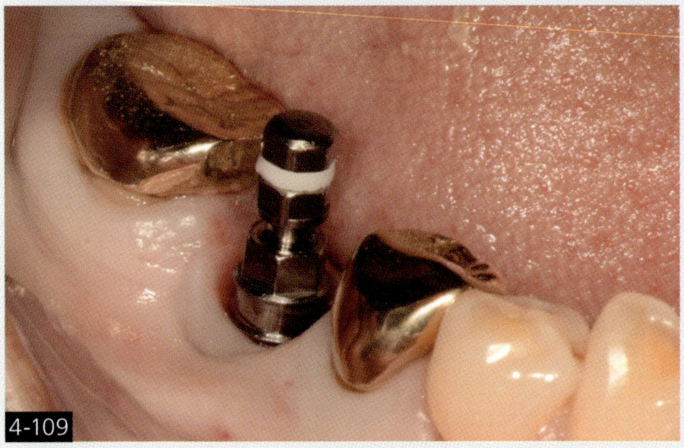

4-109

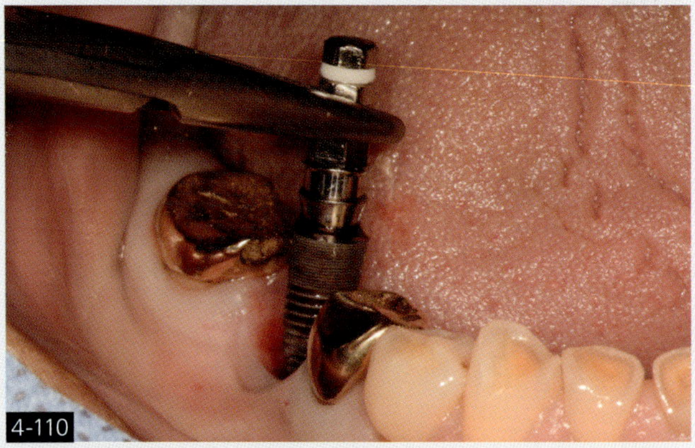

4-110

When an implant becomes mobile due to separation from the alveolar bone, it can be easily removed using a ratchet fixture adaptor in a reverse rotation **(Figures 4-107, 108)**. By lifting the implant sufficiently with reverse rotation, it can then be easily extracted using a mount or healing abutment. Since it is difficult to grip the fixture directly, using such instruments is very convenient **(Figures 4-109, 110)**.

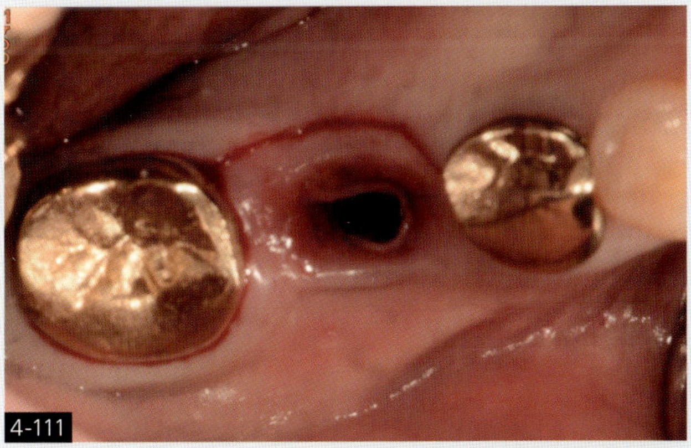

4-111

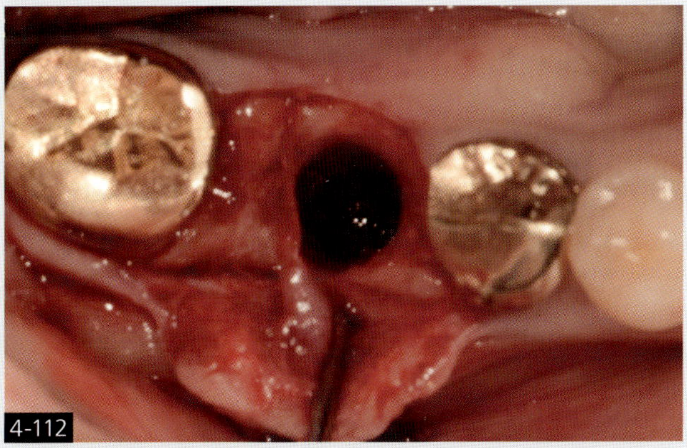

4-112

To prevent the proliferation of epithelial cells around the implant and the formation of periodontal pockets, various methods can be employed. One approach is to wait approximately two months until the soft tissue has completely healed, although this may extend the treatment duration for the patient. After a lingual incision, the flap must be cleanly separated from the alveolar bone **(Figures 4-111, 112)**.

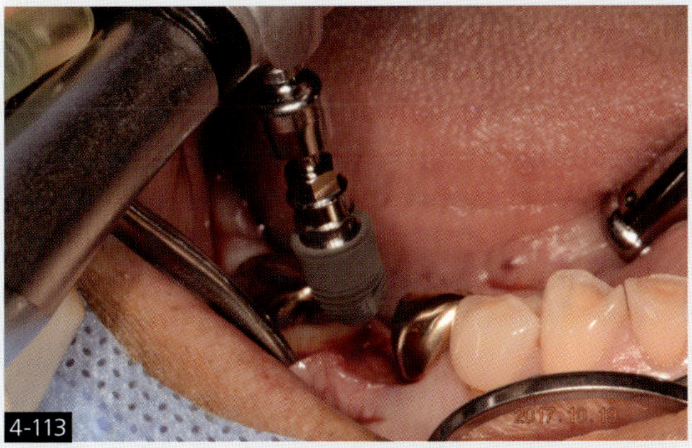

4-113

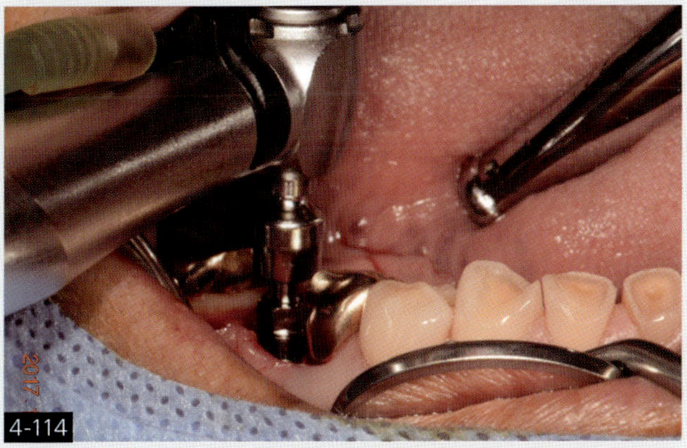

4-114

The existing product has a diameter of 5.0 mm, so the hole was judged to be slightly larger than 5.0 mm. A 6.0 mm diameter implant is being placed **(Figures 4-113, 114)**.

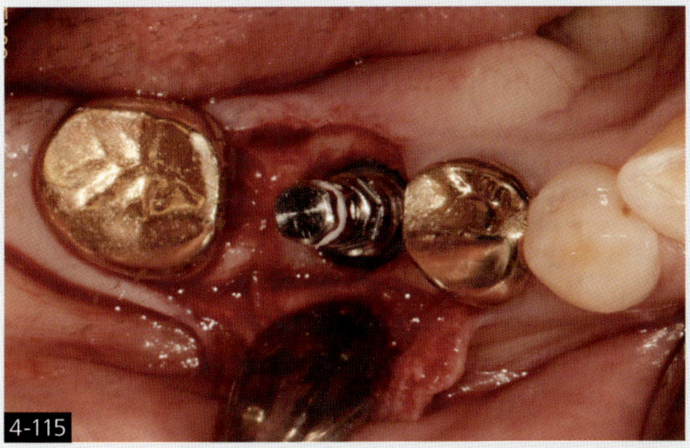

4-115

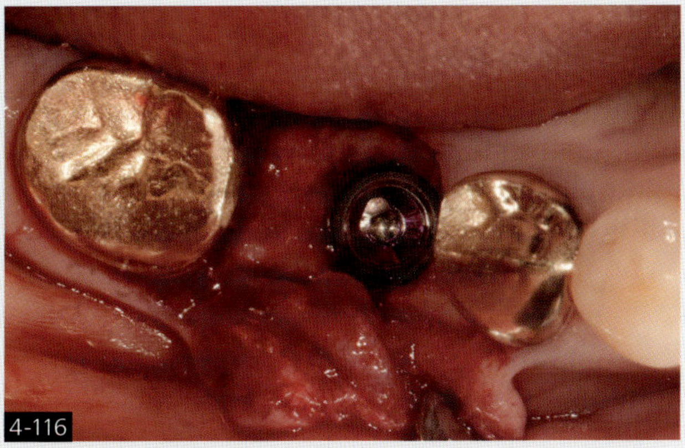

4-116

The diameter of the implant (fixture) was larger than the hole, allowing for sufficient initial stability **(Figures 4-115, 116)**. This surgical method cannot be used if the width of the alveolar bone is insufficient. At this point, it is crucial to lower the fixture top adequately.

This has two significant implications: first, it ensures that the soft tissue is effectively covered, and second, it increases the amount of attached gingiva. By placing a thicker implant deeply, the alveolar bone will rise to the top of the implant, converting the upper gingiva into attached gingiva, which is very advantageous for periodontal health (this will be explained graphically later).

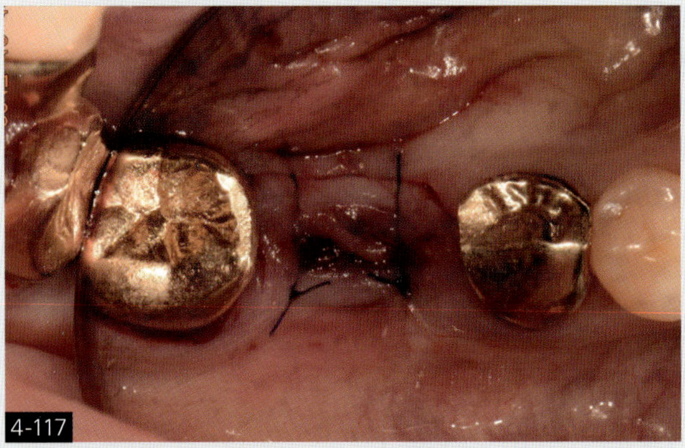
4-117

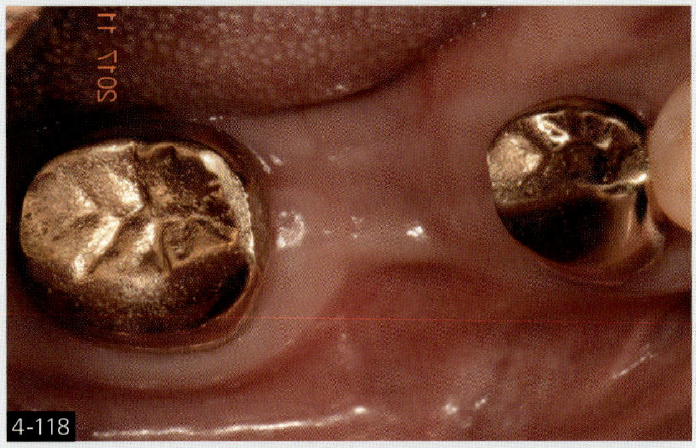
4-118

The images show the condition immediately after surgery and four weeks post-healing **(Figures 4-117, 118)**. Since all soft tissue around the implant was used to cover the surgical site, the soft tissue is completely closed. Even if epithelial cells are present internally, they will degenerate and disappear.

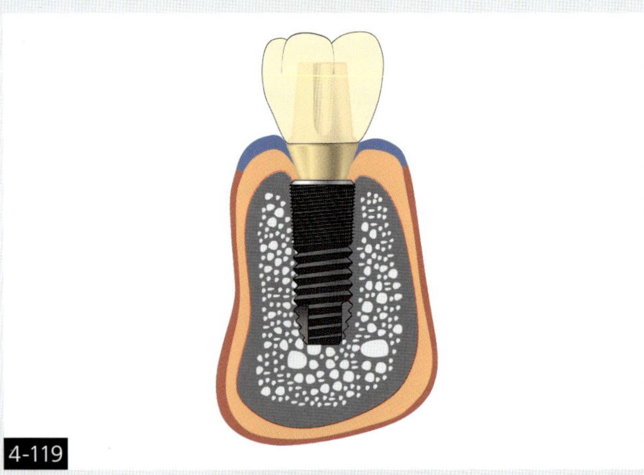
4-119

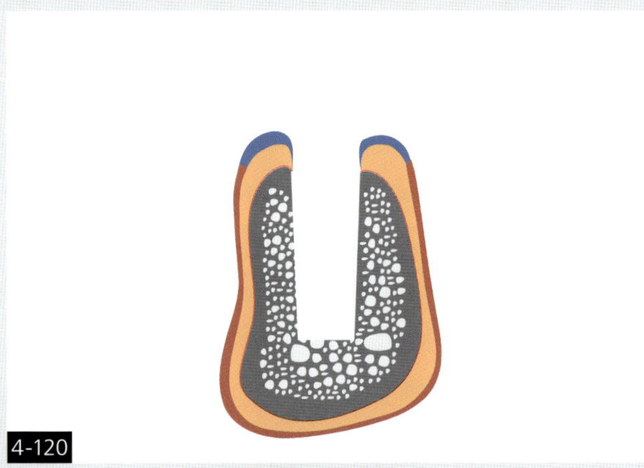
4-120

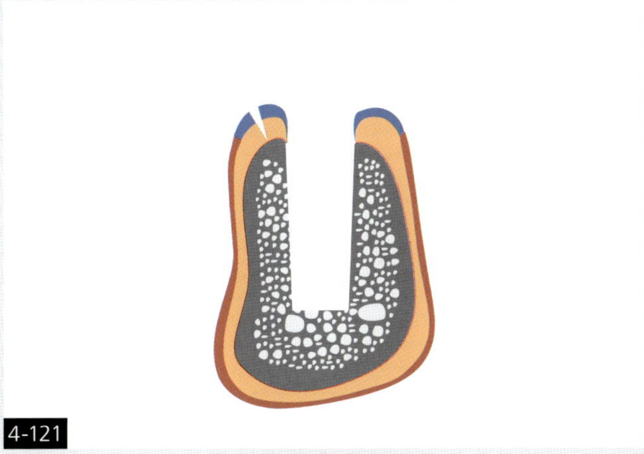

4-121

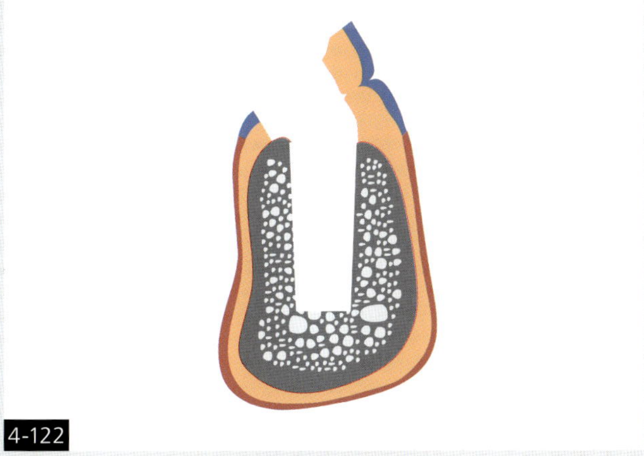

4-122

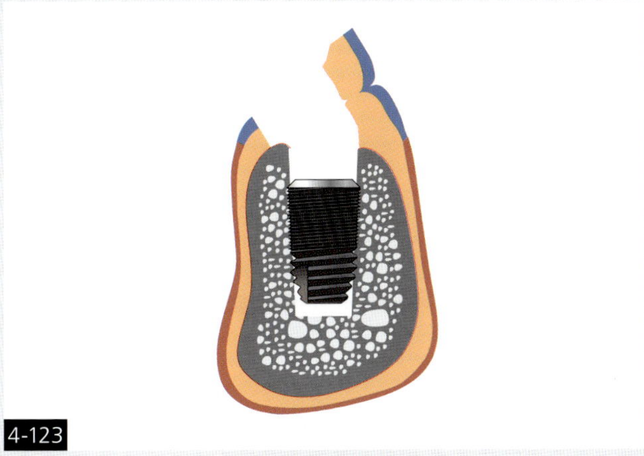

4-123

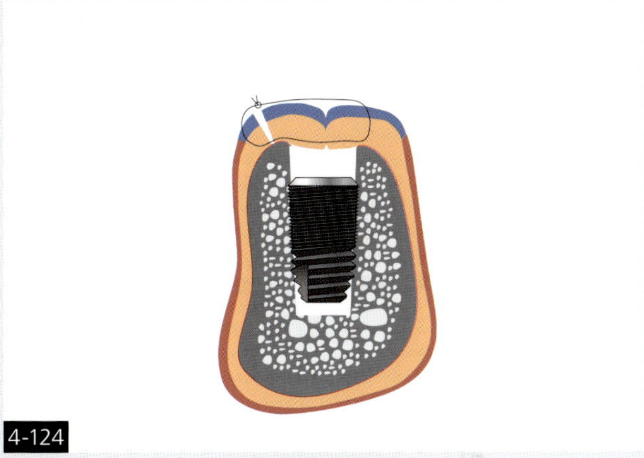

4-124

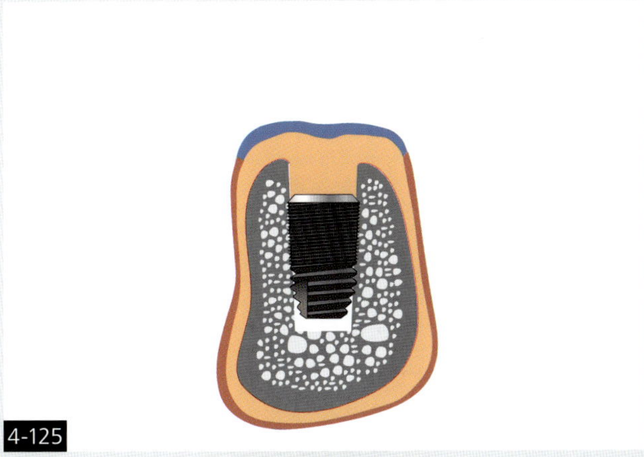

4-125

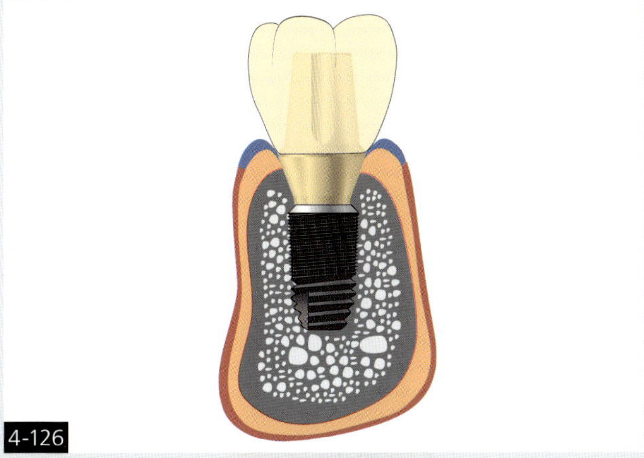

4-126

To help understand the concepts of this case, a graphical explanation is provided **(Figures 4-119~126)**. After removing all soft tissue between the alveolar bone and the implant, a 6.0 mm implant can be placed immediately. However, to prevent any remaining epithelial cells from forming periodontal pockets, this surgical method was chosen. Readers are encouraged to pay attention to the fate of the epithelial cells in the gingiva, as this will facilitate a better understanding of the surgery.

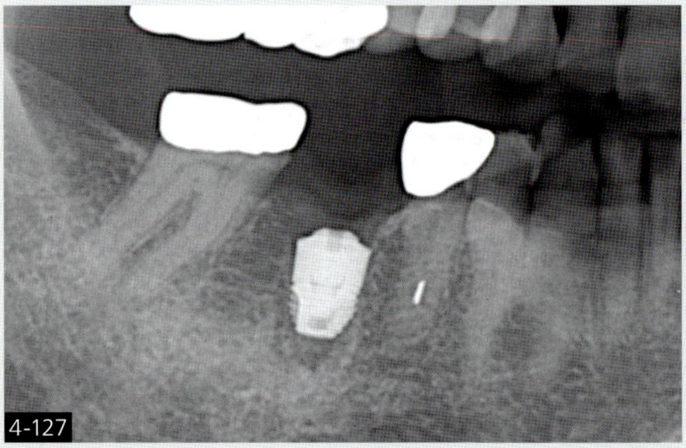

4-127

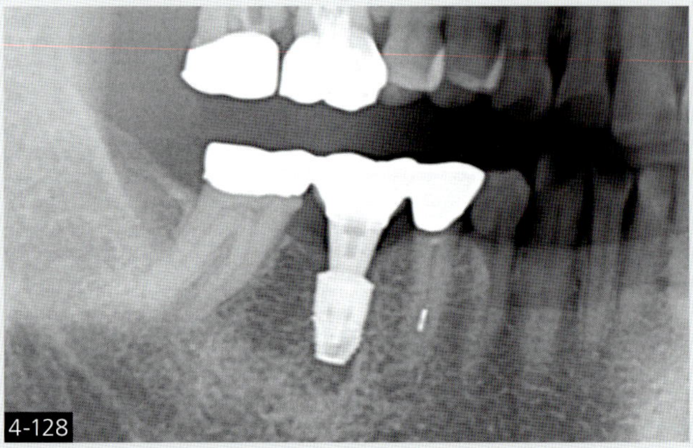

4-128

The images show the condition after the implant replacement **(Figure 4-127)** and after the prosthesis has been placed **(Figure 4-128)**. The alveolar bone has proliferated and is in contact with the abutment, which is very significant.

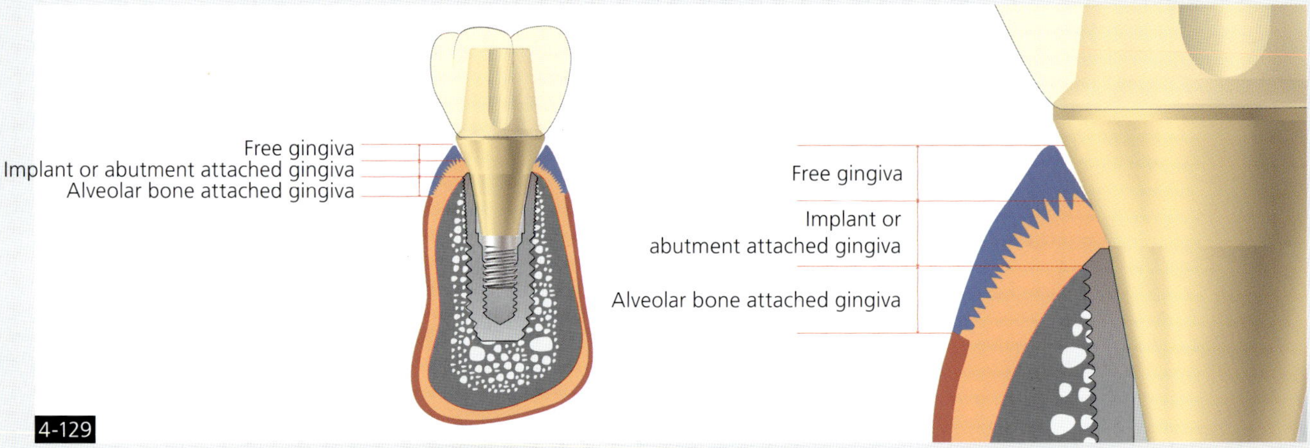

4-129

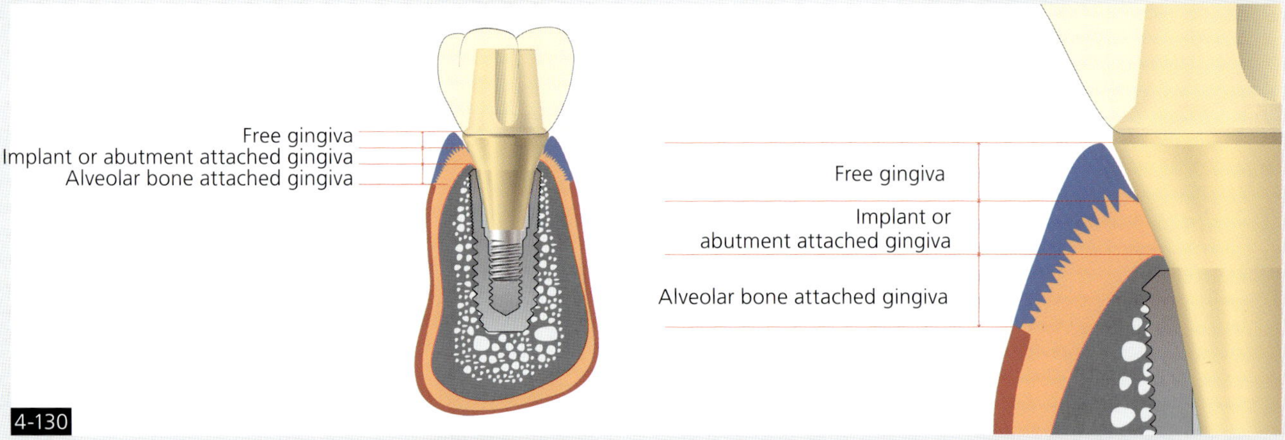

4-130

Figure 4-129 shows the fixture top aligned with the bone top, while **Figure 4-130** shows the fixture top positioned below the alveolar bone. As seen in the graphics, when the fixture top is placed deeply below the alveolar bone **(Figure 4-130)**, the alveolar bone grows up to the top of the fixture, increasing the amount of bone-attached gingiva and creating very favorable periodontal conditions. This setup effectively defends against bacterial invasion, resulting in a very healthy state for the implant procedure. The phenomenon of the alveolar bone growing above the fixture top and contacting the abutment will be discussed further later.

In cases where implants are extracted due to peri-implantitis and mechanical issues, four surgical methods aimed at preventing peri-implantitis were examined, focusing on achieving initial stability of the implant and preventing the formation of periodontal pockets. These methods can be summarized as follows:

1. An incision is made on the palatal side to displace the periodontal pocket and inflammatory tissue laterally, ensuring that the abutment is in contact with connective tissue rather than epithelial cells. If the width of the alveolar bone and gingiva is sufficient, an implant with a diameter larger than the prepared site is placed to achieve stability. Conversely, if the width of the alveolar bone and gingiva is insufficient, it is considered that a longer implant, within the limits allowed by anatomical structures such as the inferior alveolar nerve canal, can be placed approximately 2-3 mm deeper to achieve stability.

2. Instead of placing a thicker implant after removal, autogenous bone in a crescent shape is grafted into areas with insufficient alveolar bone to achieve stability during implantation. (It is not strictly necessary for the graft to be crescent-shaped. In the author's experience, a trephine drill (typically with an inner diameter of 1.8 mm and an outer diameter of 2.5 mm) is often used to harvest autogenous bone, resulting in cylindrical grafts. The key is to ensure maximum stability between the autogenous bone and the implant. The grafted autogenous bone serves to create attached gingiva, thereby preventing the occurrence of peri-implantitis.)

3. In cases where the upper part of the implant is fractured, surgery is performed after soft tissue healing. (Specifically, the upper part of the implant is covered with soft tissue, followed by the removal and re-implantation of the implant. This approach effectively prevents the formation of periodontal pockets.)

4. After implant removal, the soft tissue that has grown between the alveolar bone and the implant is utilized for coverage purposes.

Chapter 5 Response of Alveolar Bone After Implant Prosthesis

1. Recovery of Alveolar Bone After Implant Prosthesis

Loss of marginal bone can lead to gingival recession or the formation of periodontal pockets. Therefore, to some extent, preventing the loss of marginal bone during implant procedures can help suppress the occurrence of peri-implantitis. We have often been educated that the loss of marginal bone after implant procedures is a physiological and normal response. However, there are studies suggesting that marginal bone can actually increase after implant procedures, although these studies have not gained widespread acceptance. In the author's experience, the marginal bone in most implant procedures shows an increase in both quantity and quality. Additionally, the alveolar bone comes into contact with the abutment as well as the implant (in most cases where the implant is placed deeply).

To illustrate this concept for readers who may find it unfamiliar, let us examine a clinical case where the fixture top is positioned below the alveolar crest, leading to the proliferation of alveolar bone above the implant. This patient had their existing implant removed due to peri-implantitis, and the alveolar bone was allowed to heal **(Figure 5-1)**. After waiting for two months and reopening the site, it was observed that the alveolar bone lost due to peri-implantitis had not fully recovered. Although the fixture top was placed slightly deeper, the area around the fixture top still exhibited bone loss **(Figure 5-2)**. While some clinicians prefer to perform bone grafting, the author does not do so in such cases, believing that the empty space surrounded by autogenous bone will eventually fill with autogenous bone.

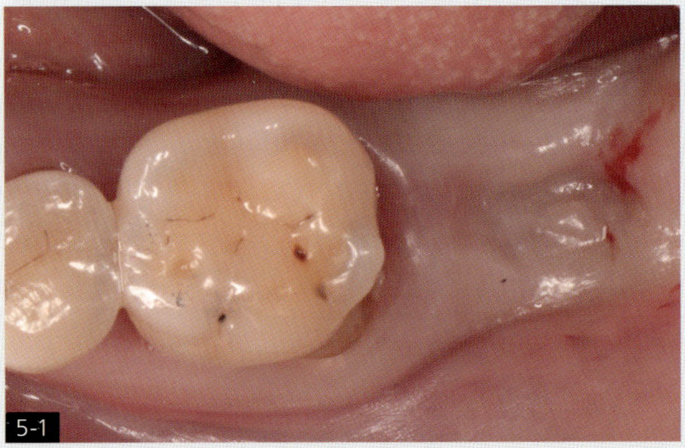
5-1

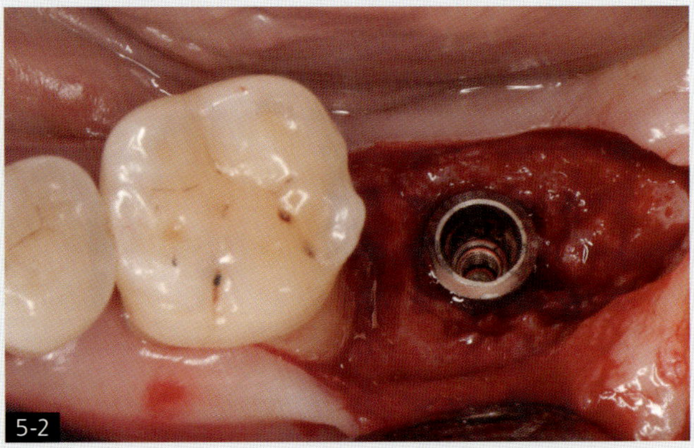
5-2

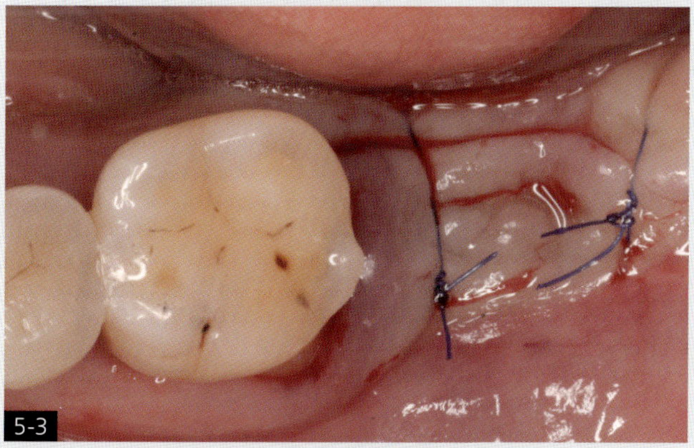

5-3

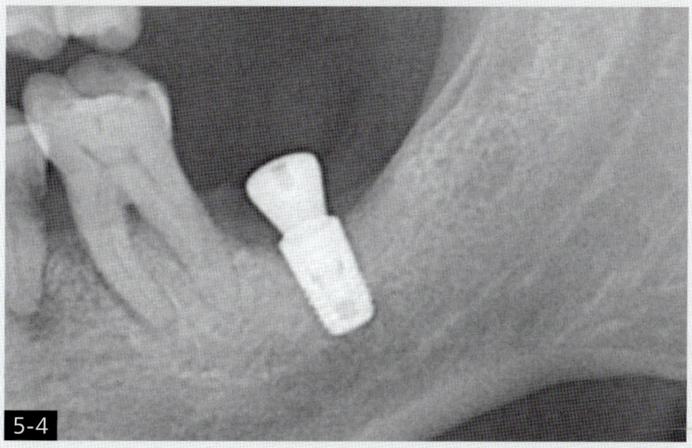

5-4

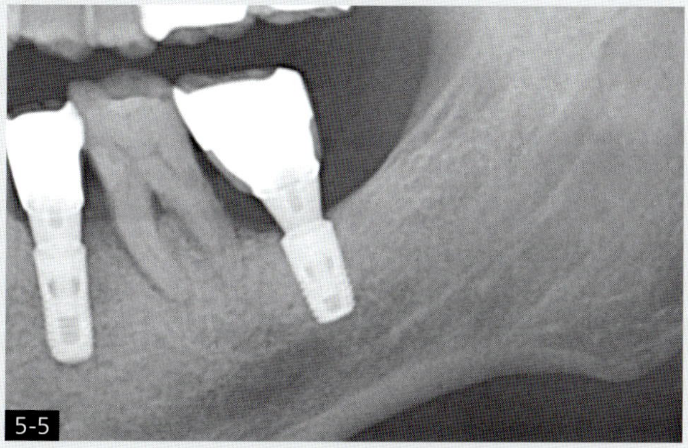

5-5

Figures 5-1~5 illustrate that the surgery was completed without bone grafting, and subsequent secondary surgery was performed, yet the alveolar bone had still not recovered **(Figure 5-4)**. The right X-ray shows that after the prosthesis, the alveolar bone has proliferated to cover the fixture top area **(Figure 5-5)**. Such bone response occurs only after the following processes have been completed: after secondary surgery, the final abutment must be secured, and a temporary restoration must be placed, followed by the re-tightening of the abutment screw. Furthermore, the abutment should not be removed from the implant. If these conditions are met, the alveolar bone will proliferate upwards until the final prosthesis is placed.

Repeatedly attaching and detaching various components for impressions at the fixture level can hinder the upward growth of alveolar bone. This repeated detachment disrupts the mucosal seal, allowing bacterial invasion, which leads to gradual recession of the gingiva and alveolar bone. The author believes that separating the abutment after it has been secured is not advisable, thus impressions for implant prosthetics are taken at the abutment level.

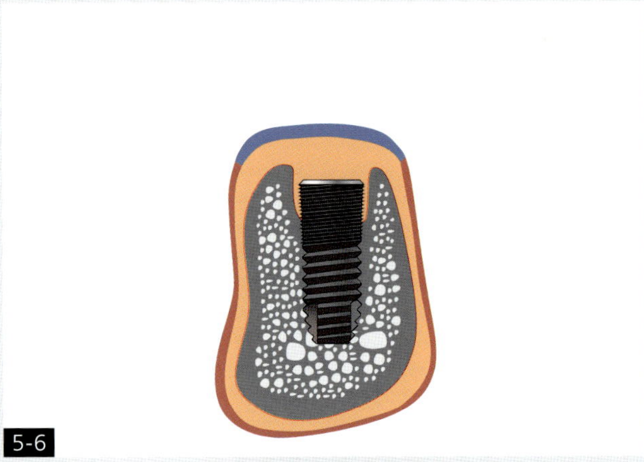

5-6

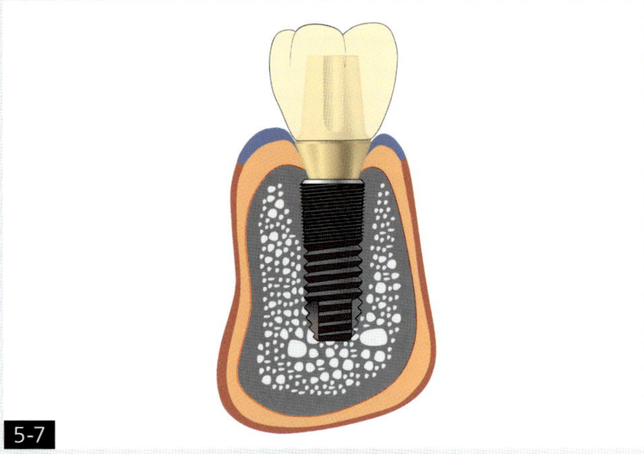

5-7

When the implant is placed below the margin of the bone defect, the alveolar bone fills in, positioning the upper part of the implant beneath the alveolar bone **(Figures 5-6, 7)**.

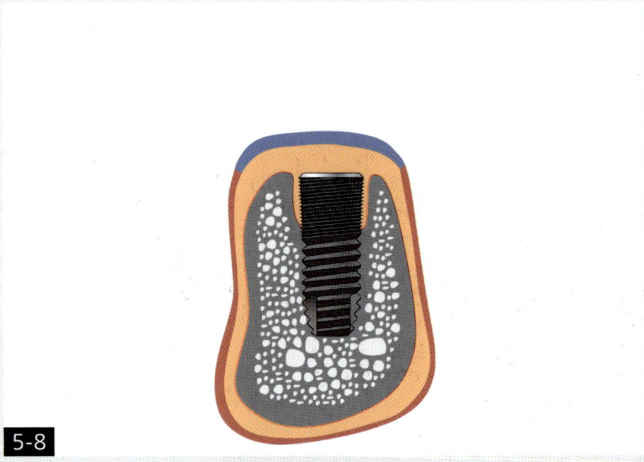

5-8

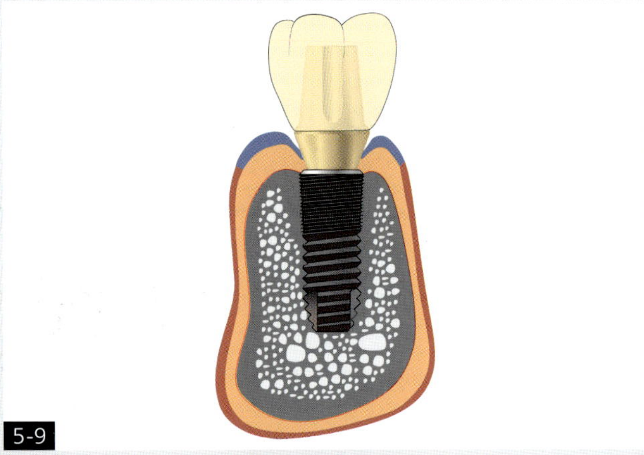

5-9

The intra-bone defect will eventually fill with autogenous bone. By positioning the implant according to the anticipated height of the healing bone, the top of the implant and the top of the alveolar bone will eventually align **(Figures 5-8, 9)**. When the positions of the marginal bone and the implant are aligned, the upper part of the implant may slightly protrude above the alveolar bone due to the tendency for marginal bone loss as the intra-bone defect fills with autogenous bone.

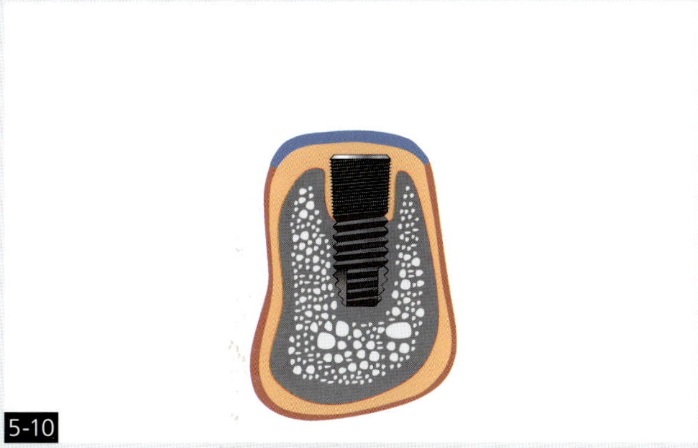

5-10

The fixture top is positioned too high

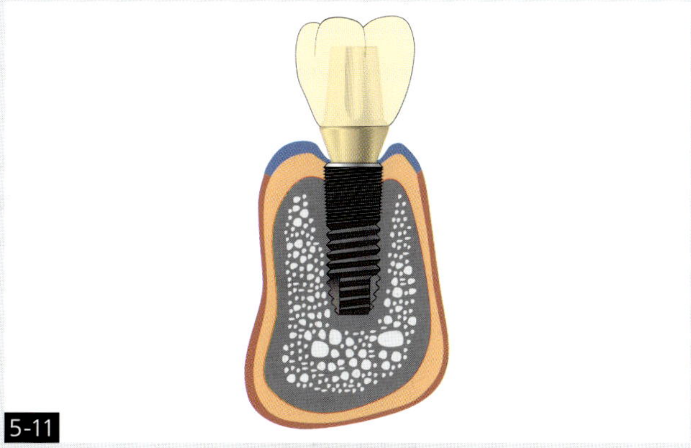

5-11

The fixture top is located above the healed alveolar bone

If the fixture top is positioned too high, it will ultimately be located above the alveolar bone **(Figures 5-10, 11)**. In Astra-type implants, such positioning of the fixture top can lead to various complications and even peri-implantitis, which should be avoided.

Let us examine another clinical case with radiographic images.

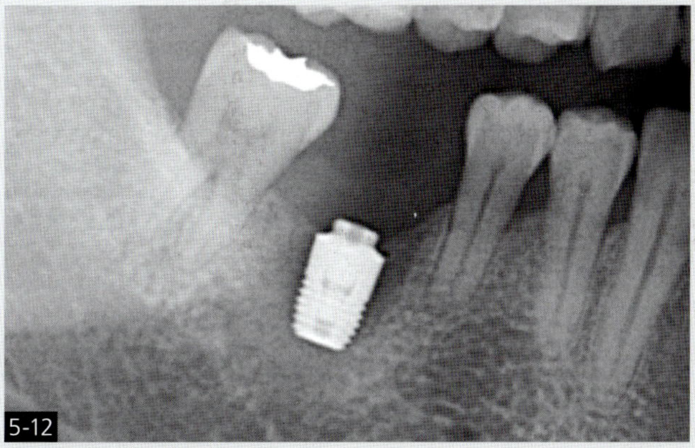

5-12

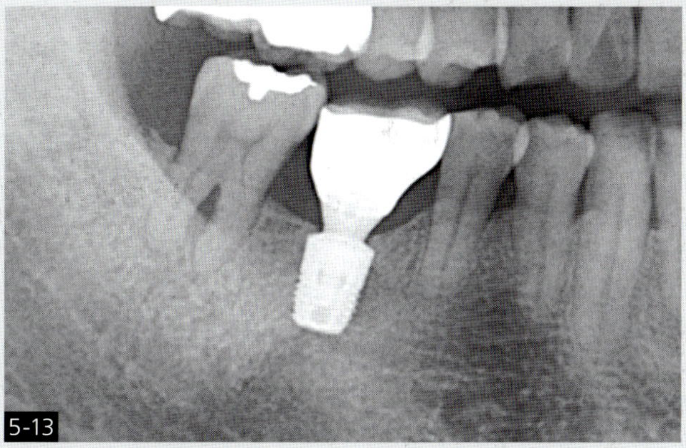

5-13

Figures 5-12 and **5-13** show images taken eight years post-implantation, demonstrating similar results **(Figures 5-12, 13)**. When the fixture top is positioned below the alveolar bone, the alveolar bone tends to cover the fixture top.

At this point, it is essential that the width of the alveolar bone is sufficient, and that there is gingiva present on the buccal and lingual sides. Now, readers can understand the periodontal implications of positioning the fixture top deeply.

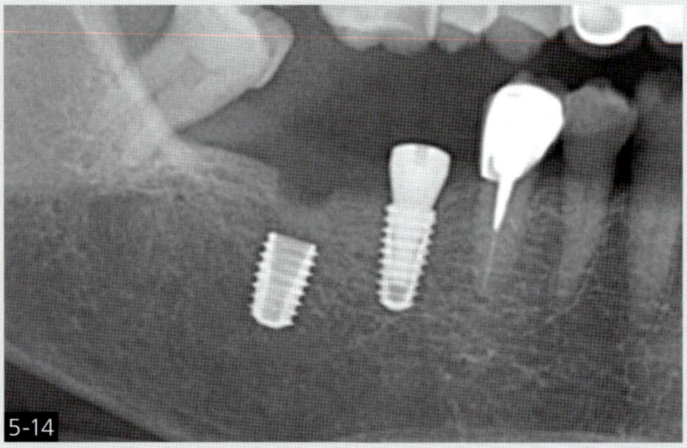
5-14

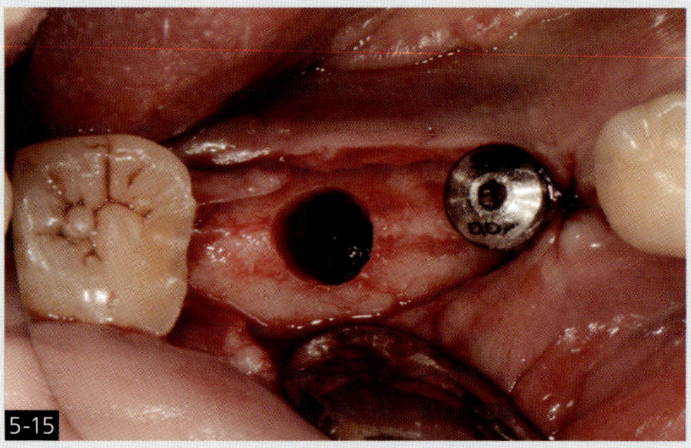
5-15

If the bone marrow is empty, placing the fixture too deeply can lead to the loss of initial stability, causing the fixture to sink **(Figures 5-14, 15)**. Therefore, great care must be taken when positioning the fixture top below the marginal bone.

2. Surgical Techniques for Alveolar Bone Recovery in the Posterior Region

When peri-implantitis occurs, the alveolar bone deteriorates, and inflammatory granulation tissue and epithelial tissue proliferate downward. We have explored the concepts and techniques to address this issue. Now, we will investigate the clinical procedures necessary to eliminate periodontal pockets during immediate implant placement after the extraction of periodontally affected natural teeth.

Additionally, we will review clinical cases of re-implantation after implant removal to aid in enhancing the clinical skills of the readers. The procedure of extracting periodontally affected natural teeth and immediately placing implants is fundamentally similar to the procedure performed after the removal of implants affected by peri-implantitis.

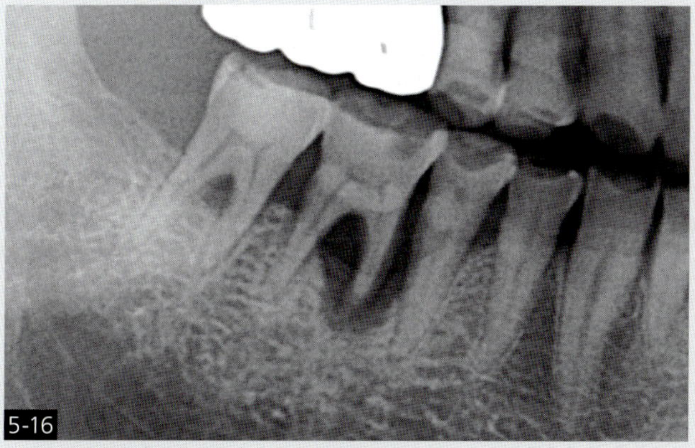
5-16

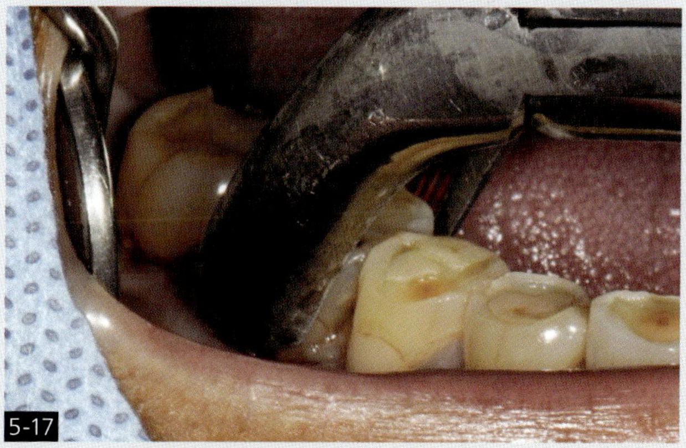
5-17

After extracting the periodontally affected tooth #46, it was decided to proceed with the implant procedure (Figures 5-16, 17). During the diagnostic process, we noted significant alveolar bone loss at the mesial root of tooth #46, as well as the downward proliferation of inflammatory granulation tissue and epithelial tissue. We also understand that placing an implant without appropriate treatment can lead to the formation of periodontal pockets and subsequent peri-implantitis. Therefore, one of the surgical methods mentioned earlier must be employed.

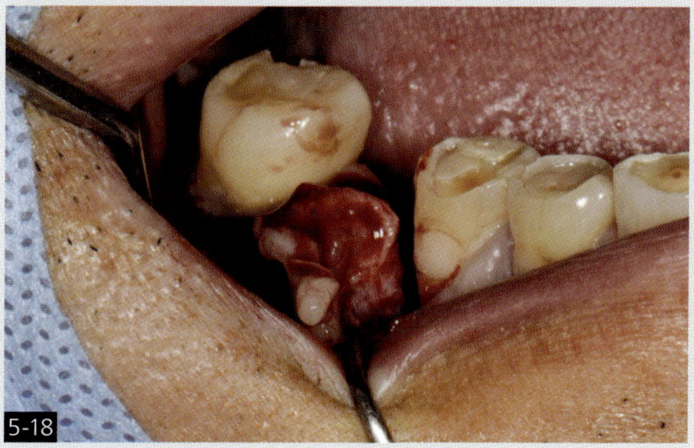
5-18

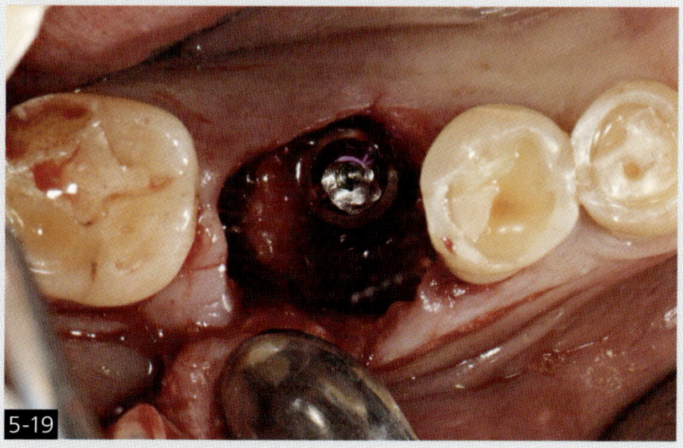
5-19

An incision was made on the lingual side of the extraction site, and both the gingiva and the granulation and epithelial tissues were completely removed **(Figure 5-18)**. No incision was made on the buccal side, leaving the granulation and inflammatory tissue attached to the buccal gingiva. My preferred position for immediate implant placement after the extraction of a mandibular molar is on the lingual side adjacent to the mesial root extraction site. This preference varies depending on the shape and inclination of the tooth, but I favor this area because it allows for a more ideal prosthetic restoration and facilitates initial stability, making the surgery much simpler. Additionally, by placing the implant slightly upright on the lingual side compared to the natural tooth inclined lingually, the screw access hole of the crown will eventually align with the center of the prosthetic restoration on the buccal-lingual side. The implant was placed in the desired location **(Figure 5-19)**.

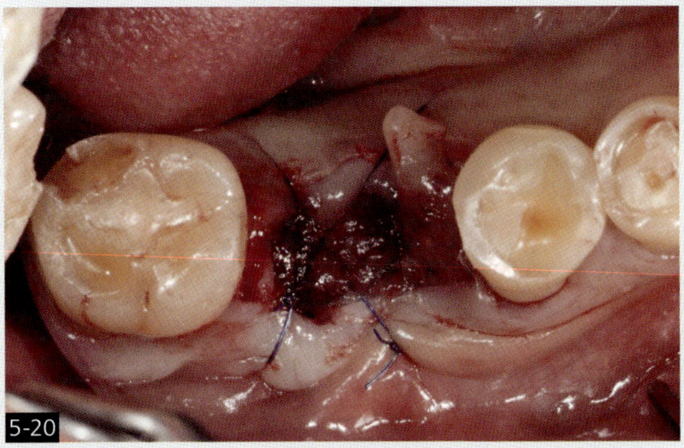
5-20

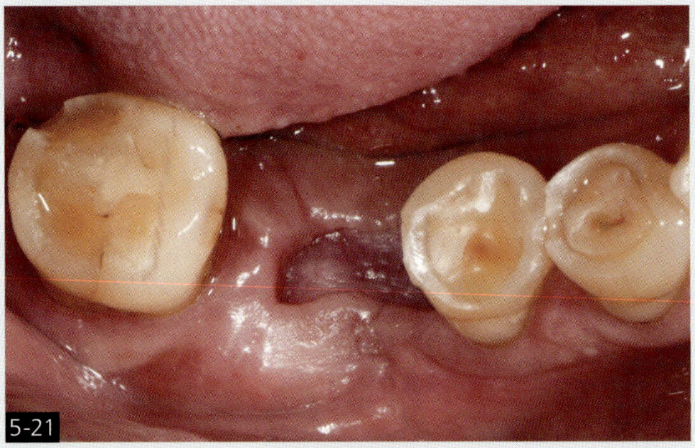
5-21

The granulation and epithelial tissues that were removed were used to cover the surgical site **(Figure 5-20)**. Since the buccal side is connected to soft tissue, this can be considered a type of pedicle graft. After approximately four weeks, it was confirmed through photographs that the implant site was completely covered with soft tissue **(Figure 5-21)**. This surgical technique can help prevent the formation of periodontal pockets around the implant.

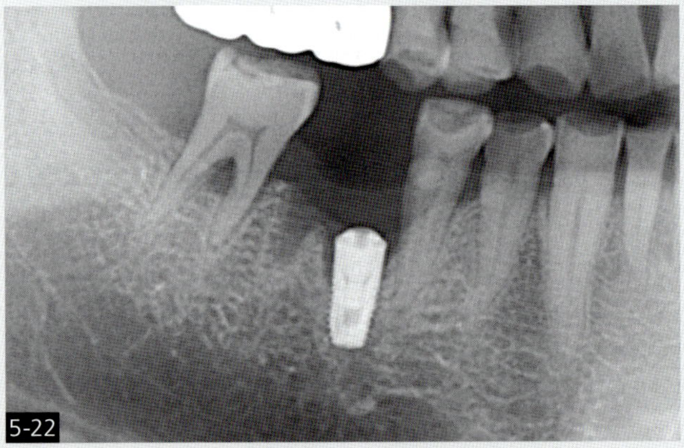
5-22

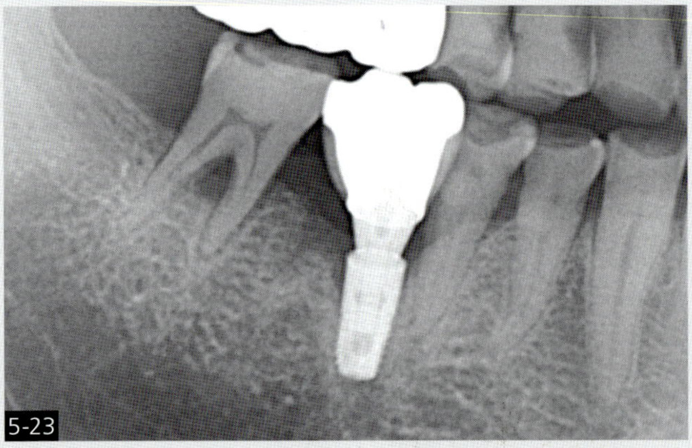
5-23

The immediate post-operative X-ray and the X-ray after prosthetic placement are shown. After 2.5 years, the alveolar bone has healed almost perfectly **(Figures 5-22, 23)**. In this case, I believe that bone grafting is not the key element of the surgery; rather, the surgical approach considering periodontal pockets is crucial. It is truly remarkable to observe that the alveolar bone of tooth #47 is gradually decreasing while the alveolar bone around implant #46 is increasing.

To make the explanation of this surgery easier, graphics have been prepared.

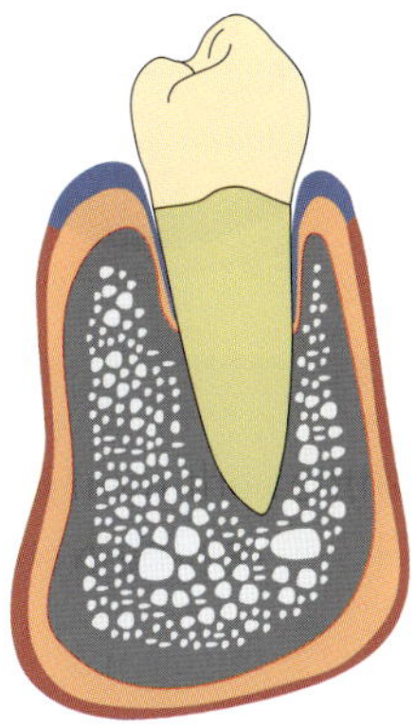

5-24

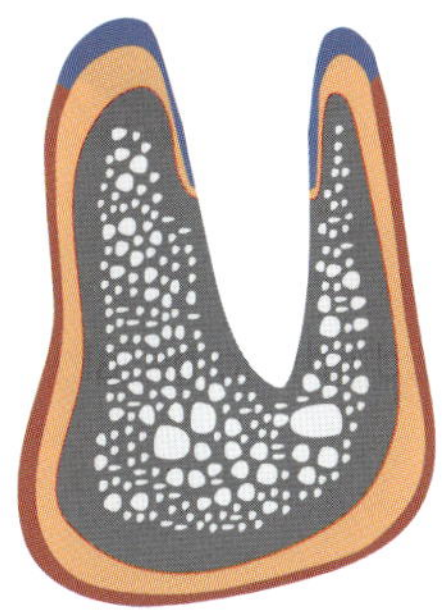

5-25

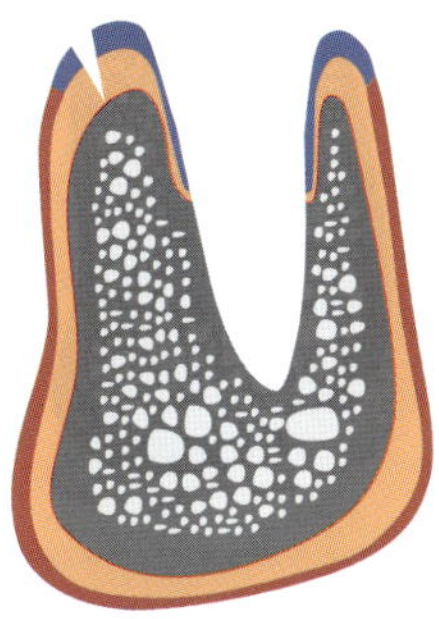

5-26

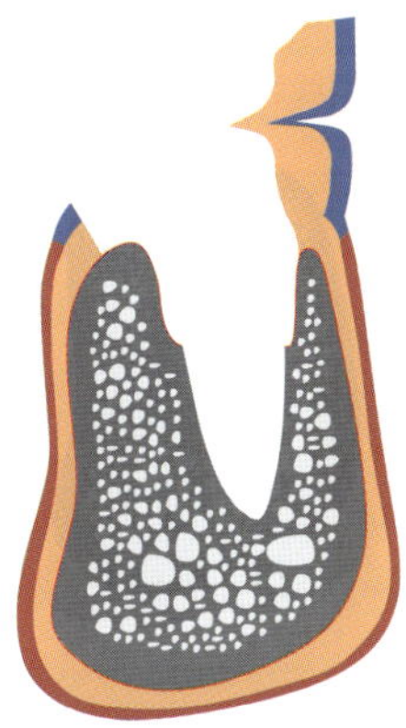

5-27

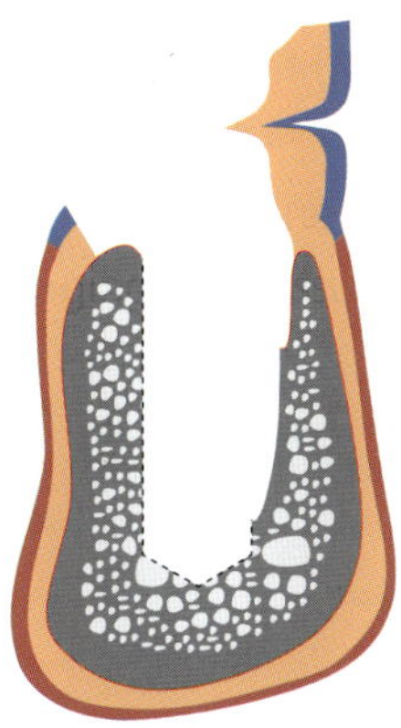

5-28

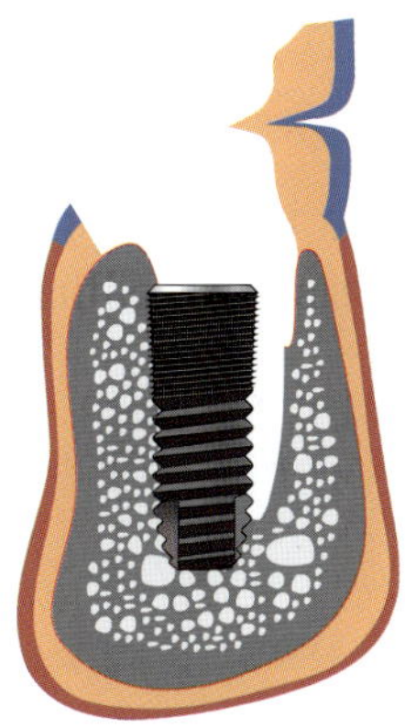

5-29

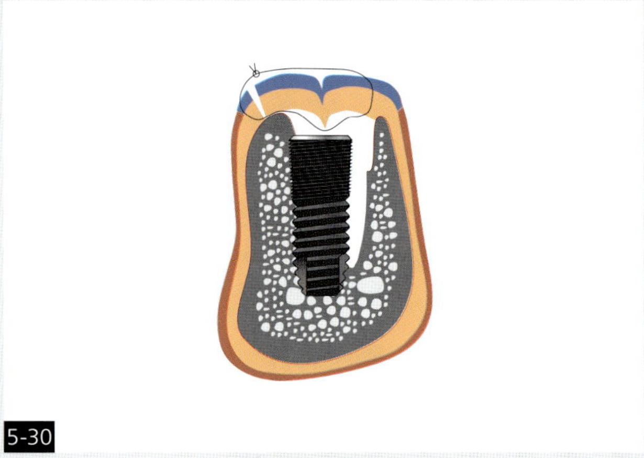
5-30

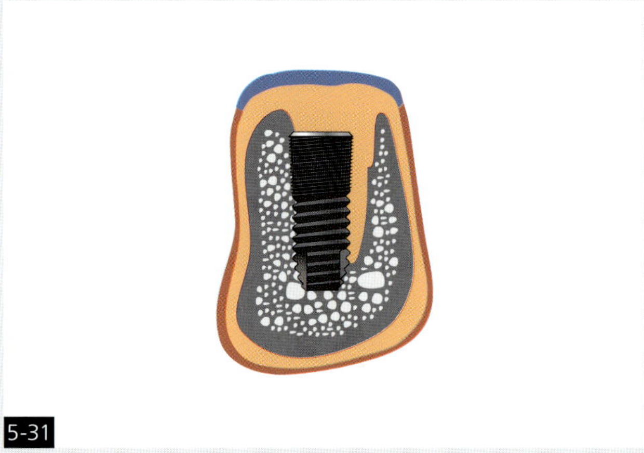
5-31

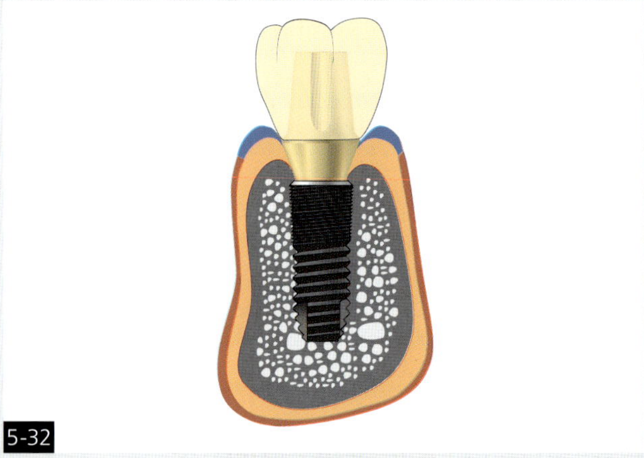
5-32

The flap management in the previously shown case is similar, allowing readers to understand easily.

This similar surgical approach can also be applied to premolars, which I would like to introduce to the readers.

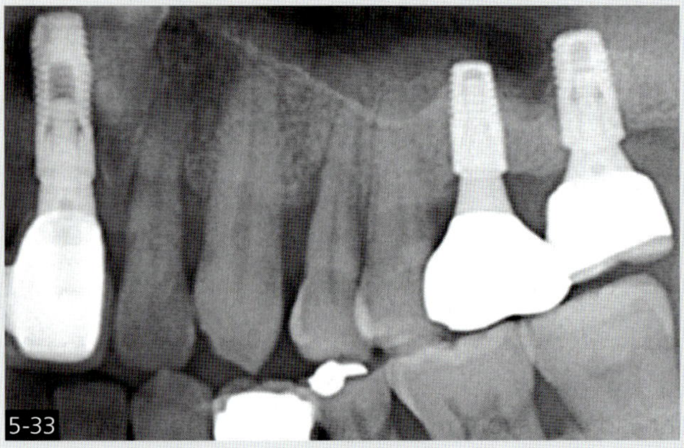
5-33

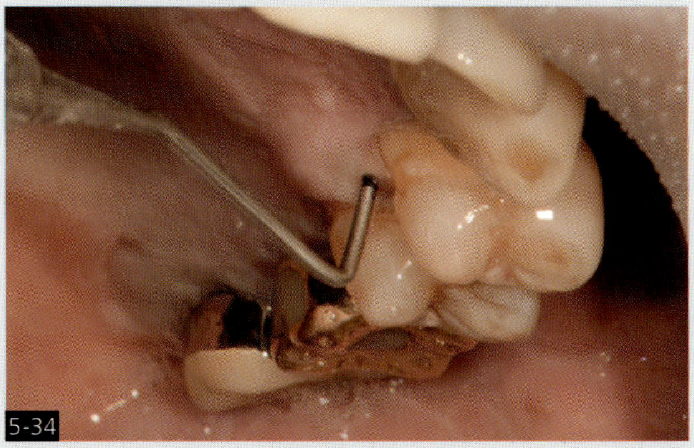
5-34

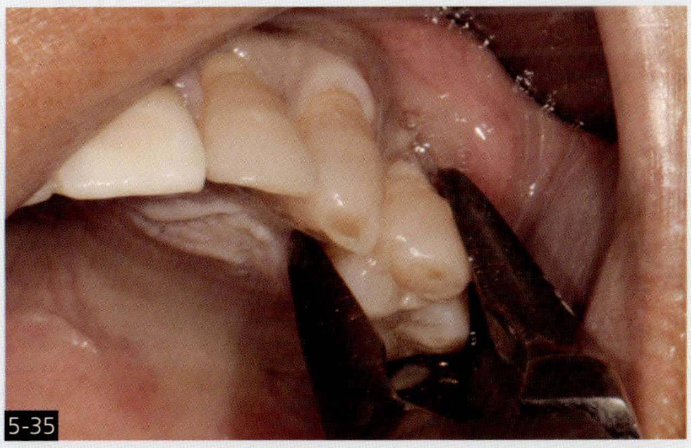
5-35

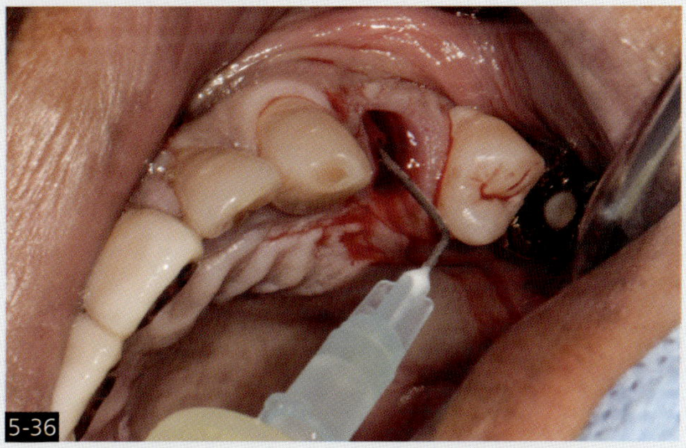
5-36

An immediate implant placement was decided after extracting tooth #24, which exhibited a deep periodontal pocket on the palatal side **(Figures 5-33, 34)**. I wash the contaminated extraction socket with a tetracycline antibiotic solution before placing the implant immediately **(Figures 5-35, 36)**.

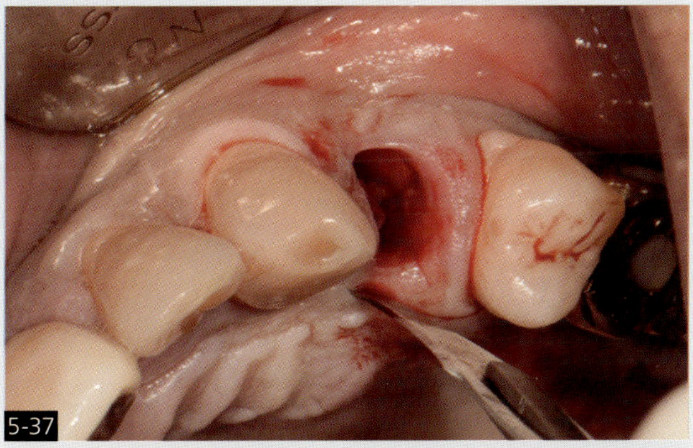
5-37

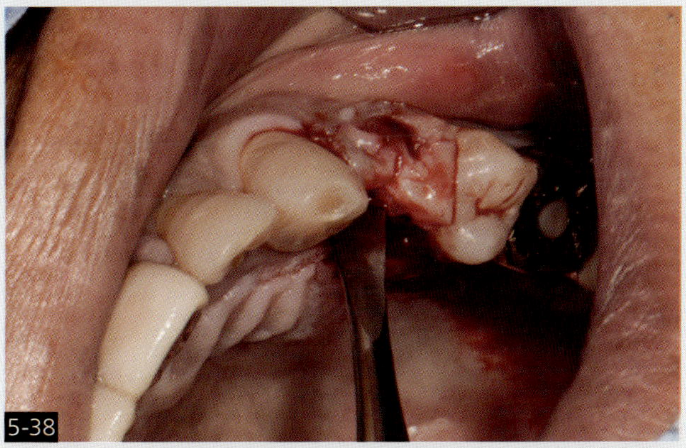
5-38

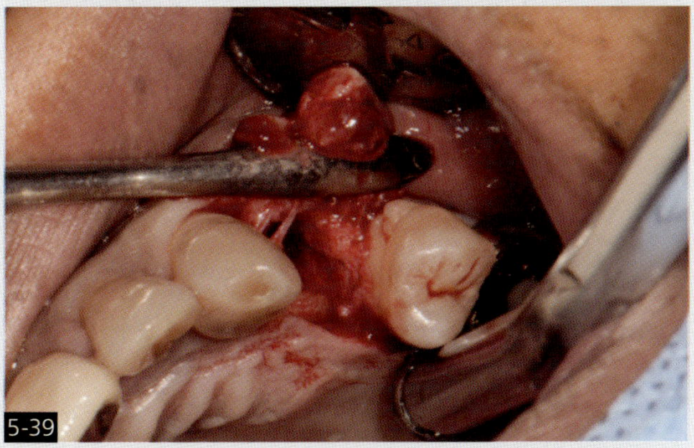
5-39

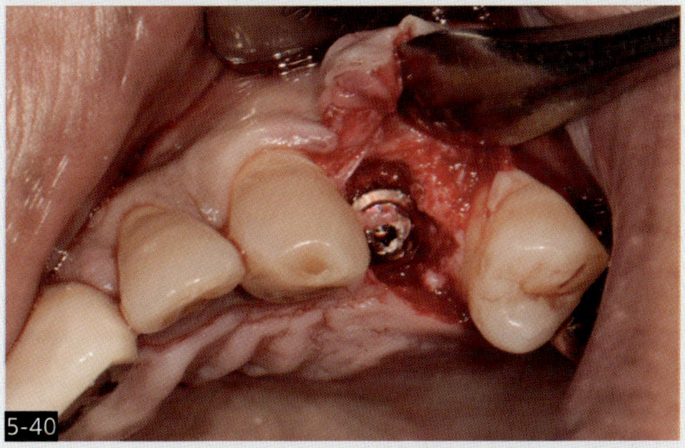
5-40

As previously described, an incision is made. A buccal incision is placed to avoid including the extraction socket, and an incision is made at the gingival sulcus adjacent to the tooth **(Figure 5-37)**.

As I have mentioned, it is preferable to reflect the soft tissue without scraping it, giving the sensation of scraping the alveolar bone instead. The buccal alveolar bone is usually very thin. If the buccal alveolar bone is fully exposed, excessive loss of buccal bone may occur postoperatively. Therefore, it is advisable to elevate the flap only to the extent necessary to visualize the buccal bone margin. If there is a periodontal pocket on the buccal side, the soft tissue in that area should also be detached from the alveolar bone **(Figure 5-39)**.

In my case, after extracting a maxillary premolar, I position the implant as far palatally as possible (within the limits allowed by the prosthetics) **(Figure 5-40)**.

I aim to place the implant palatally without breaking the palatal alveolar bone, and sometimes I intentionally create a palatal fenestration at the top of the implant. While this may lead to a bone defect on the buccal side, I usually do not perform bone grafting at this time. Since buccal bone typically resorbs after surgery, if the implant is positioned centrally in the extraction socket or on the buccal side, there may be a situation where there is no alveolar bone on the buccal side after healing.

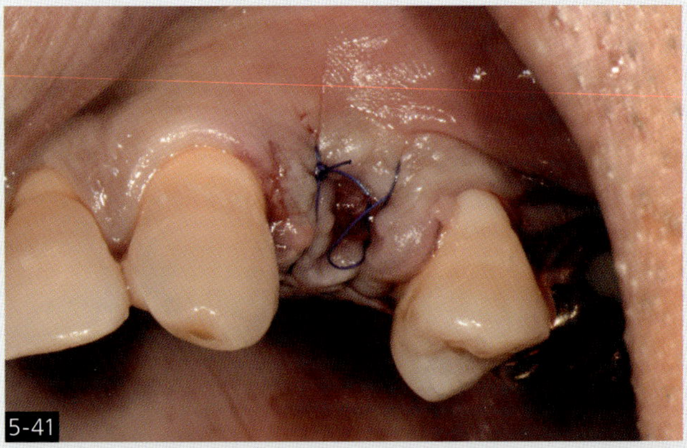

5-41

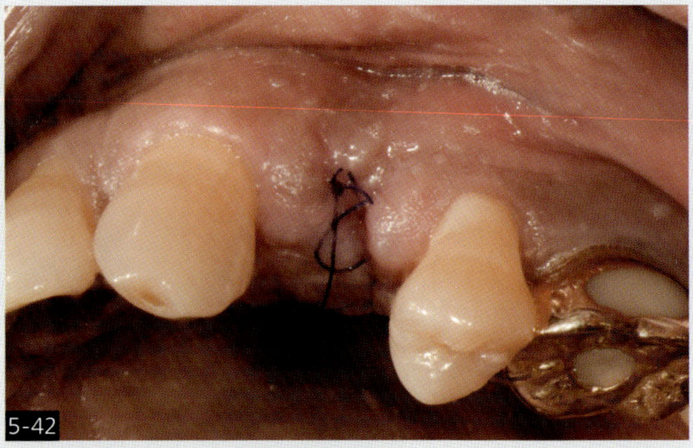

5-42

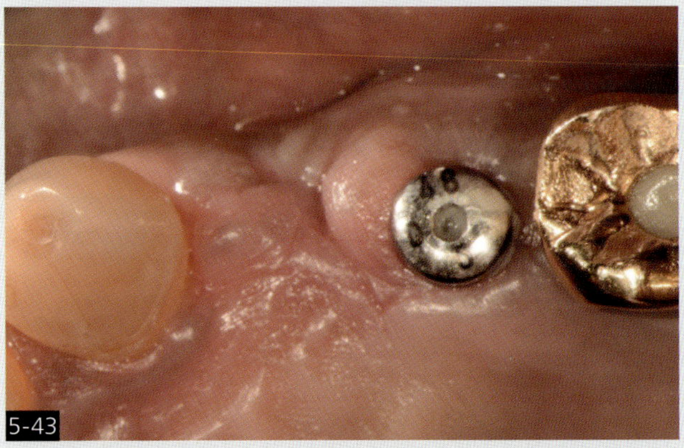

5-43

The inflammatory granulation tissue and epithelial tissue that formed the periodontal pocket were used to cover the extraction socket **(Figure 5-41)**. The postoperative appearance after one week is shown in **Figure 5-42**, and after four weeks, the surgical site was completely covered with soft tissue **(Figure 5-43)**. Tooth #25 was also in poor condition, so an immediate implant was placed after extraction. In the case of tooth #25, since the periodontal pocket was not deep, I was not concerned about the formation of a pocket after implant placement, so I directly attached the healing abutment.

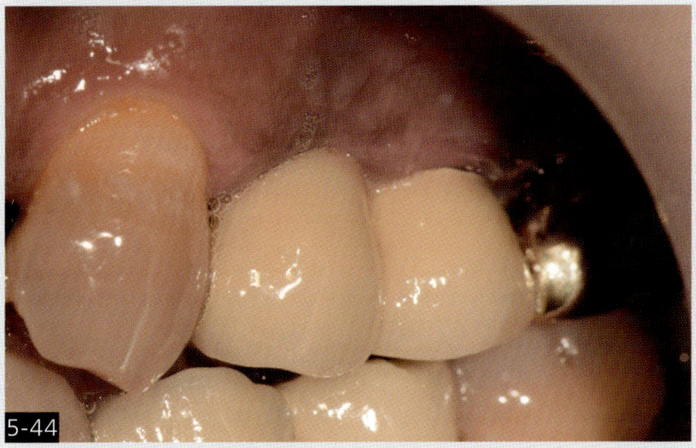

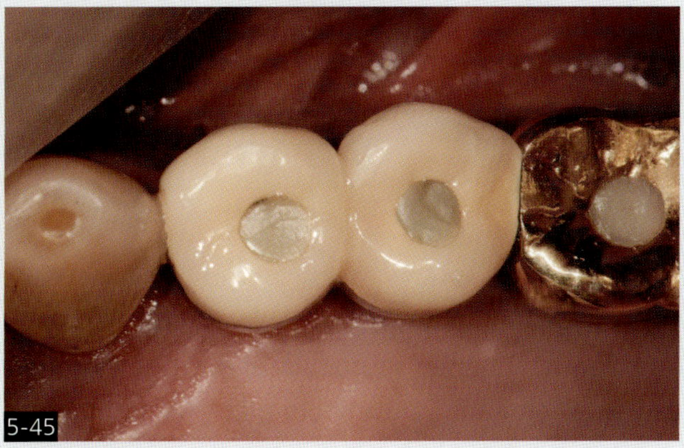

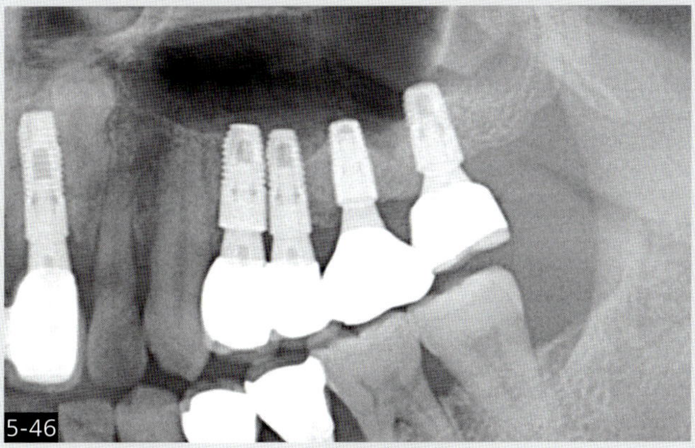

After extracting a periodontally affected natural tooth and placing an implant, there were no issues, and all treatments were successfully completed **(Figures 5-44, 45)**. There was no loss of alveolar bone, and peri-implantitis did not occur. The radiographic image shows the condition four years post-treatment **(Figure 5-46)**. Although the distance between the two implants appears close on the radiograph, this is not the case in the actual clinical photographs.

3. Maxillary Molar Implant Repair Case

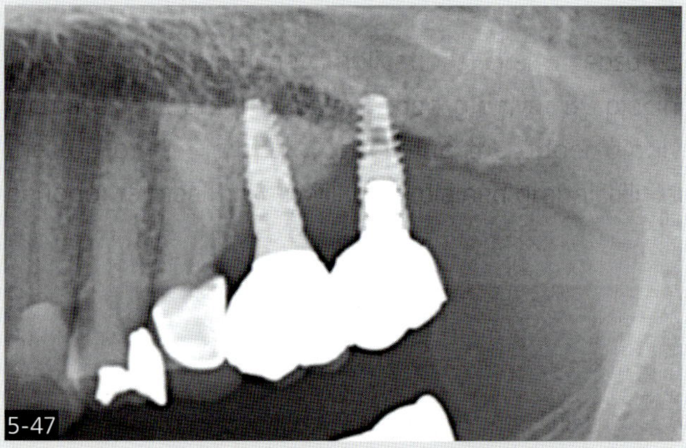

5-47

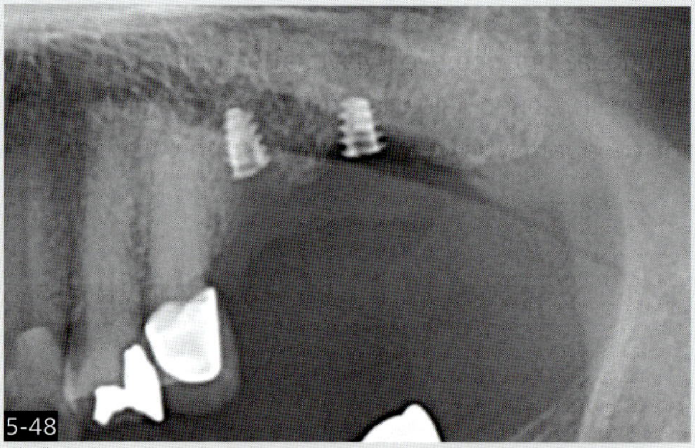

5-48

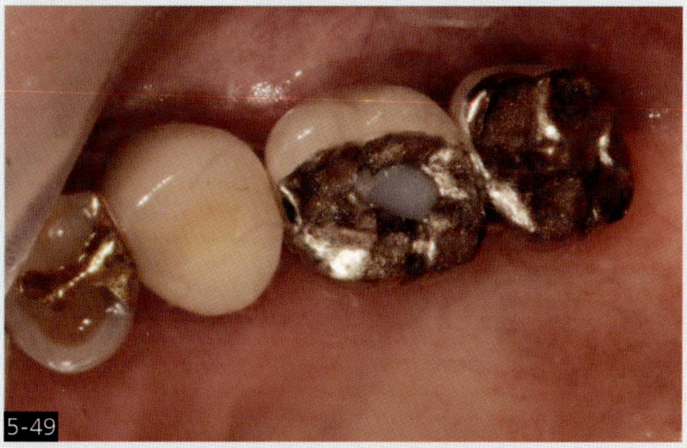

5-49

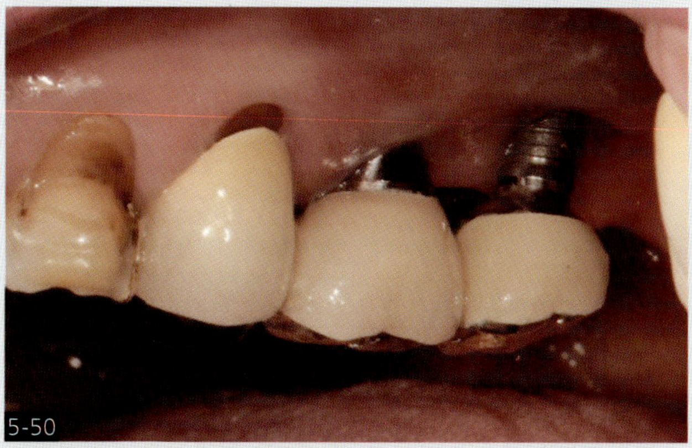

5-50

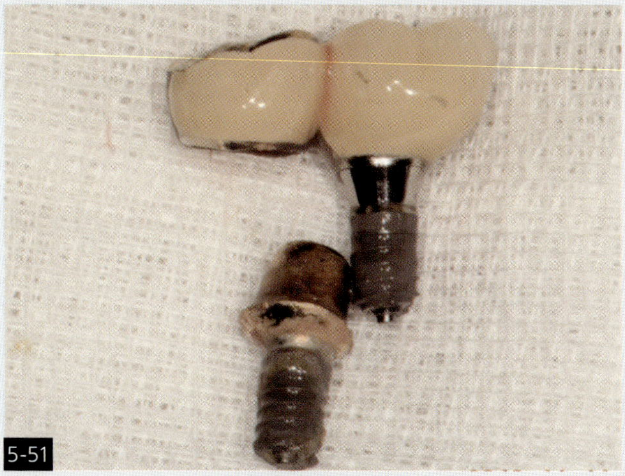

5-51

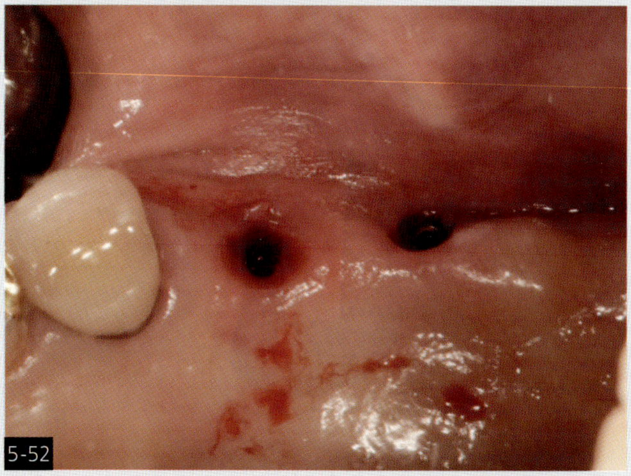

5-52

Implant #27 shows excessive alveolar bone loss **(Figure 5-47)**. Peri-implantitis occurred, and ultimately, both implants fractured **(Figures 5-48, 51, 52)**. In the clinical photograph taken before the fracture, excessive gingival recession can be observed **(Figure 5-50)**. It is unlikely that the implant placement surgery was performed in such a state from the beginning. In my opinion, the drilling for implant placement was done on the buccal side rather than centrally between the gingiva and alveolar bone, resulting in thin buccal bone that subsequently resorbed after surgery. The loss of buccal alveolar bone led to gingival recession, resulting in significant exposure of the upper portion of the implant.

When implants are placed in the maxillary molar region solely based on prosthetic considerations, such outcomes frequently occur. Therefore, I compromise between the ideal prosthetic position and the biologically ideal position. To place the implant centrally in the gingiva, I drill slightly more palatally than the aforementioned situation. Typically, this results in a less favorable prosthetic situation, so I tilt the fixture top significantly towards the buccal side to ensure that the screw hole aligns with the center of the crown.

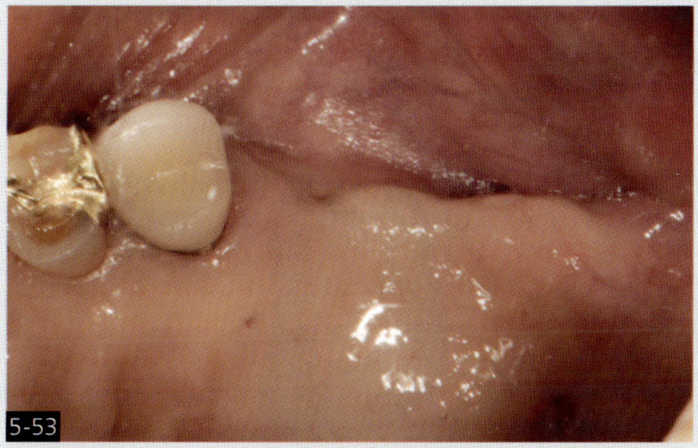
5-53

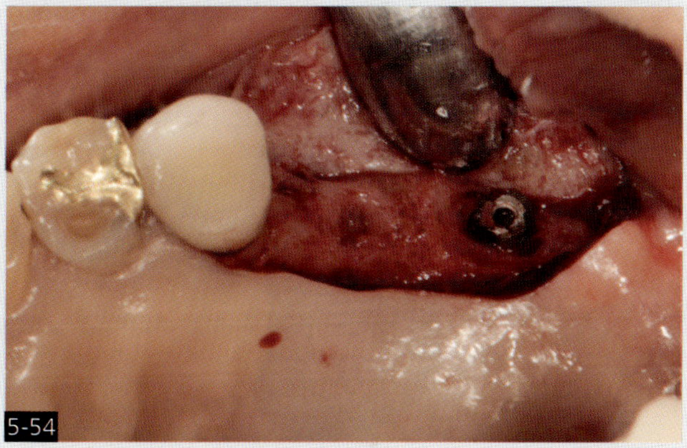
5-54

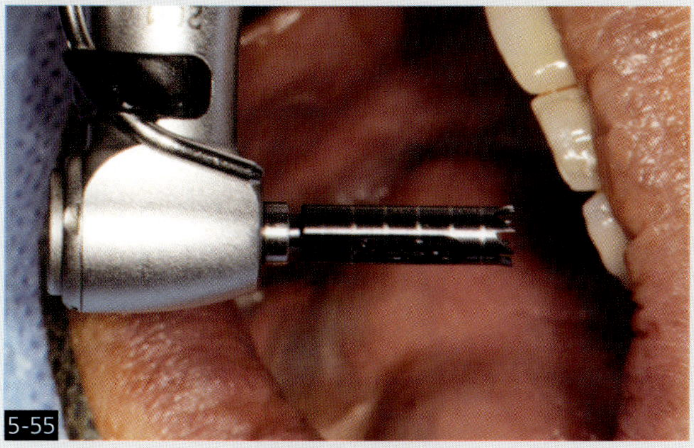
5-55

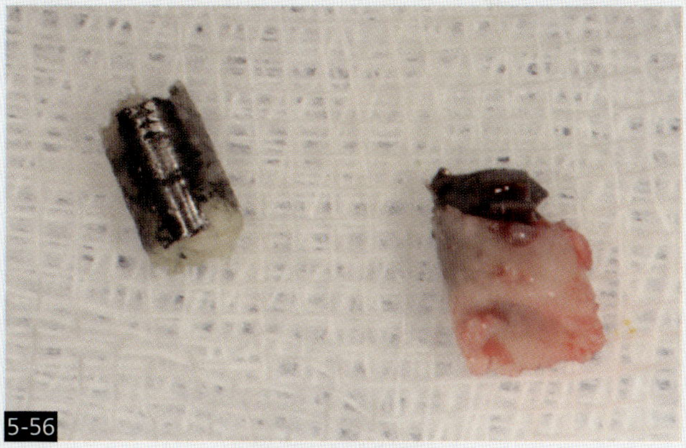
5-56

After waiting approximately two months, it can be seen that the soft tissue has completely covered the area (Figure 5-53). The fractured remnants of the implant need to be removed, and a new implant must be placed. Implant #26 became difficult to remove as it was buried in the alveolar bone (Figure 5-54). A trephine drill was used to remove the fractured implant fragment. Using a trephine drill with an inner diameter of 4.0 mm and an outer diameter of 5.0 mm, the diameter of the hole formed after the removal of the implant was 5 mm. Implant #26 was covered with autogenous bone, resulting in a significant amount of alveolar bone adhering to the fractured piece (Figures 5-55, 56).

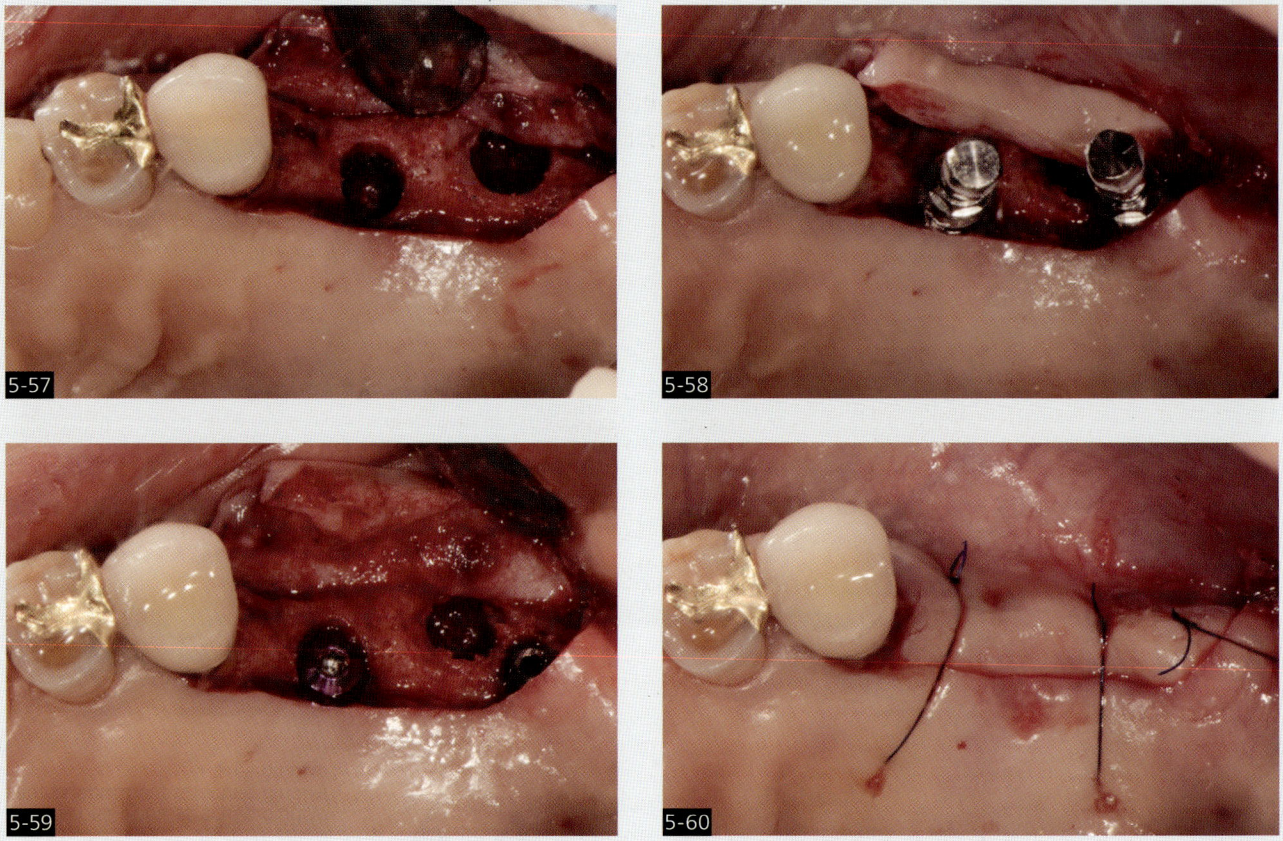

5-57 5-58 5-59 5-60

After removing the fractured implant, the 5 mm diameter hole can be observed **(Figure 5-57)**. In the case of implant #26, the placement position was appropriate, so a 4.5 mm diameter implant was reinserted into the area. For implant #27, it was placed slightly more palatally. To utilize more alveolar bone, implant #27 was positioned slightly posterior to its original location. Since placing implant #27 further back could lead to it being outside the gingival margin, it was tilted slightly mesially. This positioning and angling of implant #27 aimed to maximize the use of alveolar bone while ensuring it remained within the gingival envelope **(Figure 5-58)**. It can be seen that implant #27 was moved palatally and posteriorly from its original position. The implant must be moved palatally to ensure that there is gingiva on the buccal side; if it is placed in the original position, there may be no gingiva on the buccal side, leading to the risk of peri-implantitis again **(Figure 5-59)**.

For implant #26, the hole created after removing the fractured piece has a diameter of 5 mm, while the diameter of the newly placed implant is 4.5 mm. It is not possible to achieve initial stability by placing a smaller diameter implant into a larger hole. Therefore, in such cases, it is necessary to drill deeper after removing the implant. Drilling should extend at least 2 mm deeper to achieve initial stability at the apex of the fixture. Since stability must be obtained from such a short length, under-drilling should be considered during the drilling process. There is typically about a 0.5 mm gap between the top of the fixture and the alveolar bone, which will be filled with autogenous bone, so there is no need for concern. It is quite natural for a defect surrounded by autogenous bone to be filled with autogenous bone, as has been observed in previous cases.
Although it was possible to remove the fractured piece and place the implant at the same position and angle

immediately after the fracture, I chose to wait for the soft tissue to heal before placing the implant. This decision was based on the possibility of needing to adjust the placement of implant #27 and potentially grafting additional buccal bone. If bone grafting is required after placing the implant on the buccal side, flap coverage becomes crucial, so I waited for the soft tissue to heal. Ultimately, it turned out that waiting for soft tissue healing was unnecessary, but that was my original intention. I encourage readers that if an implant fractures and bone grafting is anticipated, waiting for the soft tissue to close before surgery can make flap management much easier, as demonstrated in this case.

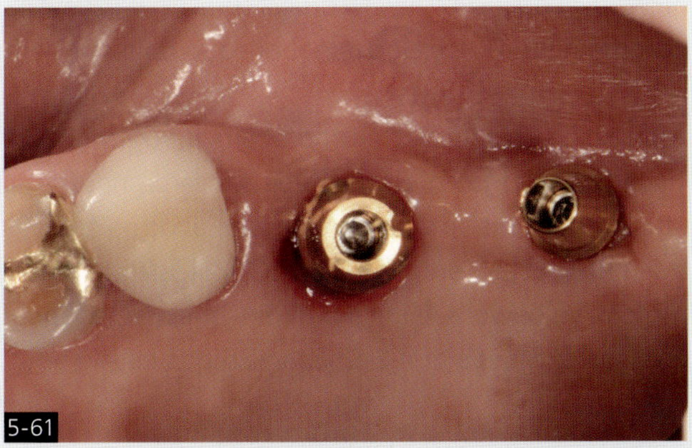

5-61

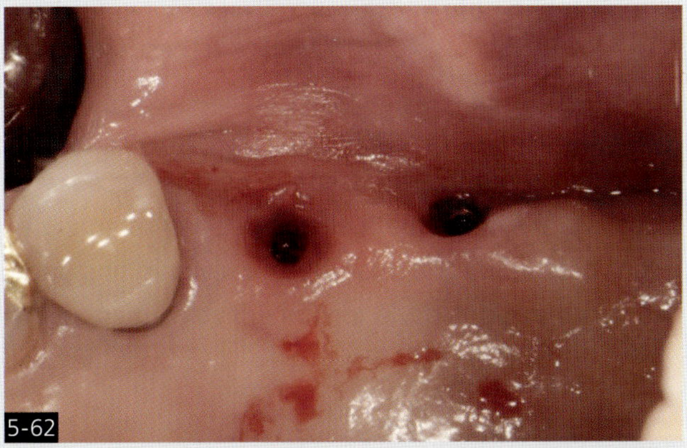

5-62

The implant was placed palatally to allow for the development of gingiva on the buccal side **(Figure 5-61)**. Comparing the clinical photograph taken immediately after the implant fracture **(Figure 5-62)** shows a significant difference.

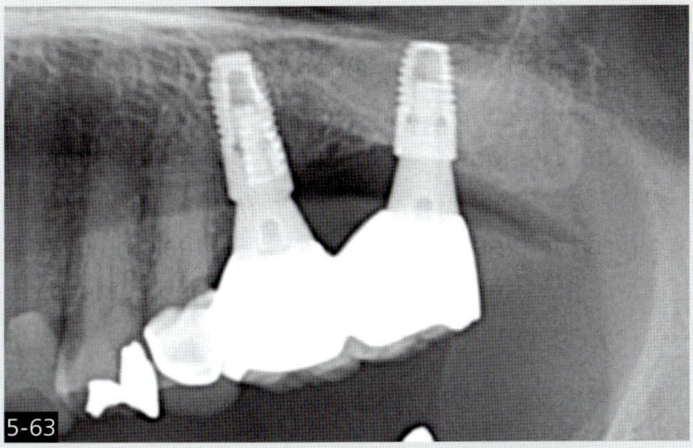

5-63

Radiographically, satisfactory treatment results can be observed. This patient has had no issues five years post-surgery. This clinical case highlights the importance of gingiva in implant surgery and the significance of the type of implant used. I believe that whether an implant fractures or not is greatly influenced by its macroscopic design.

4. Various Clinical Cases of Alveolar Bone Recovery

When there is an alveolar bone defect, most practitioners consider bone grafting alongside implant placement. However, I have consistently emphasized that intraosseous defects can heal spontaneously over time and have presented related clinical cases. I would like to present several cases that demonstrate that such occurrences are not random but can happen consistently.

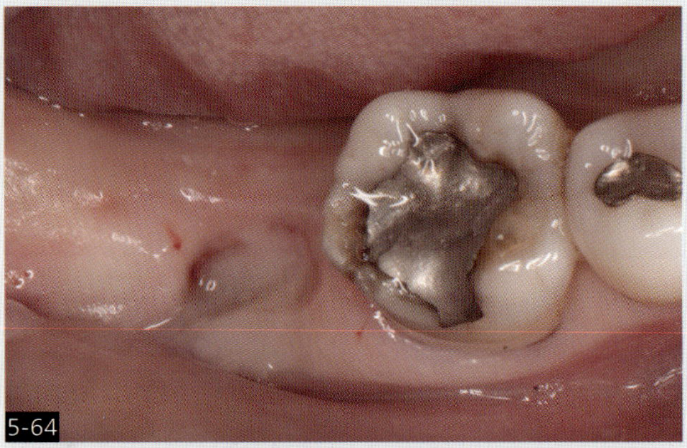

5-64

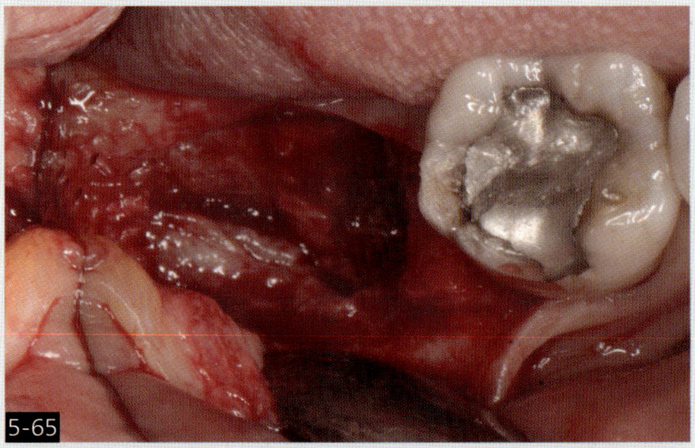

5-65

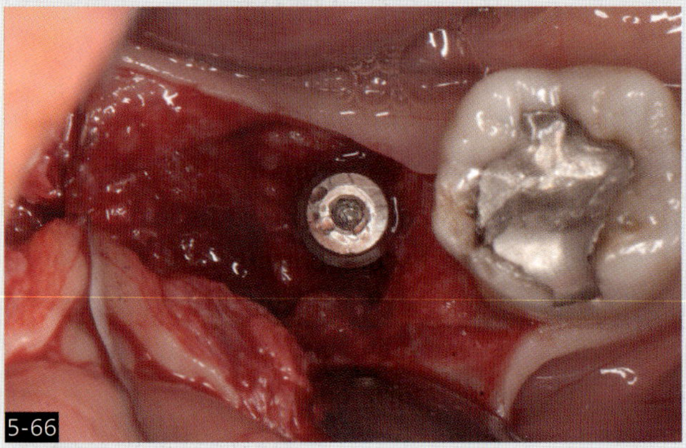

5-66

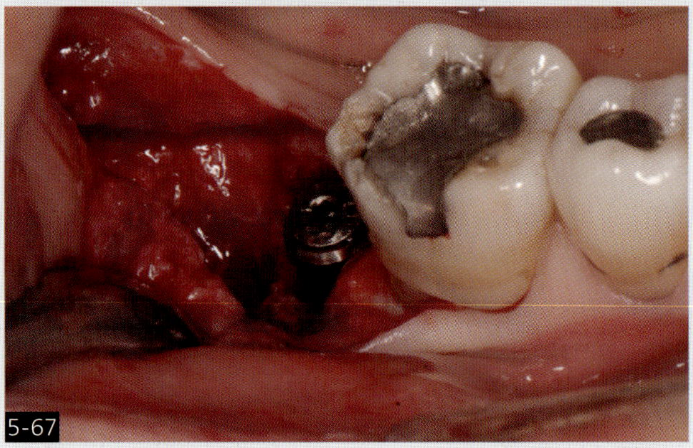

5-67

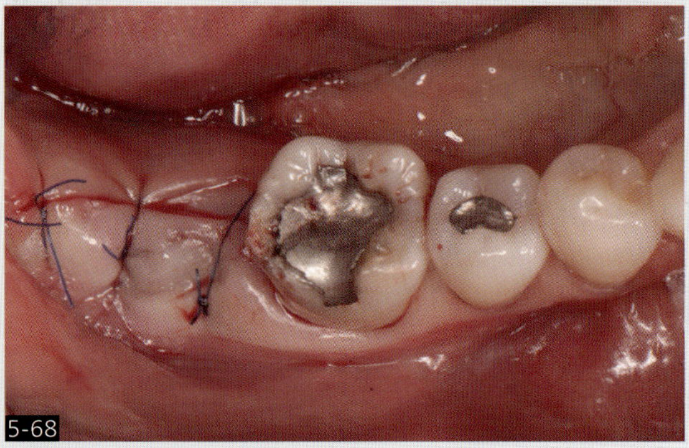

5-68

Approximately two months have passed since the extraction of a tooth due to periodontitis **(Figure 5-64)**. A flap was raised to expose the alveolar bone for implant placement, but the bone defect had not healed at all **(Figure 5-65)**. Even after implant placement, a significant bone defect remained **(Figures 5-66, 67)**. In many cases, dentists tend to perform bone grafting. It is difficult to shake off the notion that the treatment for a bone defect is bone grafting.

There is a principle commonly used in animal experiments known as the critical defect size. This principle states that when creating a circular bone defect using a trephine drill, defects with a diameter of 8 mm or less heal spontaneously, while larger defects do not heal on their own. Given that the diameter of the implant (fixture) is 5 mm, it can be inferred that the defect behind the implant is greater than 5 mm. Despite the presence of a very large bone defect, the area was sutured without bone grafting **(Figure 5-68)**.

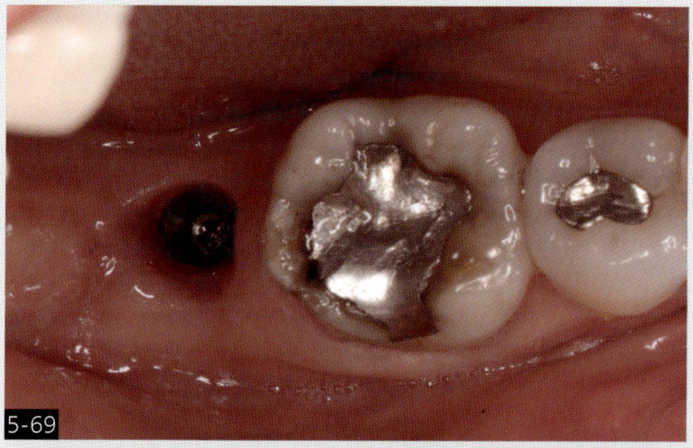
5-69

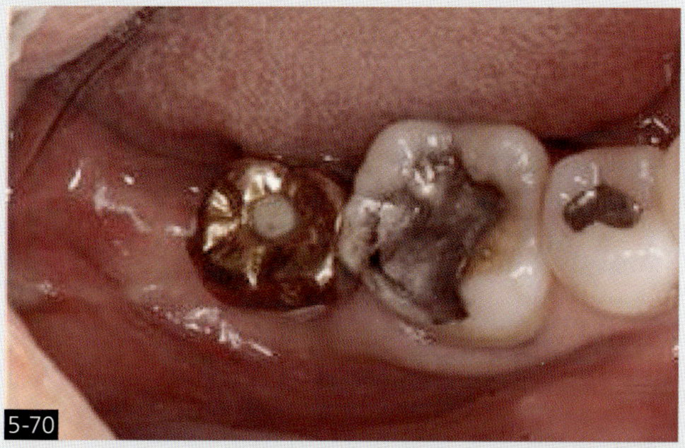
5-70

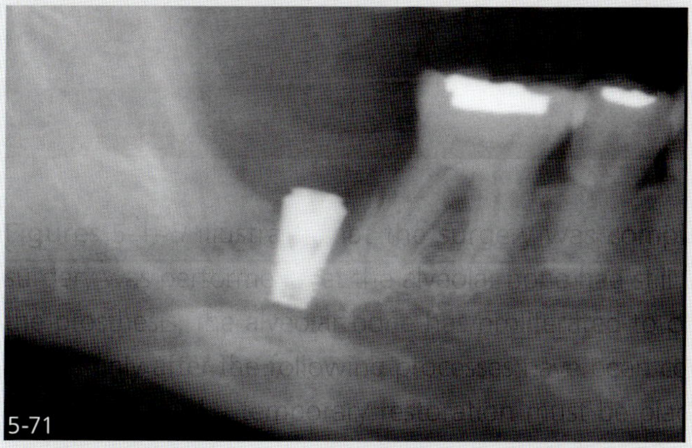
5-71

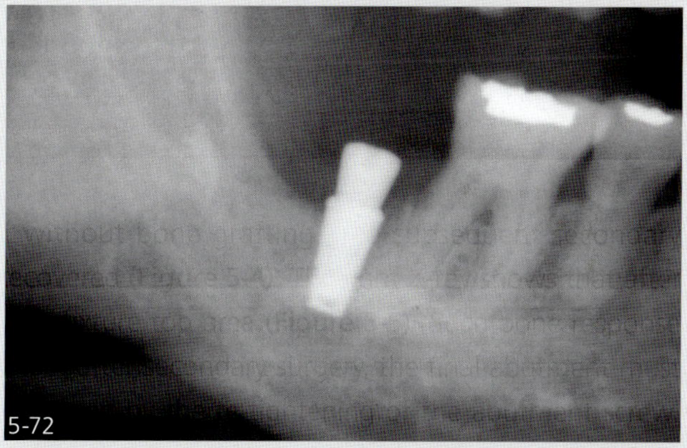
5-72

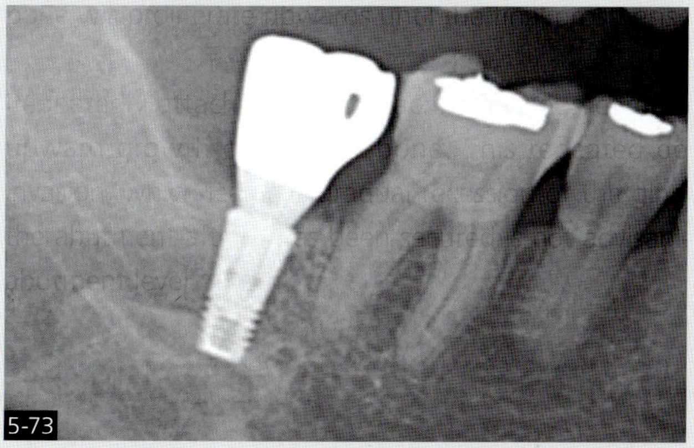
5-73

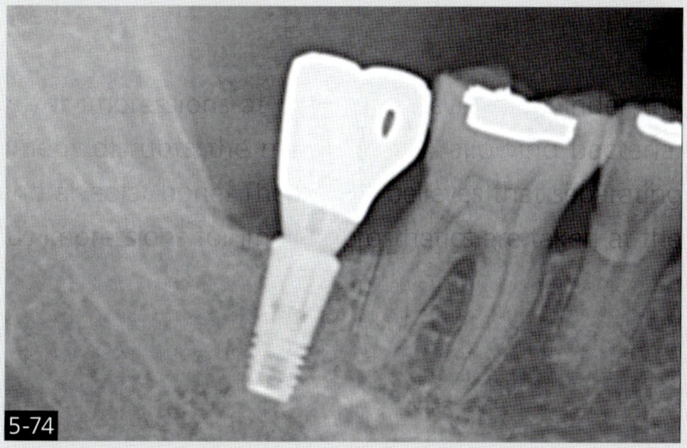
5-74

After the secondary surgery, the prosthetic work was completed **(Figures 5-69, 70)**. **Figure 5-71** shows the condition one week after implant placement, indicating that no graft material was placed in the bone defect. Figure 5-72 shows the condition after the secondary surgery, where the bone defect appears to be partially filled with autogenous bone.

Figure 5-73 shows the condition two years after the completion of the prosthesis, demonstrating that the bone defect has completely healed with autogenous bone. Although there was no alveolar bone grafting, healing occurred successfully. Figure 5-74 shows the condition six years post-prosthesis, where the alveolar bone has risen to the top of the implant. While the appearance may be influenced by the angle of the radiographic image, it is believed that sufficient alveolar bone regeneration has occurred beyond that difference.

I rarely perform bone grafting. However, it is essential to carefully observe the shape of the bone defect. Intrabony defects, or contained defects, which are surrounded by autogenous bone, tend to fill with alveolar bone over time. For clinical success, it is crucial to achieve sufficient stability from below the defect during surgery; otherwise, the implant may become loose and fail under prosthetic load. While there are many considerations and challenges in such clinical cases, I want to emphasize that it is generally more common for the quantity and quality of alveolar bone to increase rather than decrease after implant placement and prosthetic work.

Let's examine another clinical case where alveolar bone fills spontaneously after implant placement. Due to the fracture of the mesial root of tooth #46, significant bone loss occurred. An implant was placed immediately after extraction without bone grafting. The top of the fixture was positioned slightly below the height of the adjacent alveolar bone. In this case, a healing abutment was attached simultaneously with the implant placement. Determining the position of the implant top immediately after extraction is crucial. I believe that it is not always advisable to place the implant too deeply; generally, I estimate the healing state of the alveolar bone after extraction and place the implant about 1 mm deeper than that. If the SLA surface becomes contaminated, that area will not achieve osseointegration, leading to the formation of a periodontal pocket. The formation of a periodontal pocket can result in peri-implantitis, preventing the filling of the defect with autogenous bone. Additionally, after the extraction of a natural tooth, the alveolar ridge tends to undergo slight atrophy. For these two reasons, I prefer to place the top of the fixture slightly below the crestal bone (about 1 mm) during immediate implant placement.

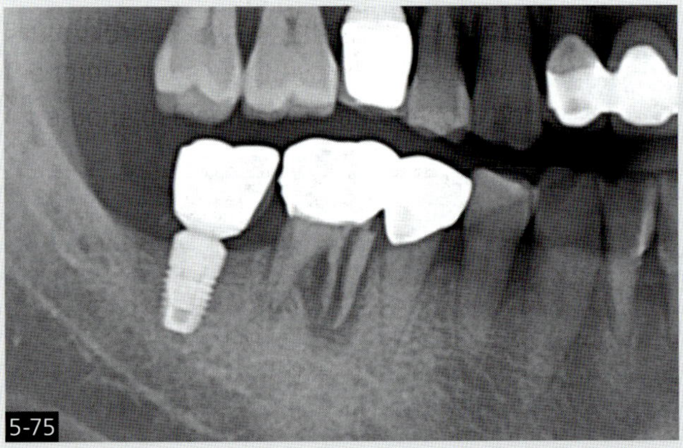

5-75

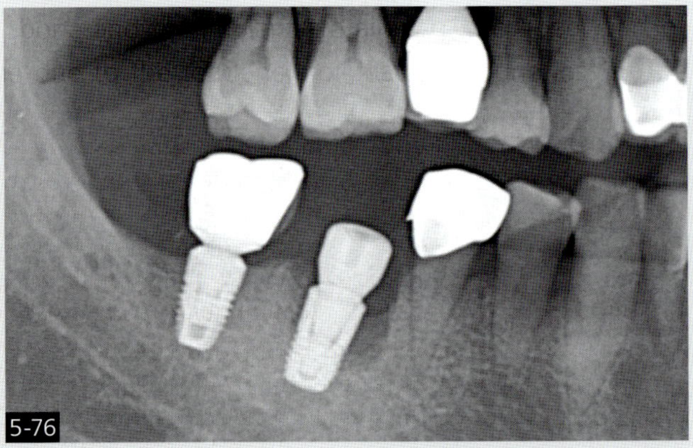

5-76

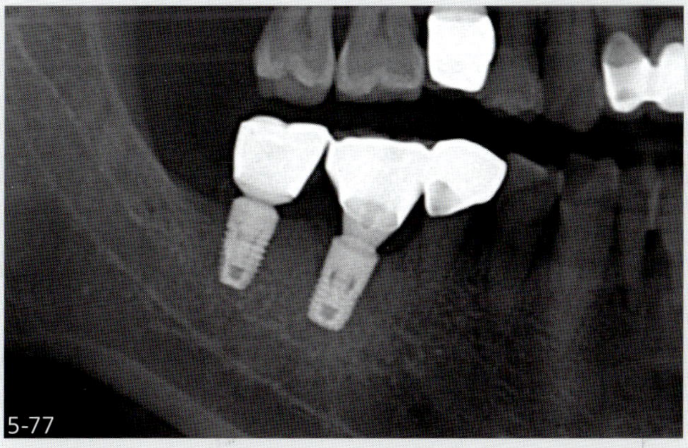

5-77

Figure 5-75 show the bone loss due to the fracture of the mesial root of tooth #46. An implant was placed immediately after extraction (Figure 5-76), and approximately one year later, the alveolar bone had recovered to the level of the fixture top (Figure 5-77).

This has been graphically represented for easier understanding.

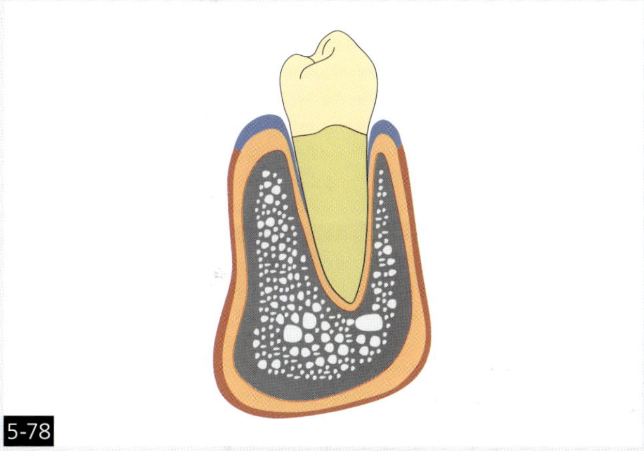

5-78

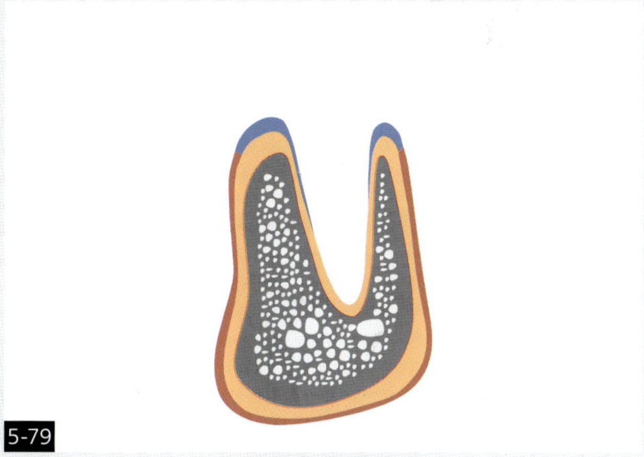

5-79

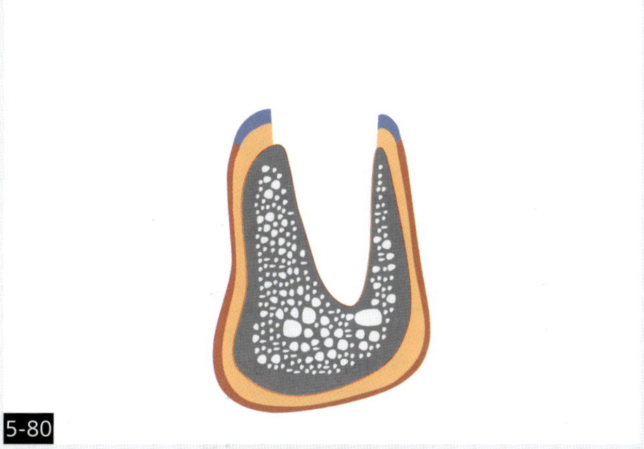

5-80

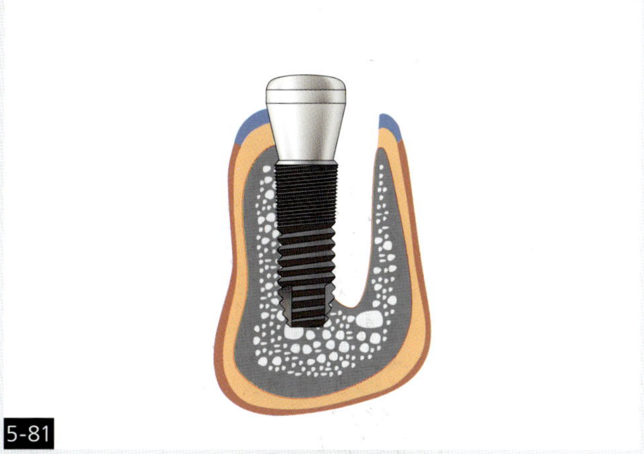

5-81

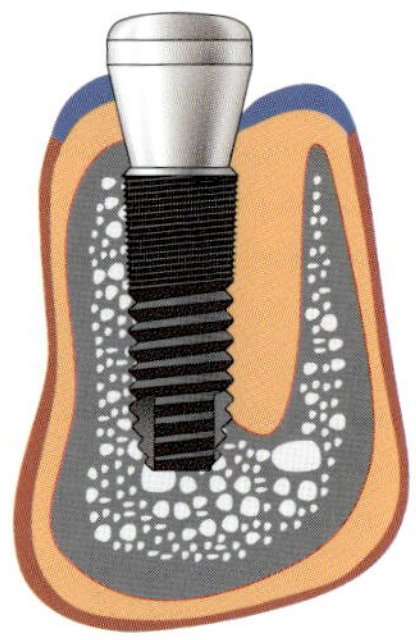

5-82

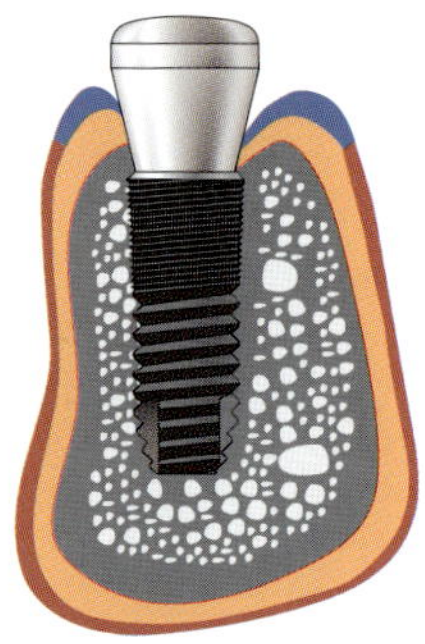

5-83

Severe bone loss is observed due to periodontitis in the natural tooth caused by the fracture of the mesial root **(Figure 5-78)**. After extraction **(Figure 5-79)**, the inflammatory tissue and epithelial tissue forming the periodontal pocket were thoroughly removed **(Figure 5-80)**. An implant was placed, and a healing abutment was attached **(Figure 5-81)**. The epithelial cells adhered to the healing abutment **(Figure 5-82)**, defending against bacterial invasion from the outside, allowing the inflammation within the bone defect to resolve and normal healing to occur **(Figure 5-83)**.

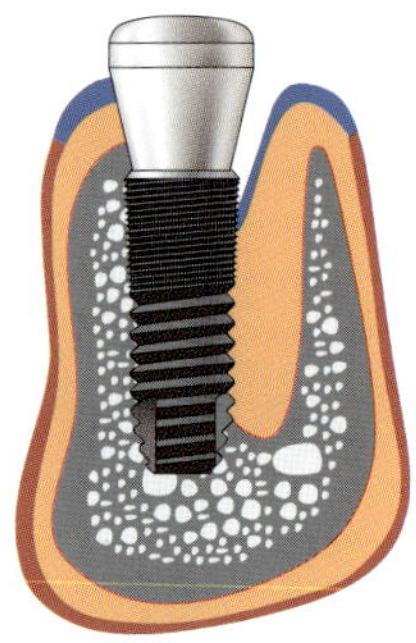

5-84

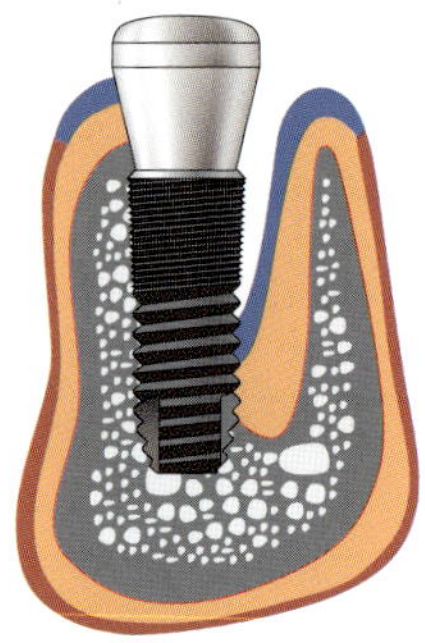

5-85

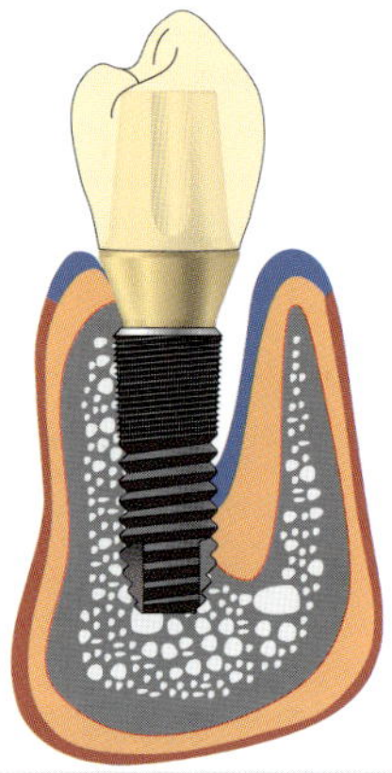

5-86

If the epithelial cells proliferate downward **(Figure 5-84)** or if the SLA implant surface becomes contaminated, the epithelial cells will not attach to the healing abutment. Instead, the epithelium will proliferate downward, causing the SLA surface of the implant to be located within the periodontal pocket, which can deepen enough to create peri-implantitis **(Figure 5-85)**. The alveolar bone will also fail to achieve osseointegration with the contaminated implant surface, retreating a certain distance. As a result, it may appear that nothing has happened, but an environment conducive to peri-implantitis has already been established since the implant placement stage **(Figure 5-86)**.

It is crucial to manage the inflammatory and epithelial tissues when natural teeth are affected by periodontitis. Sometimes, it may be impossible or uncertain to achieve a clean excision of these soft tissues. In such cases, it is advantageous to delay implant placement after extraction, as described below.

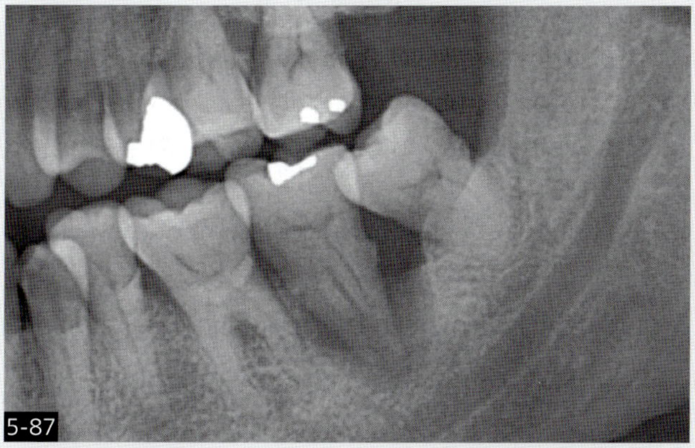

5-87

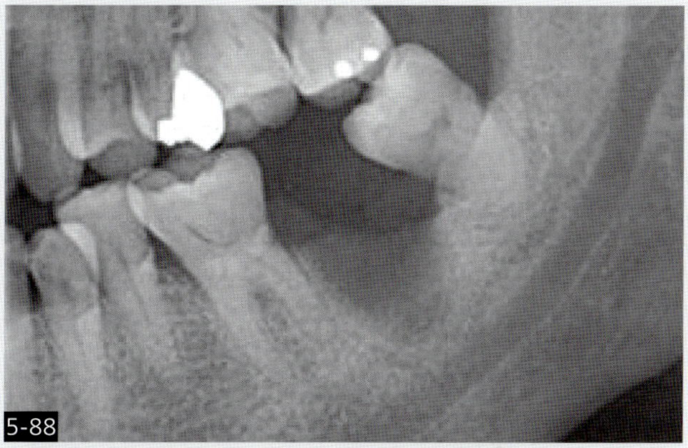

5-88

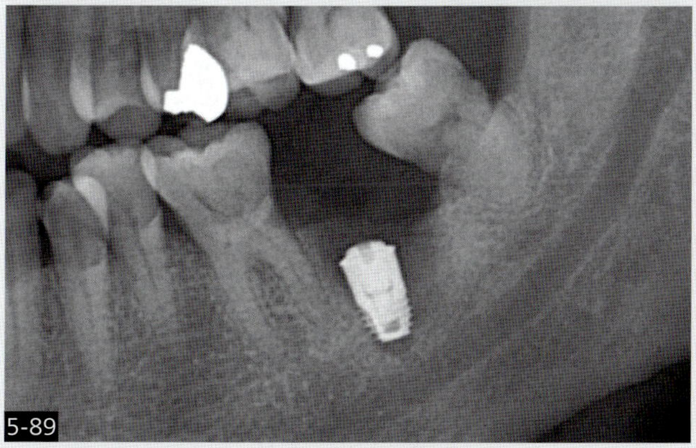

5-89

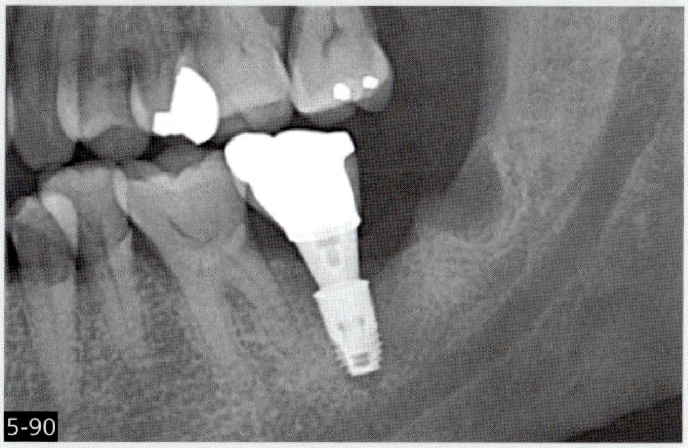

5-90

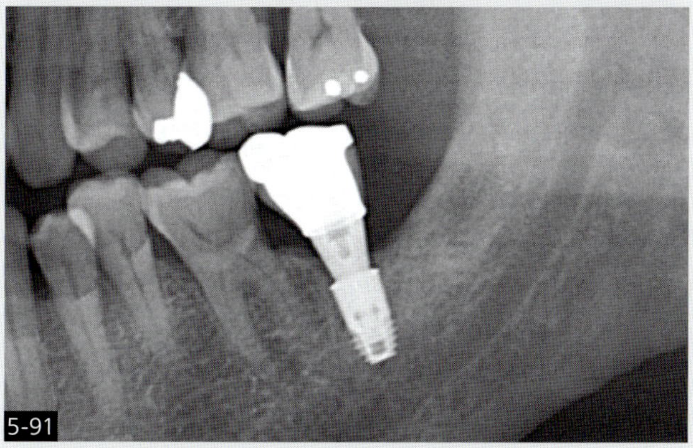

5-91

Severe alveolar bone loss and deep periodontal pockets were observed due to periodontitis in a natural tooth **(Figures 5-87, 88)**. Due to the difficulty in managing the soft tissues after extraction and the challenge of achieving initial stability at the root apex, delayed implant placement was performed two months after extraction **(Figure 5-89)**. Three months after placement, the prosthetic treatment was completed **(Figure 5-90)**, and approximately 2.5 years later, the alveolar bone had healed almost perfectly **(Figure 5-91)**. This clinical case serves as a reminder that when epithelial cell attachment and mucosal seal are formed on the abutment, the underlying alveolar bone heals completely.

Let's explore another case to understand how this surgical concept facilitates alveolar bone healing.

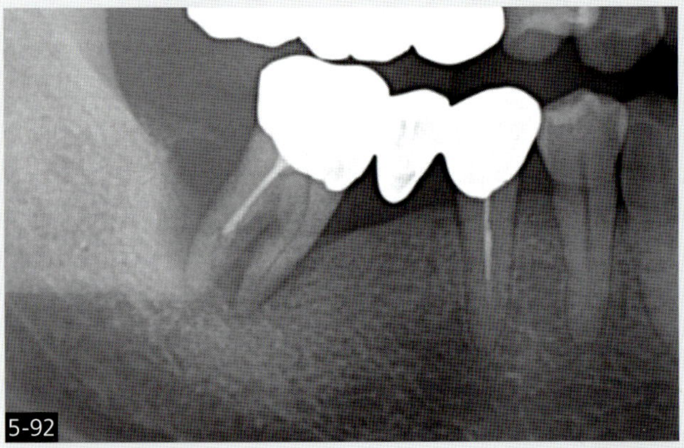

5-92

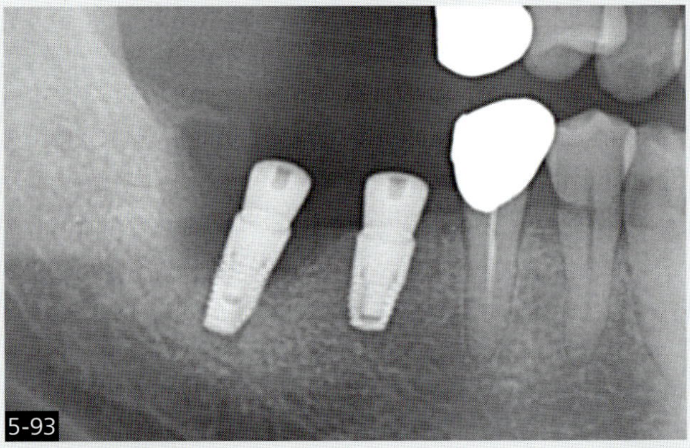

5-93

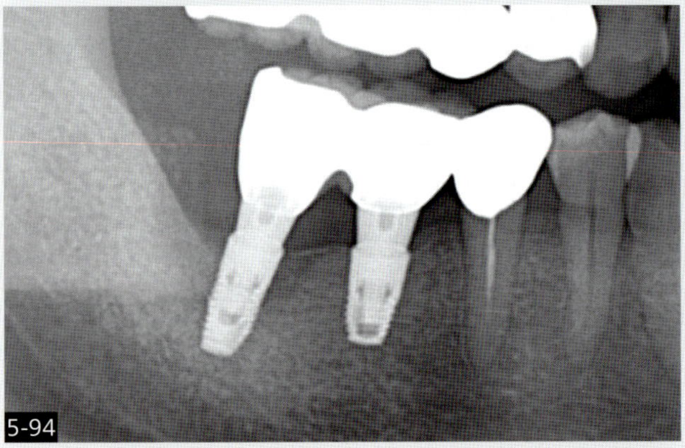

5-94

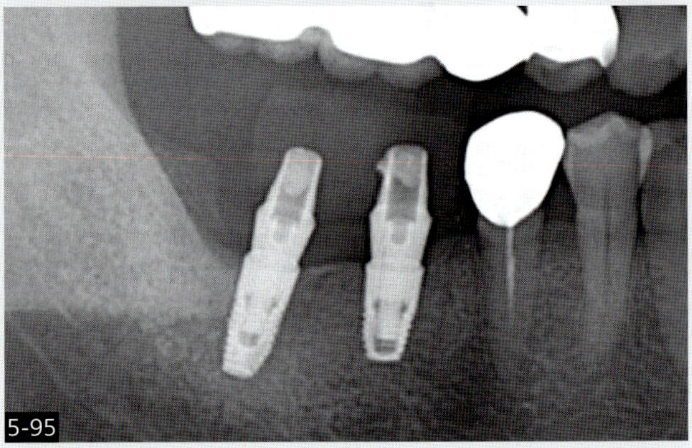

5-95

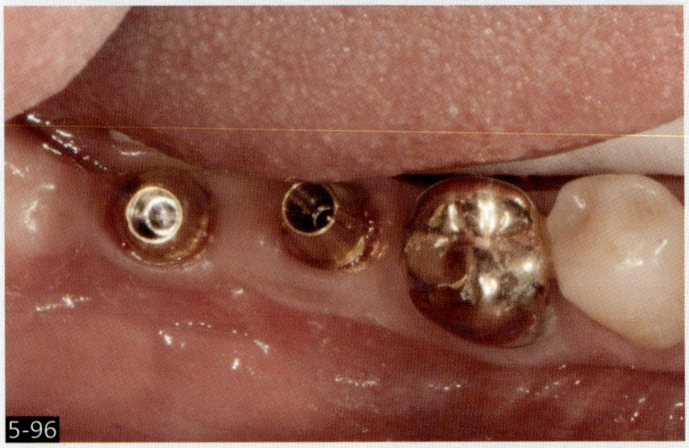

5-96

Due to severe periodontitis in tooth #47, implants were placed in the areas of teeth #46 and #47 after extraction **(Figures 5-92, 93)**. By the time the prosthetic work was completed, significant healing of the alveolar bone had occurred, although it was not complete **(Figure 5-94)**. **Figure 5-95** shows the condition about 1.5 years post-surgery, where the alveolar bone has nearly healed. This demonstrates that autogenous bone can heal without bone grafting, as the surgical technique allowed for epithelial cell attachment to the healing abutment rather than the implant itself.

Let's examine a few more cases where the quantity and quality of alveolar bone increased.

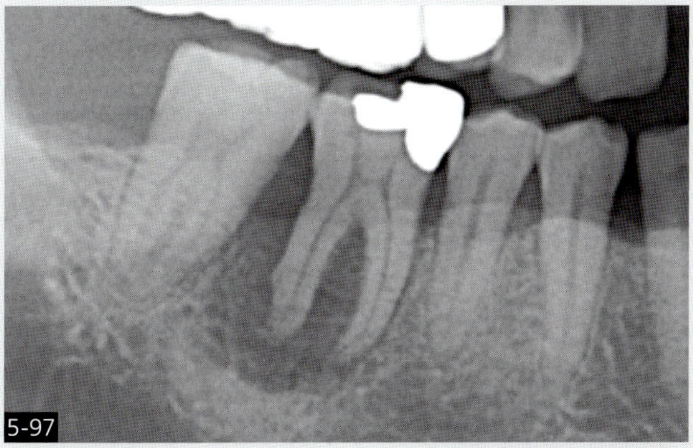
5-97

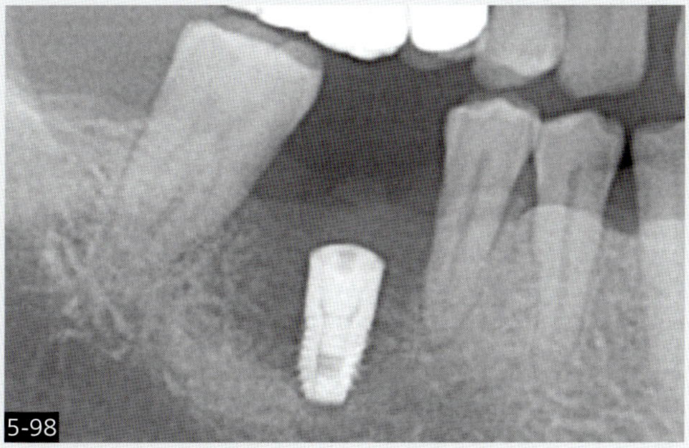
5-98

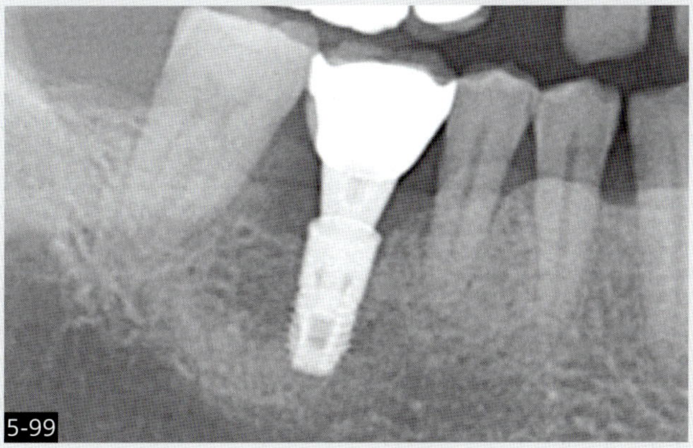
5-99

Tooth #46, which had periodontitis, was extracted **(Figure 5-97)**, and an implant was placed two months later **(Figure 5-98)**. Approximately one year after the implant prosthesis was placed, the quantity and quality of the alveolar bone had increased **(Figure 5-99)**.

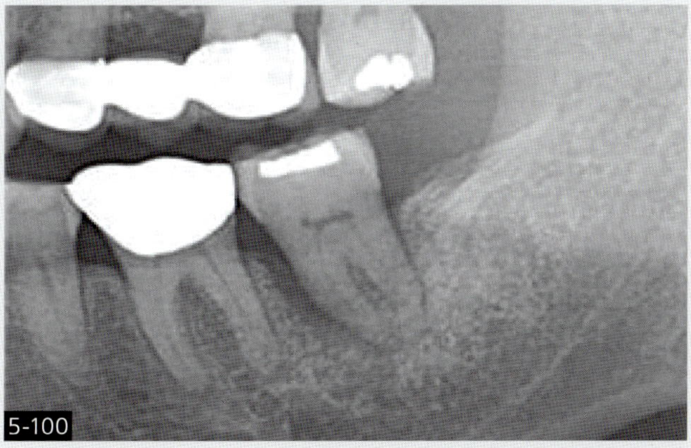
5-100

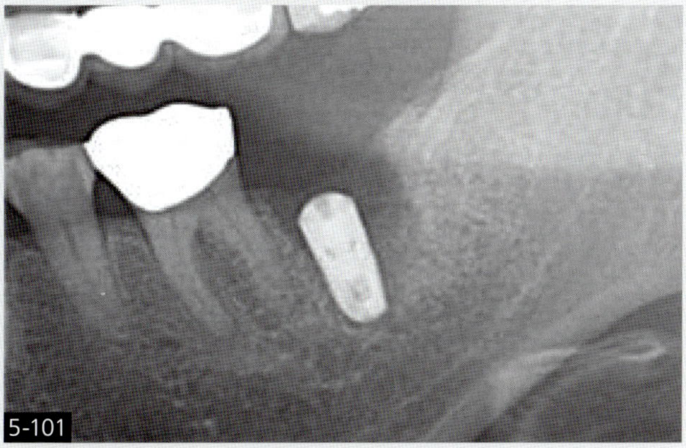
5-101

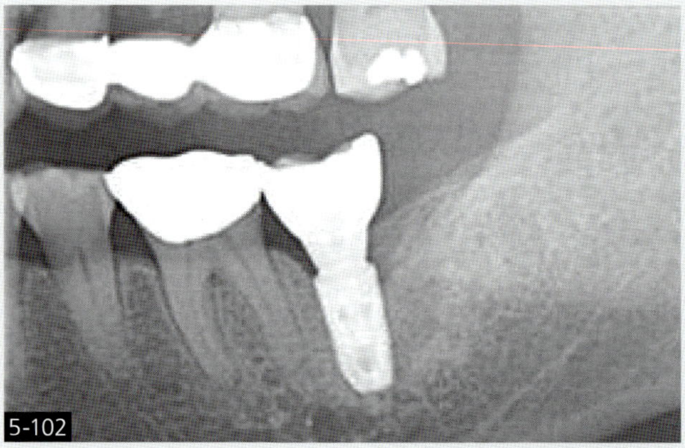

5-102

Tooth #37 was extracted due to periodontitis **(Figure 5-100)**. An implant was placed two months after extraction **(Figure 5-101)**, and about 1.5 years post-placement, the alveolar bone had healed almost perfectly **(Figure 5-102)**.

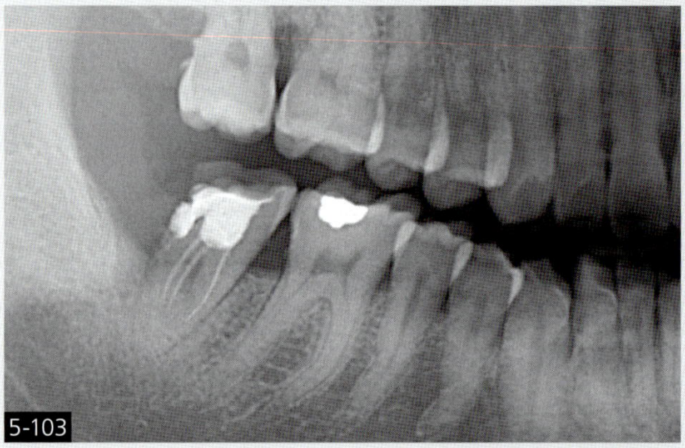

5-103

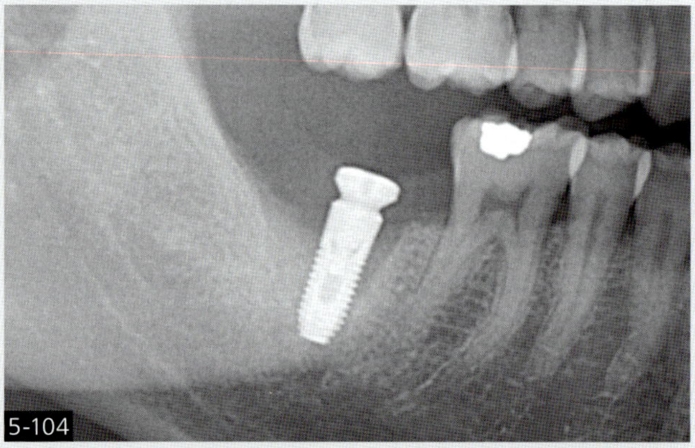

5-104

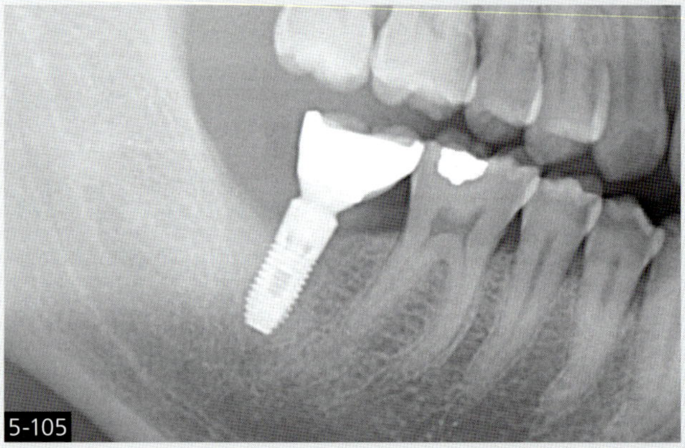

5-105

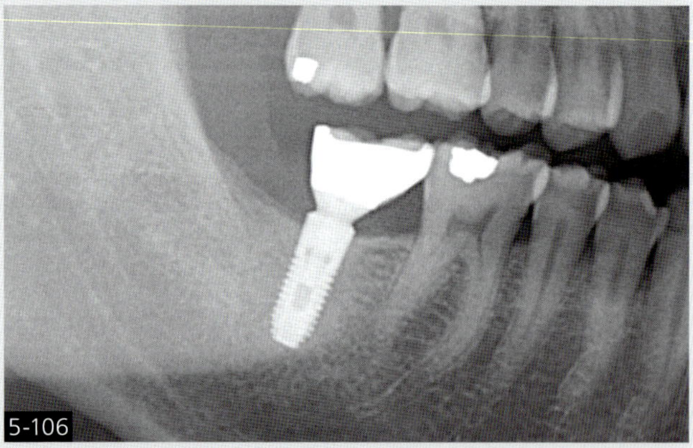

5-106

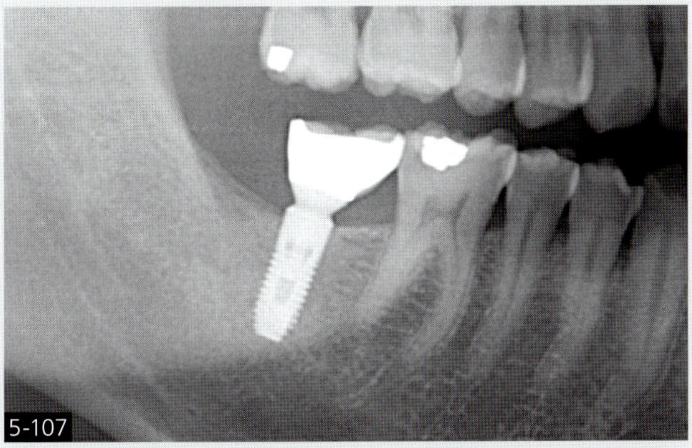

5-107

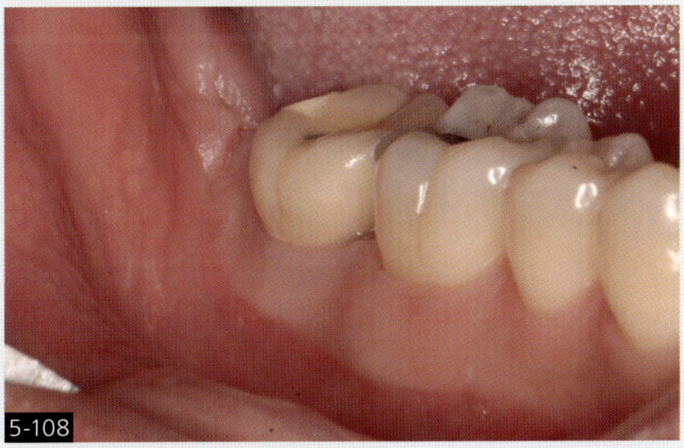

5-108

Tooth #47 had severe caries, and an implant was placed immediately after extraction **(Figures 5-103, 104)**. The fixture top was positioned too high, leading to concerns about prognosis. A high position increases the likelihood of surface contamination, which can later result in peri-implantitis **(Figure 5-104)**. However, one year after the prosthesis was placed **(Figure 5-105)**, the quantity of alveolar bone had increased **(Figure 5-106)**. After five years, the amount of alveolar bone had nearly reached the fixture top **(Figure 5-107)**, and clinically, there were no issues **(Figure 5-108)**. This is an astonishing case where the healing of the alveolar bone exceeded my expectations.

Response of Alveolar Bone After Implant Prosthesis

_ Abutment and Prosthesis

Chapter 6

1. Gold Abutment

Typically, when there is an alveolar bone deficiency, bone grafting is performed. However, I have demonstrated through numerous cases that alveolar bone can regenerate without bone grafting. The presentation of many cases is intended to convey that this phenomenon is not merely coincidental. As previously explained, this regeneration occurs when there is consideration for epithelial cell attachment and mucosal sealing. Additionally, it is crucial not to repeatedly insert and remove the abutment during prosthetic procedures. The attachment of epithelial cells to the abutment is essential to prevent bacterial invasion, allowing the underlying alveolar bone to heal normally. Occasionally, abutments made from materials that do not promote epithelial cell attachment are used, leading to peri-implantitis. Let us explore this further.

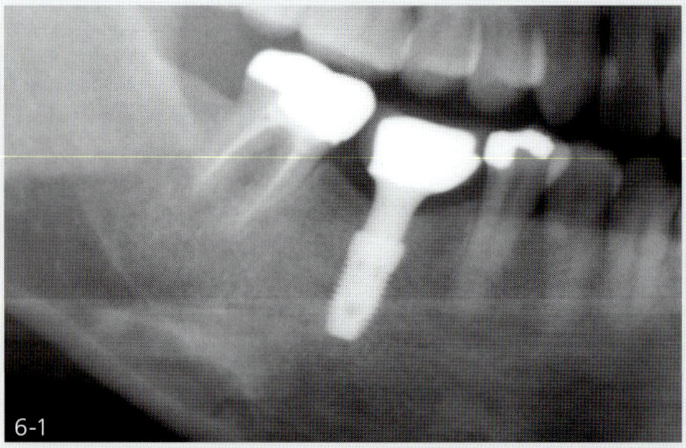

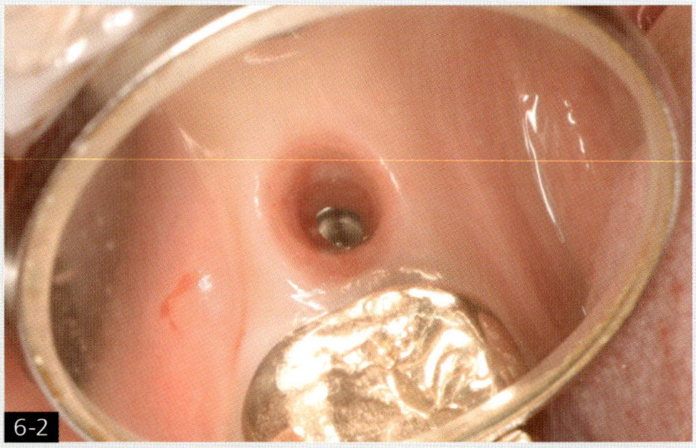

After extracting tooth number 46, an immediate implant was placed. The fixture top was positioned too deeply, resulting in direct contact between the abutment and the alveolar bone after six years **(Figures 6-1, 2)**. When the abutment is made from materials such as titanium, alumina, or zirconia that allow for osseointegration, both osseointegration and epithelial cell attachment occur, preventing harm to the underlying alveolar bone. In other words, because the abutment at the top of the implant prevents bacterial invasion, the alveolar bone can maintain its health.

Let us examine the issues that arise periodontally when materials that do not allow for epithelial cell attachment are used.

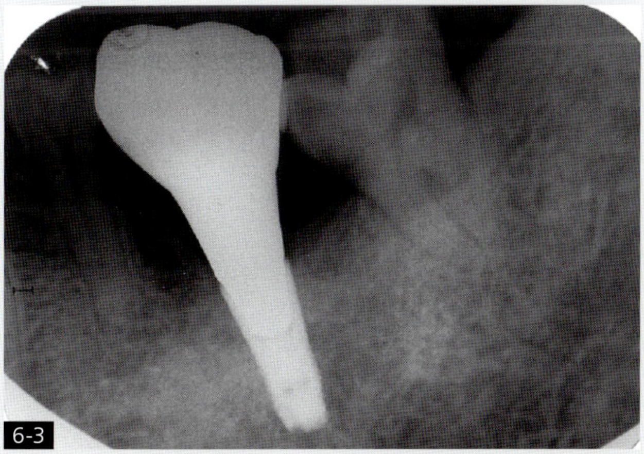
6-3

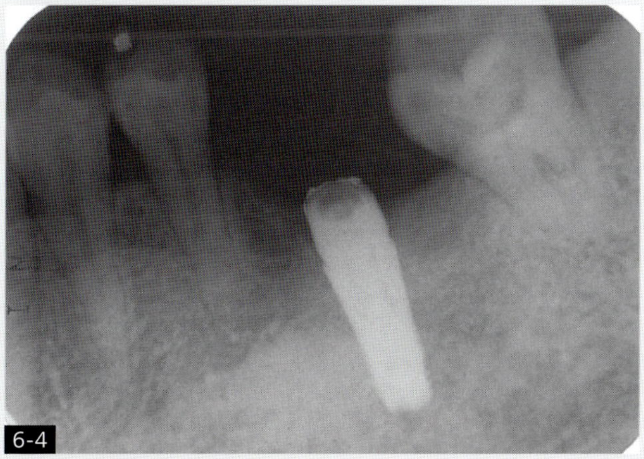
6-4

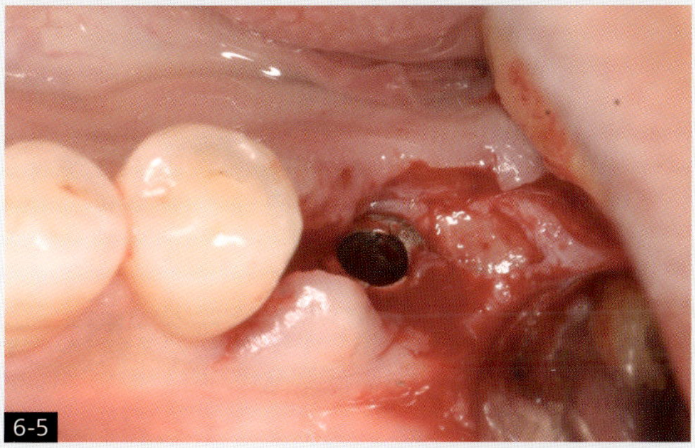
6-5

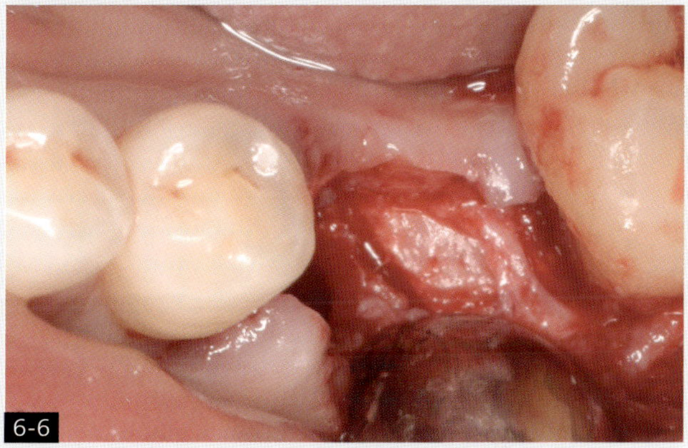
6-6

An incident occurred where the abutment of implant number 36 fractured **(Figures 6-3, 4)**. The implant was placed immediately after extraction, and the fixture top was positioned deeply. It was initially thought that the fractured abutment could be easily removed, but unexpectedly, this was not the case. Consequently, the flap had to be elevated to facilitate removal **(Figures 6-5, 6)**. Due to the lack of movement of the abutment, the boundary between the abutment and the alveolar bone was resected, allowing for the removal of the fractured abutment. Upon probing the alveolar bone, it was found that there was direct bone contact without any soft tissue interposition between the abutment and the alveolar bone **(Figure 6-6)**.

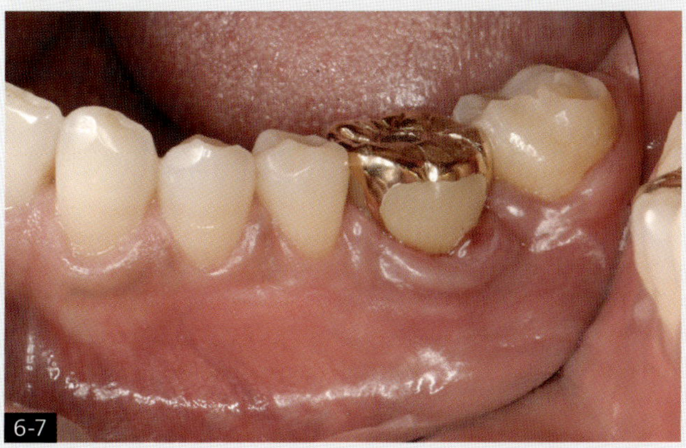
6-7

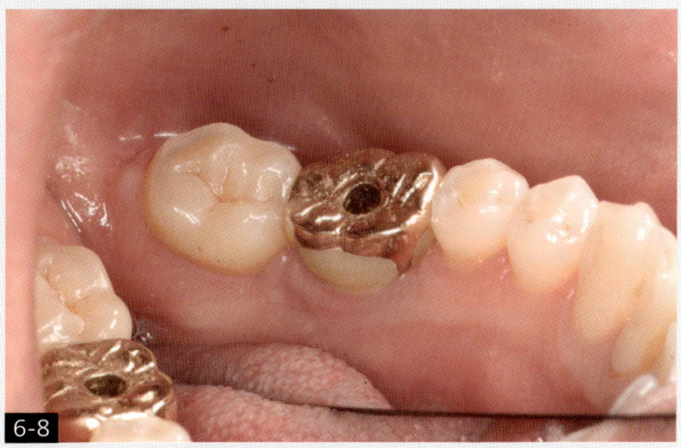
6-8

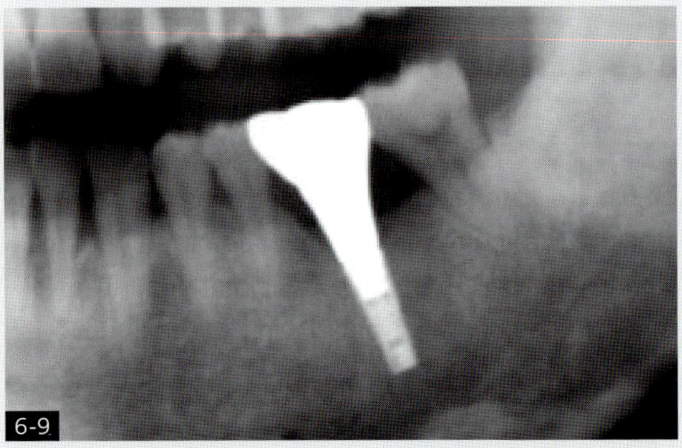

6-9

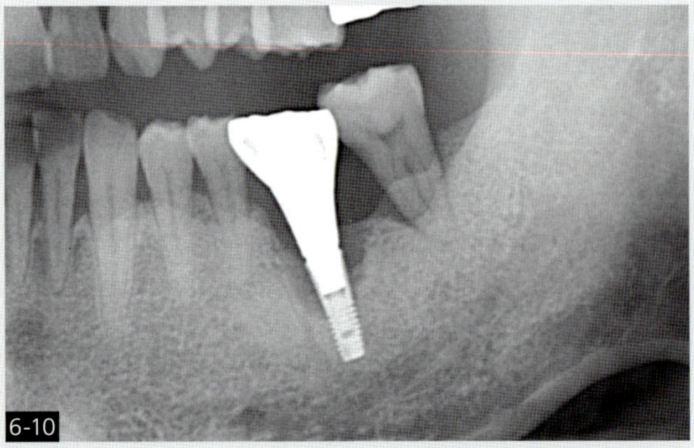

6-10

At the time of re-prosthetic treatment, the implant was positioned too deeply, making it difficult to find an appropriate abutment. Due to the lack of a long gingival height abutment, a Gold UCLA abutment was used. Subsequently, inflammation of the gingiva occurred **(Figures 6-7, 8)**, and signs of alveolar bone loss began to appear **(Figures 6-9, 10)**. Initially, there was slight marginal bone loss after using the Gold abutment, but soon significant resorption of the alveolar bone above the implant was observed.

This is attributed to the fact that the material Gold does not allow for epithelial cell attachment, preventing the formation of a mucosal seal, which leads to the deepening of the periodontal pocket. Within this deep periodontal pocket, pathogenic bacteria proliferate, resulting in peri-implantitis. To ensure the long-term prognosis of implant treatment, it is evident that abutments made from materials that do not promote epithelial attachment should not be used for deeply placed implants.

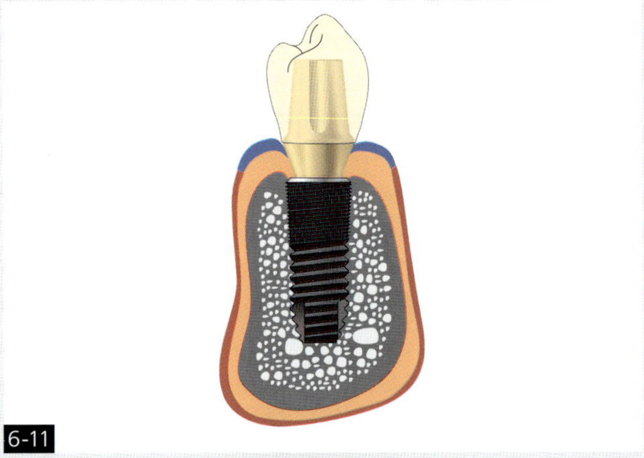

6-11

Titanium abutment

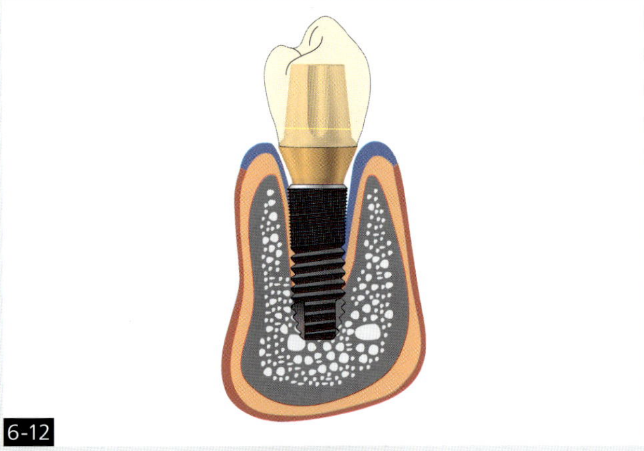

6-12

Gold abutment

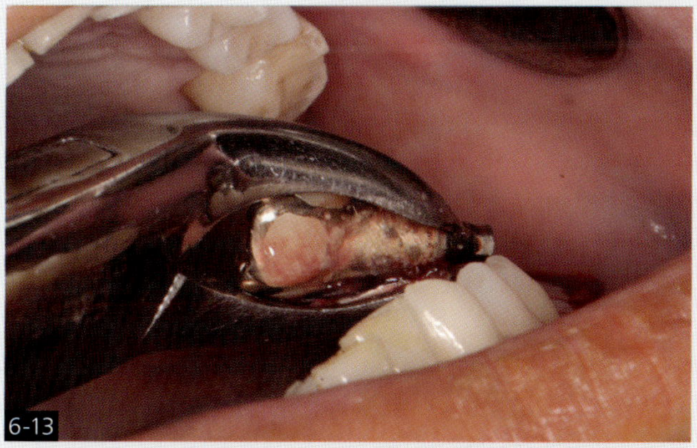
6-13

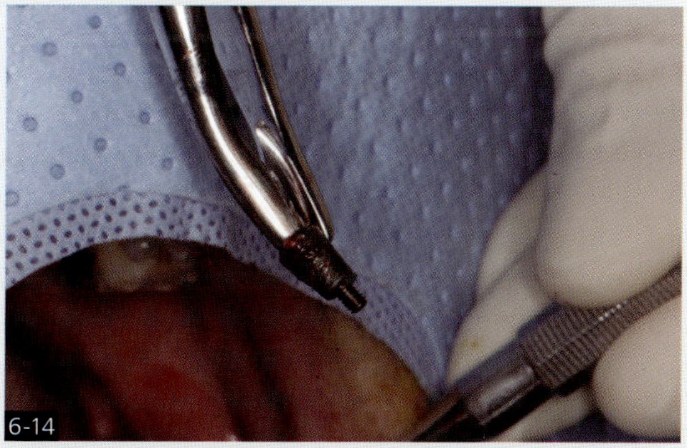
6-14

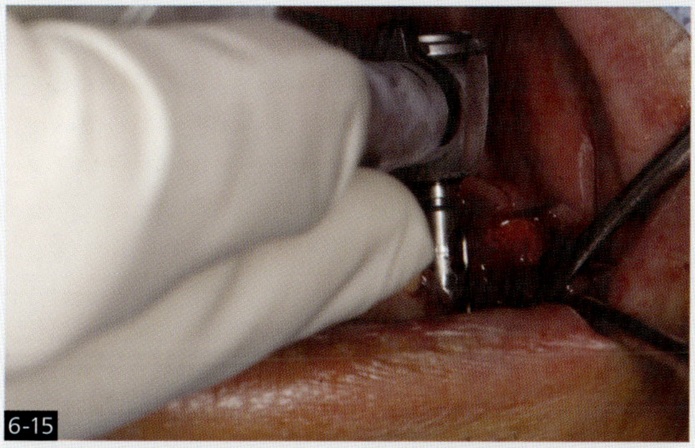
6-15

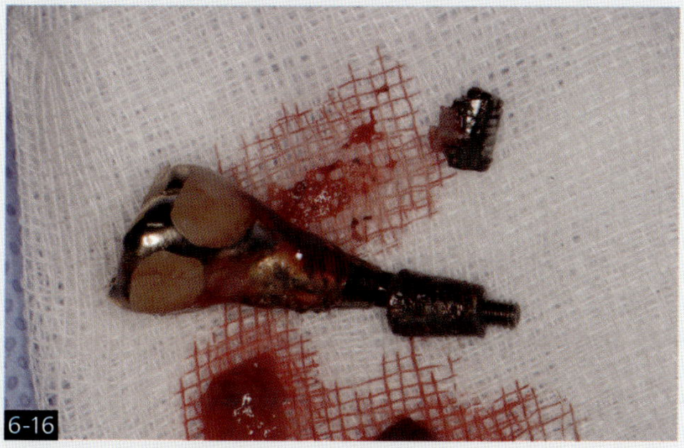
6-16

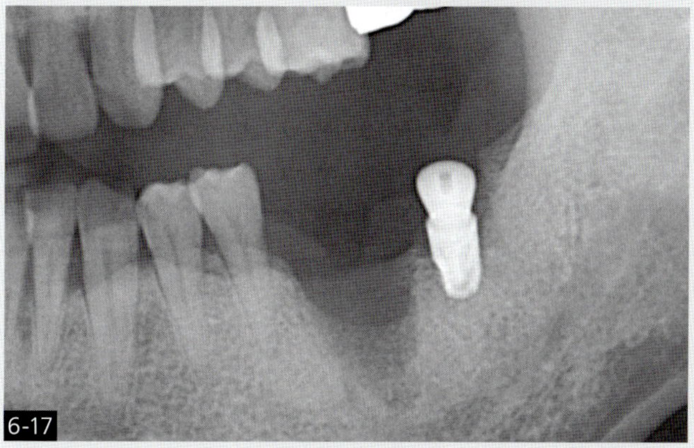
6-17

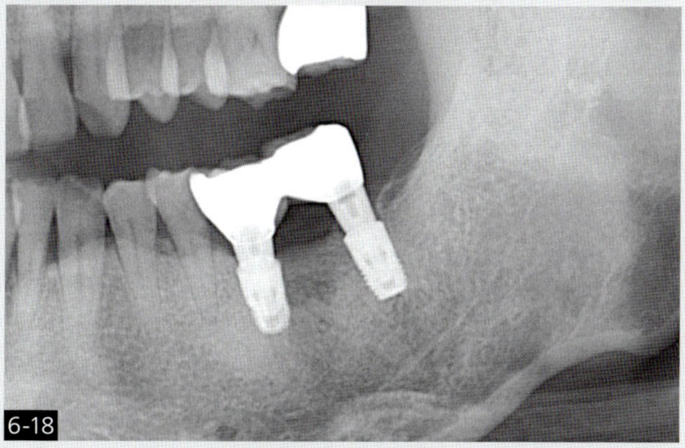
6-18

Ultimately, along with alveolar bone loss, the implant fractured **(Figures 6-13, 14)**. After removing the upper portion, the broken lower part was extracted using a trephine drill **(Figures 6-15, 16)**.

While removing implant number 36, an implant was placed in position 37. Due to the excessive bone deficiency at position 36, the decision was made to forgo implant placement and allow for further recovery of the alveolar bone. After the alveolar bone had recovered, a new implant was placed, concluding the treatment **(Figures 6-17, 18)**.

2. Margins of Prostheses

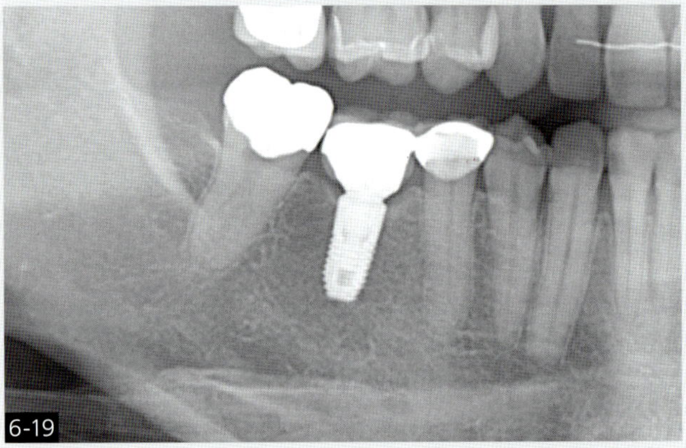
6-19

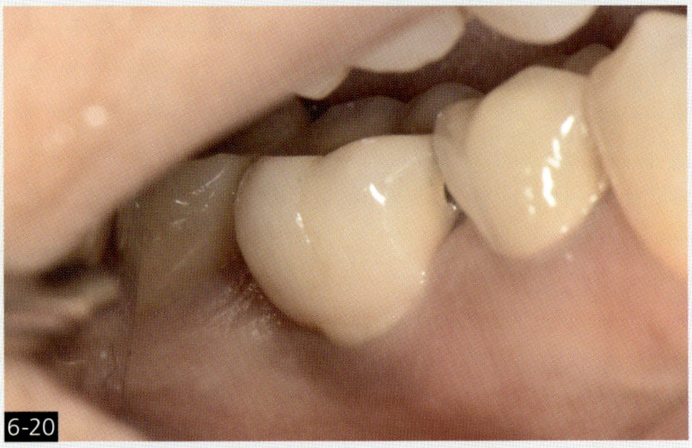
6-20

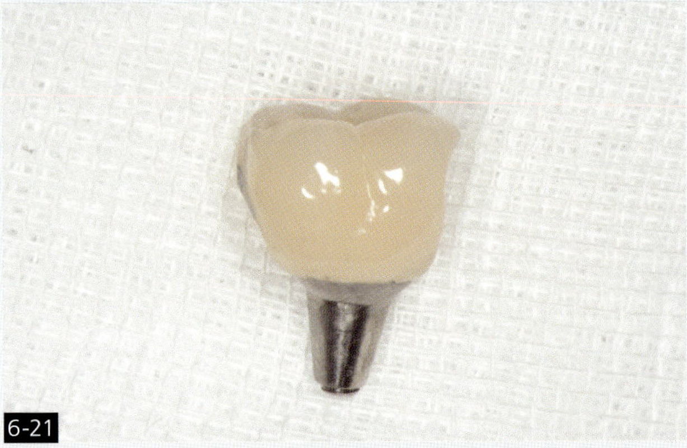
6-21

Approximately seven years after the placement of implant number 46, there was evidence of drainage on the buccal side of the implant **(Figure 6-20)**. Radiographic examination did not reveal any significant abnormalities **(Figure 6-19)**.

Given the possibility of residual adhesive remaining during the attachment of the prosthesis, both the prosthesis and the abutment were removed simultaneously, but no residual adhesive was found, and the area was clean **(Figure 6-21)**. After disinfecting and reattaching the prosthesis, a follow-up one week later showed continued drainage. It was determined that the margin of the prosthesis was positioned too subgingivally, leading to this issue, prompting a decision to replace the abutment with one that had a higher gingival height.

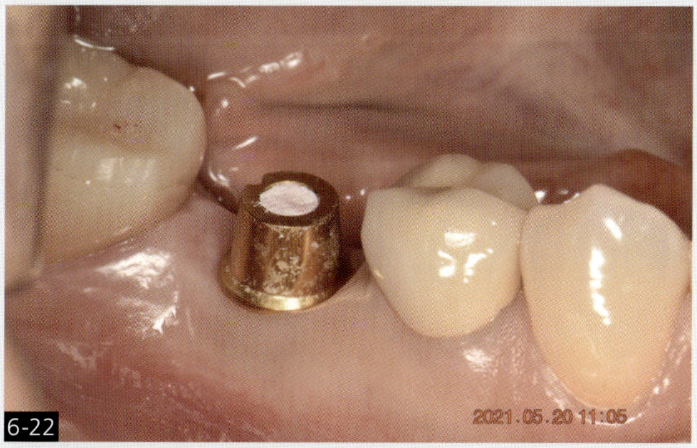

6-22

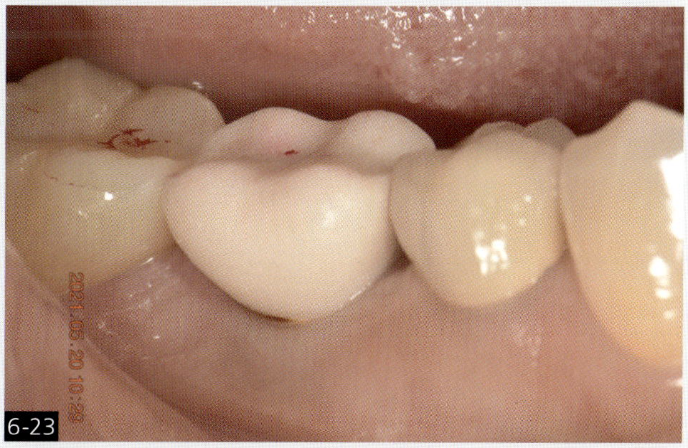
6-23

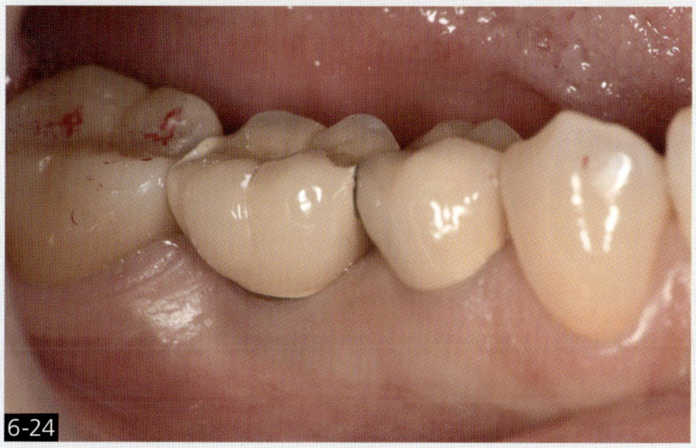
6-24

The abutment was changed from a subgingival margin to a supragingival margin **(Figure 6-22)**, and after placing a temporary crown, the situation was reassessed one week later. No further drainage was observed on the buccal side **(Figure 6-23)**. It was concluded that the problem was resolved, and the final prosthesis was completed **(Figure 6-24)**. This clinical case illustrates that using a gold abutment or placing the margin of the prosthesis too deeply subgingivally can lead to periodontal issues around the implant.

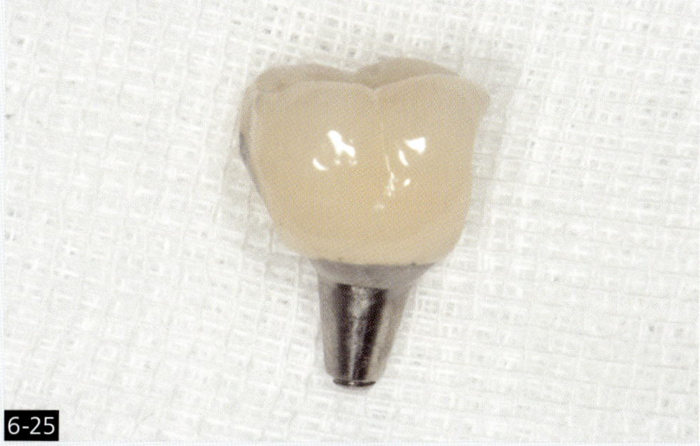
6-25

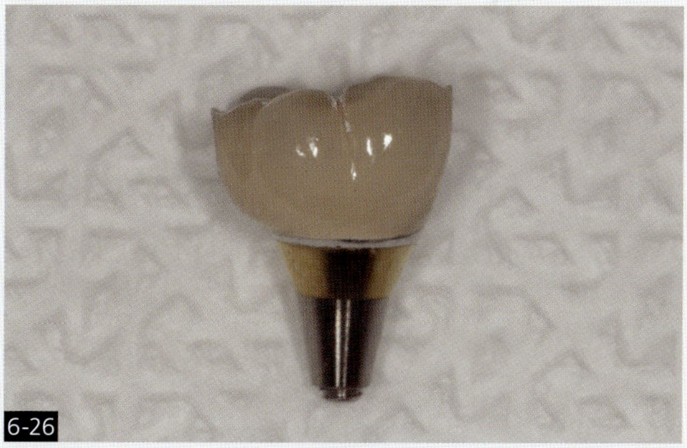
6-26

A clear difference in gingival height can be observed between the original abutment **(Figure 6-25)** and the newly placed abutment **(Figure 6-26)**. In selecting an abutment, it is fundamentally recommended that the margin be set above the gingival level, and only in unavoidable cases, such as when aesthetics are crucial or when adjusting the emergence profile, should the margin be placed subgingivally.

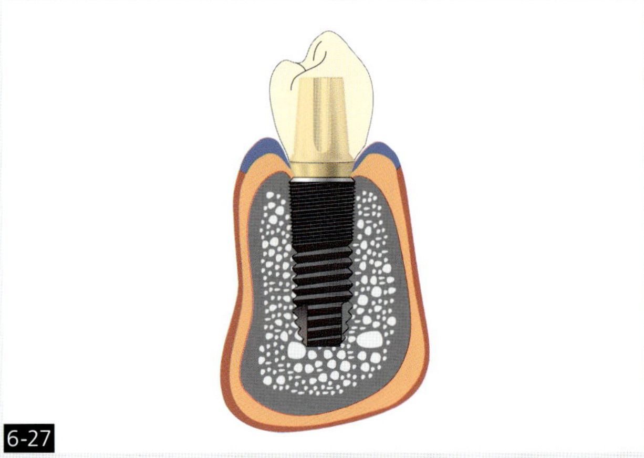

6-27

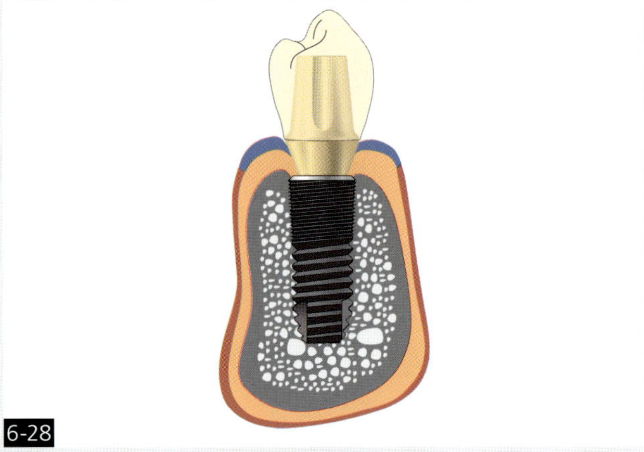

6-28

It is known that after implant placement, alveolar bone is lost annually due to bacterial invasion in the oral cavity. However, I argue that there is an increase in bone over the years. It has been established by researchers that in natural teeth, the alveolar bone recedes a certain distance from aggressive factors like calculus, which is referred to as biological width.

This concept also exists in implants, where the micro-gap between the fixture and abutment acts as an aggressive factor over time. However, this theory does not explain the phenomenon of bone increase up to the abutment. Let us consider what factors contribute to the loss of alveolar bone in implants. I believe that the margin of the prosthesis is one of these aggressive factors. In other words, I propose that the alveolar bone recedes a certain distance from the margin of the prosthesis. The following case will illustrate this point.

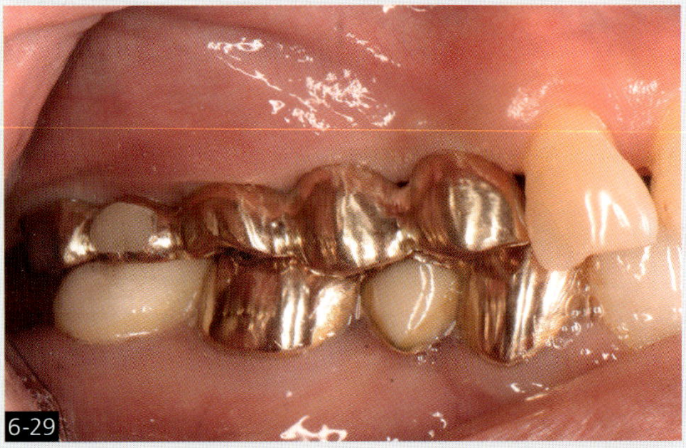

6-29

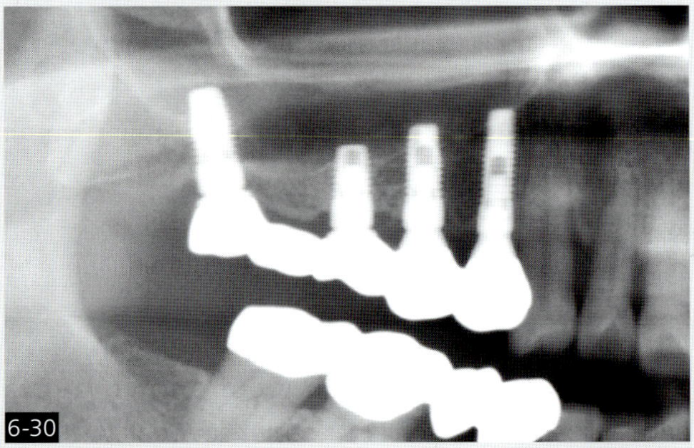

6-30

After the completion of prosthetic treatment **(Figure 6-29)**, radiographic findings ten years later showed no loss of alveolar bone in the premolar region, while some marginal bone loss was observed in the molar region **(Figure 6-30)**.

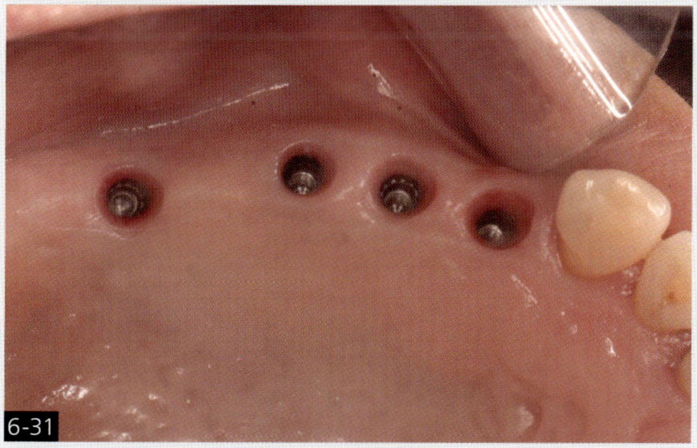

6-31

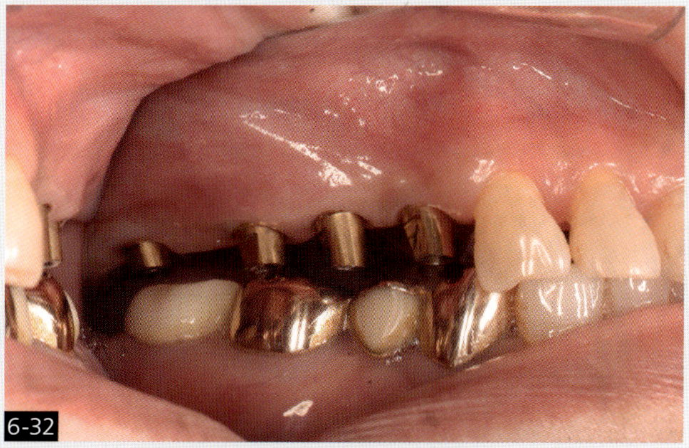

6-32

The condition during prosthetic treatment over twenty years ago is shown **(Figures 6-31, 32)**. It can be seen that there was insufficient occlusal height with the opposing tooth in the molar region. Therefore, a subgingival margin was established for the molar region, while a supragingival margin was set for the premolar region. Since epithelial cell attachment does not occur on the prosthesis, placing the margin subgingivally leads to the formation of periodontal pockets, allowing bacterial invasion, which causes the alveolar bone to recede a certain distance from this margin.

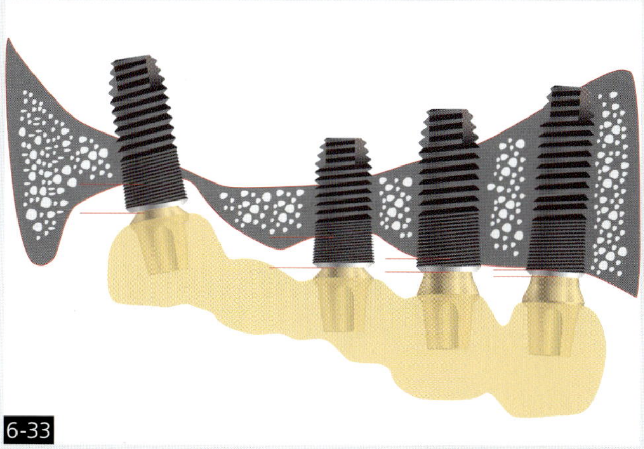

6-33

The distance between the alveolar bone and the connection is not constant

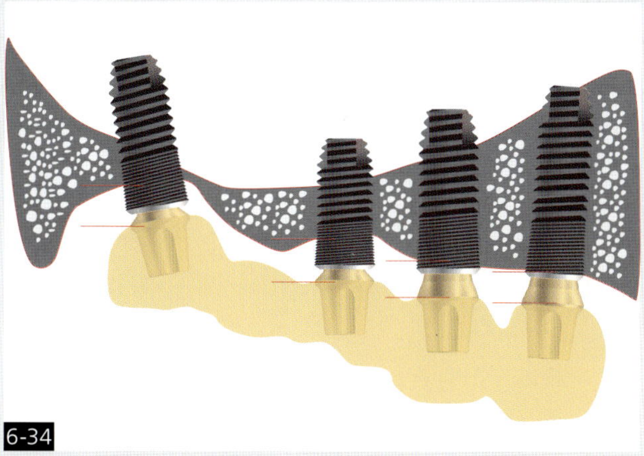

6-34

The distance between the alveolar bone and the margin of the prosthesis remains consistent.

Chapter 7

Causes of Peri-implant Marginal Bone Loss
_ Micro-gap vs. Micro-mobility

1. Micro-gap vs Micro-mobility

The loss of alveolar bone around implants has traditionally been attributed to bacteria, particularly those residing at the fixture-abutment connection, which are believed to contribute to bone destruction. However, there are claims and studies suggesting that such gaps and the bacteria within them may not be direct causes of bone resorption. Therefore, it is essential to consider whether we should focus on micro-gaps or micro-mobility in order to ensure the long-term prognosis of implants in clinical practice.

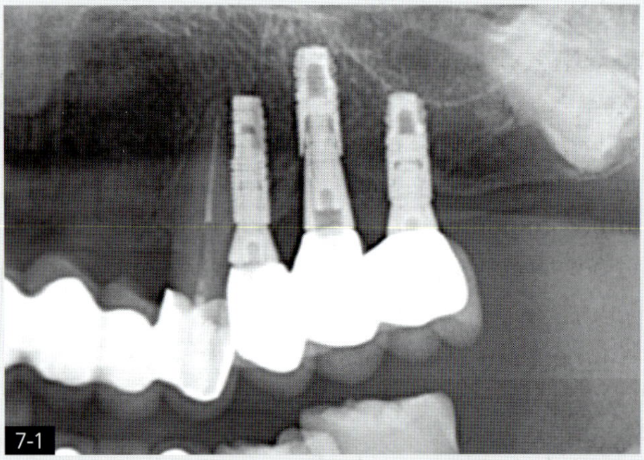

7-1

A patient has undergone implant treatment for eight years. Among the implants in the left maxilla, the central implant shows a micro-gap due to improper abutment connection. However, there is no observable bone loss (Figure 7-1). This case raises the question of whether the mere presence of a micro-gap is a direct cause of alveolar bone loss.

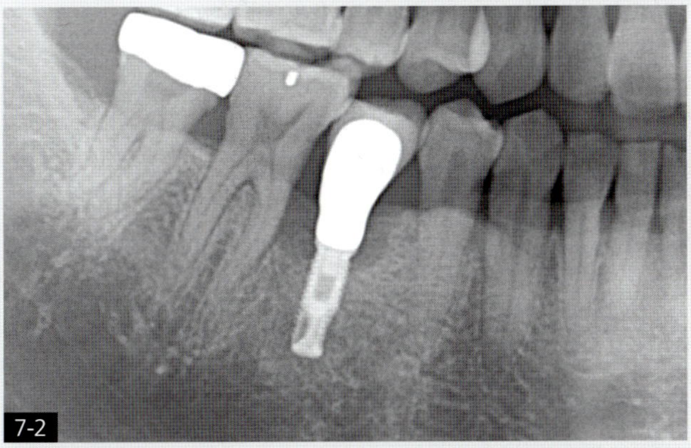
7-2

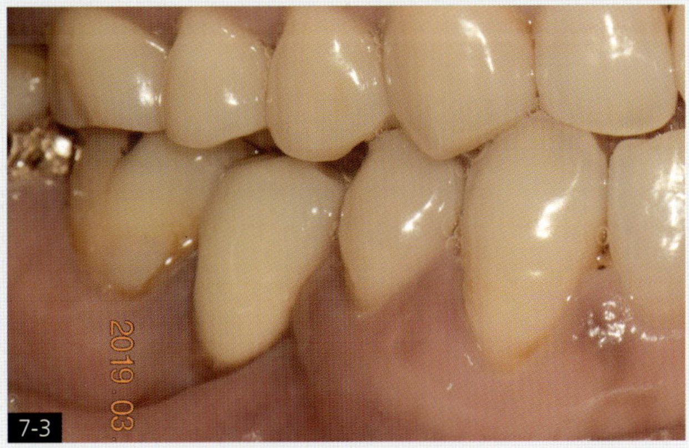
7-3

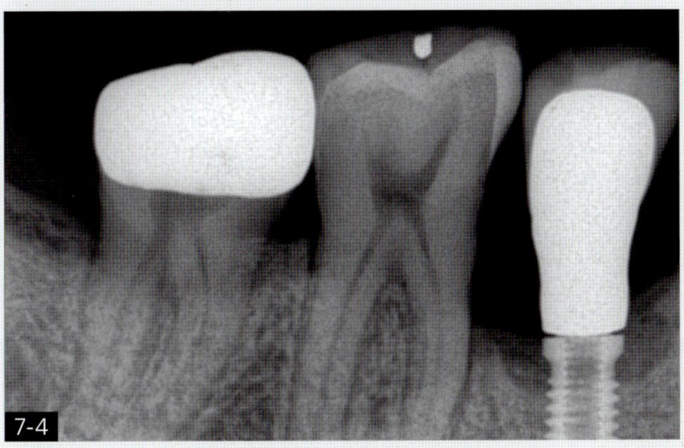
7-4

Around implant number 45, significant alveolar bone loss has occurred, accompanied by pus formation and the onset of peri-implantitis. Along with bone loss, there is also gingival recession, resulting in a notably elongated implant crown **(Figures 7-2, 3)**.

Radiographic images reveal the presence of a micro-gap, and the abutment screw was found to be loose **(Figure 7-4)**. The patient presented with complaints of crown mobility. In this case, both a micro-gap and micro-mobility are present. It is concluded that micro-mobility associated with a micro-gap contributes to the development of peri-implantitis. However, as seen in the case depicted in **Figure 7-1**, even if a micro-gap occurs in one of multiple implants, the absence of micro-mobility prevents the onset of peri-implantitis. This indicates that a micro-gap alone does not cause peri-implantitis with associated bone loss; rather, the presence of micro-mobility is necessary for the development of this condition.

There are instances where micro-mobility occurs at the abutment without resulting in bone resorption. This typically happens when micro-mobility occurs at a level significantly above the alveolar bone or gingiva. If a mucosal seal has already formed around the implant fixture, and micro-mobility occurs above this seal, further bacterial invasion is prevented, thus preventing additional bone loss. In extreme cases, if the fixture top is positioned above the gingiva, movement of the abutment does not lead to bone loss. Similarly, when non-epithelial adhering materials (such as gold or CCM abutments) are used, peri-implantitis does not frequently occur for the same reason.

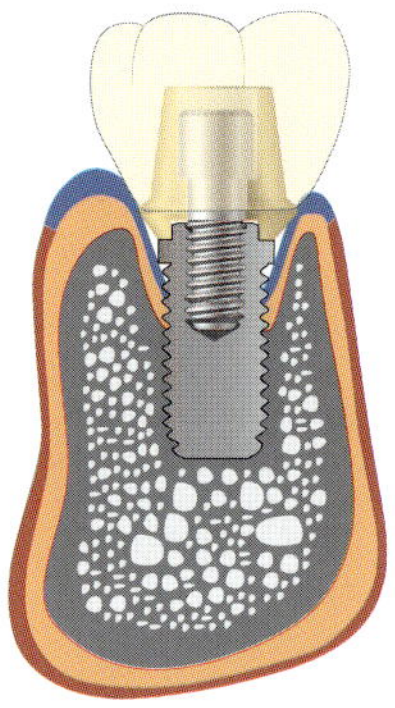

7-5

Micro-mobility at the fixture-abutment connection exists below the alveolar bone, leading to bone loss.

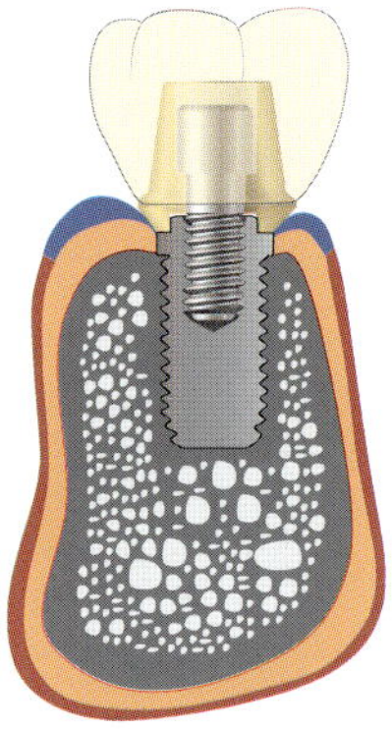

7-6

Micro-mobility at the fixture-abutment connection exists above the alveolar bone, preventing bone loss.

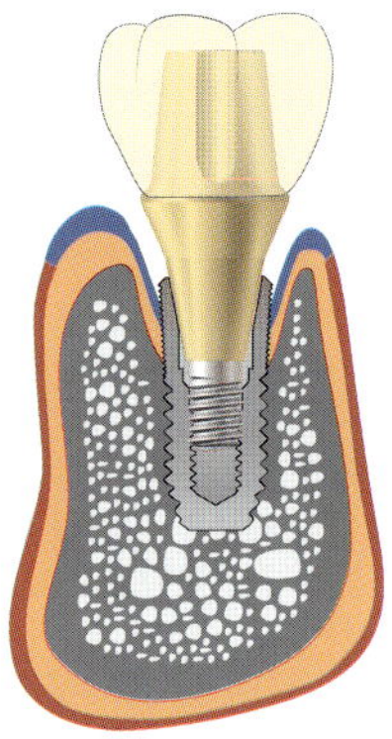

7-7

Micro-mobility at the fixture-abutment connection exists below the alveolar bone, leading to bone loss.

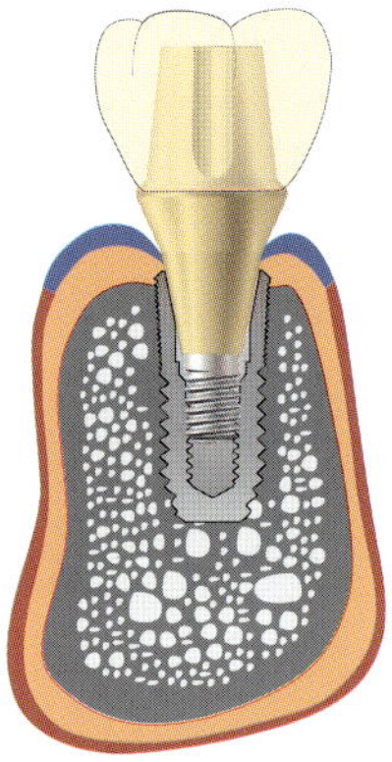

7-8

Micro-mobility at the fixture-abutment connection exists above the alveolar bone, preventing bone loss.

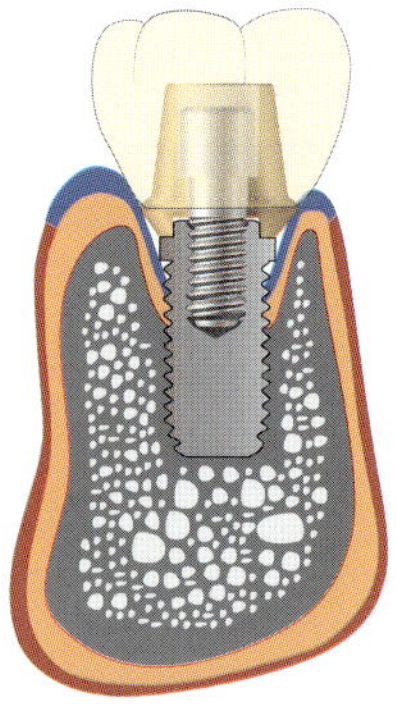

7-9

A gold abutment positioned below the alveolar bone leads to bone loss.

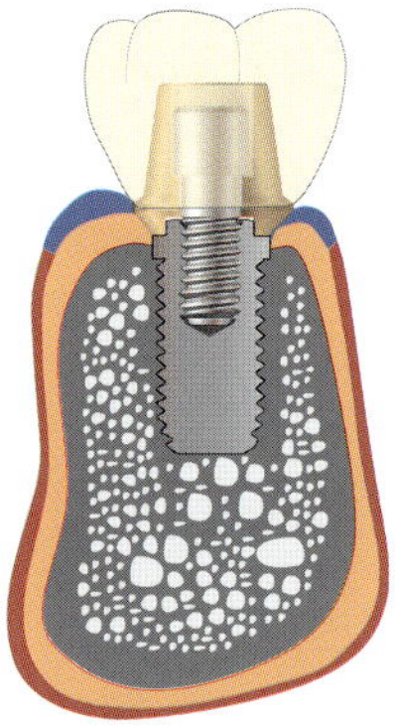

7-10

A gold abutment positioned above the alveolar bone does not lead to bone loss.

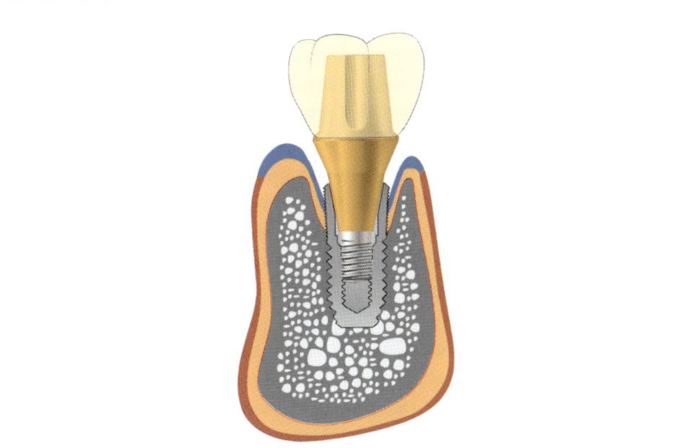

7-11

A gold abutment positioned below the alveolar bone leads to bone loss.

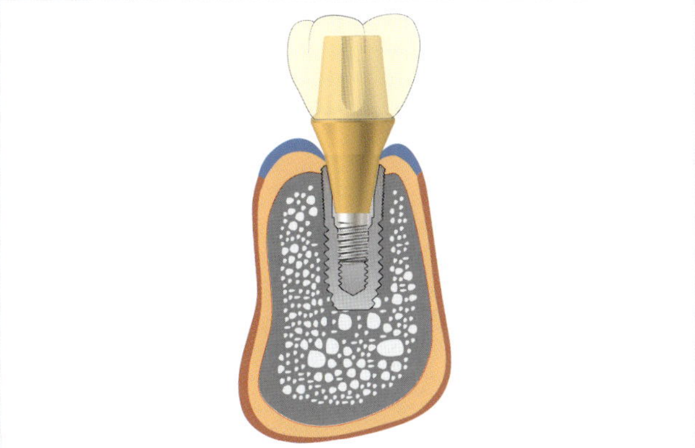

7-12

A gold abutment positioned above the alveolar bone does not lead to bone loss.

Let's examine another case regarding the response of alveolar bone to micro-gaps.

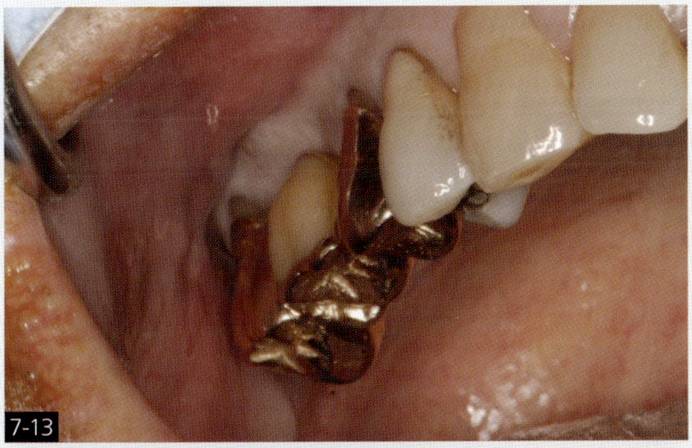

7-13

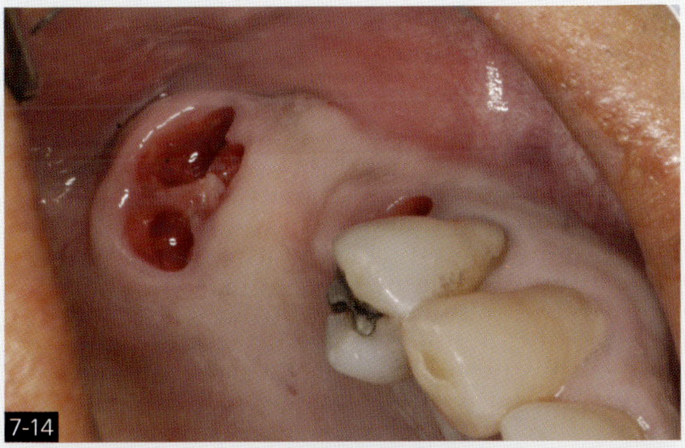

7-14

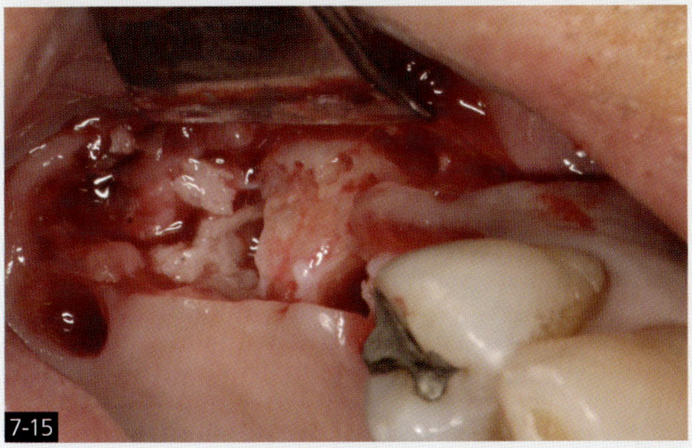

7-15

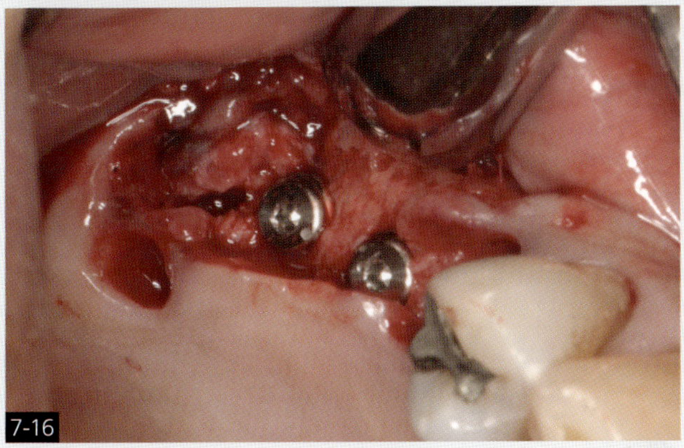

7-16

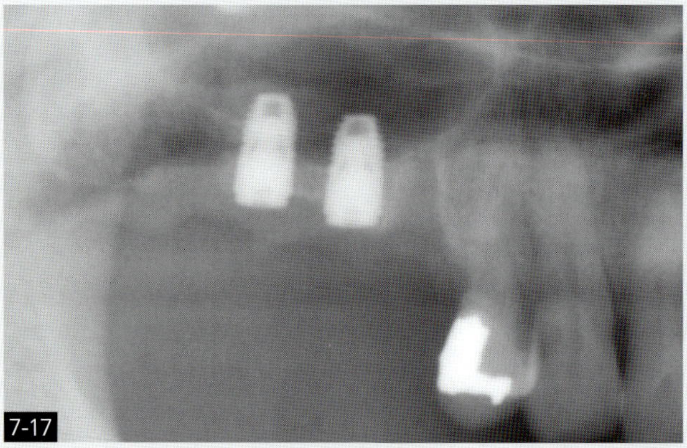

7-17

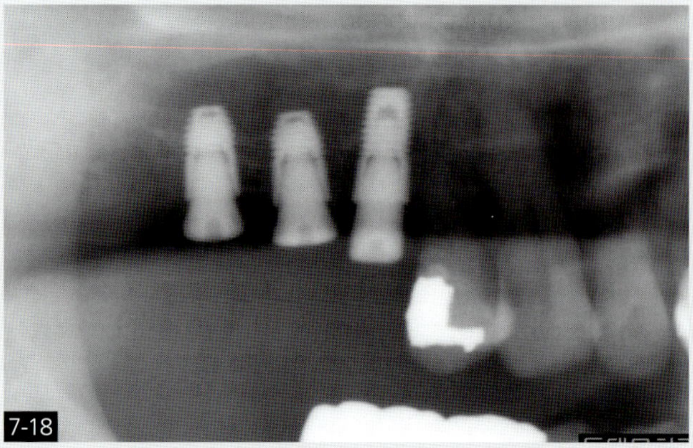

7-18

In this case, a #15-17 bridge was removed, and three implants were planned for placement. After the extraction of the bridge, implants were placed in positions 16 and 17, while implant 15 was placed after some healing had occurred **(Figures 7-13 to 7-18)**. After approximately two months, an implant was placed in the area of tooth 5, while the molar implants underwent a second surgery.

As seen in **Figure 7-18**, the healing abutment screw was unable to fully engage with the internal threads of the implant due to contact with the bottom of the internal threads, resulting in a micro-gap at the fixture-abutment connection. Despite this micro-gap persisting for six weeks, there was no observable bone loss, and clinically, there were no issues.

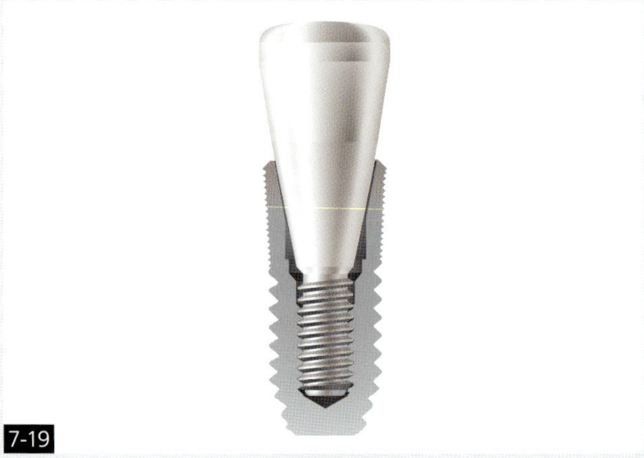

7-19

The healing abutment screw inside the implant was in contact with the bottom of the fixture's internal threads, preventing contact at the conical connection area.

Despite the six-week duration of the micro-gap, there was no bone resorption.

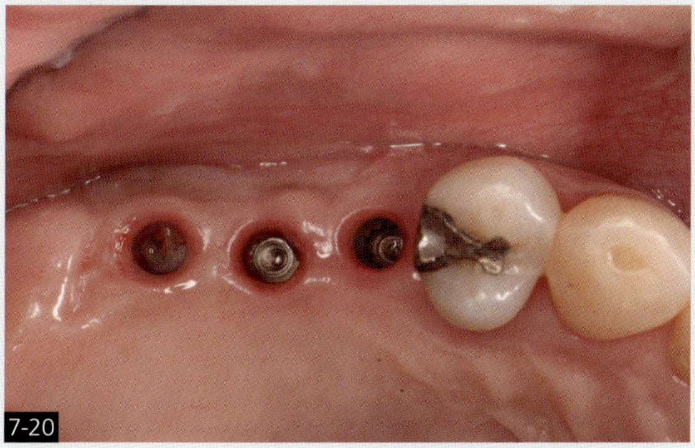

7-20

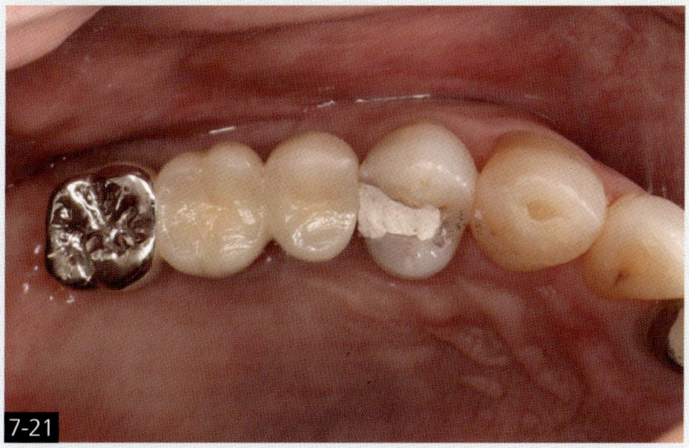

7-21

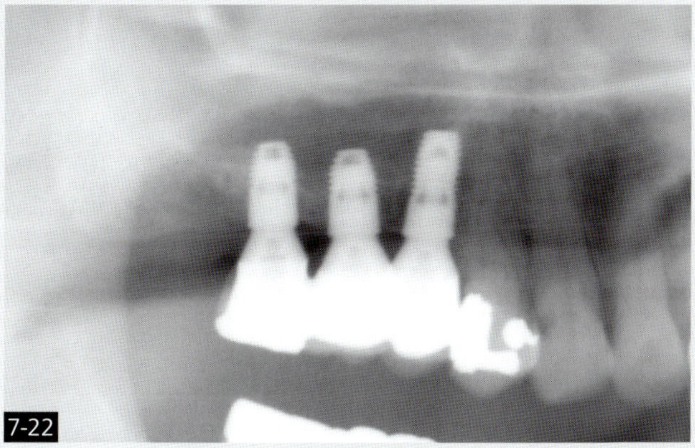

7-22

In the area of tooth 17, soft tissue had proliferated into the fixture. After removing the soft tissue that had grown into the area of tooth 16 for observation, no abnormalities were found. Tooth 15 had a healing abutment that was properly secured, showing normal gingival appearance **(Figure 7-20)**.

After the prosthesis was completed **(Figure 7-21)**, a radiographic examination five years later revealed no signs of bone loss **(Figure 7-22)**. This case illustrates that the micro-gap at the fixture-abutment connection alone does not lead to alveolar bone loss.

2. The Truth About Platform Switching

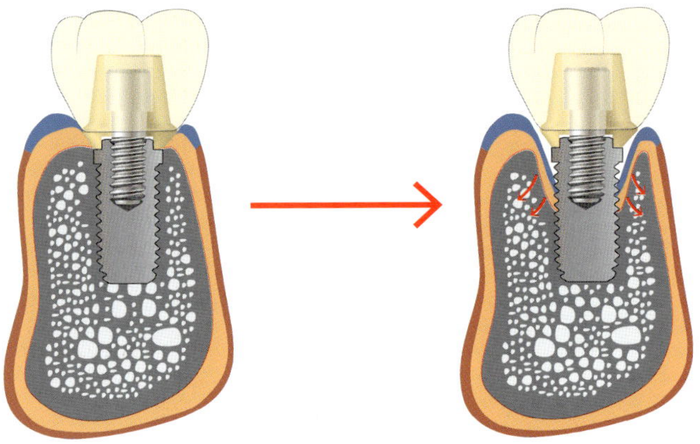

7-23

External connection-type implants often show bone loss after prosthetic placement, which is typically considered a normal bone response. The theory of platform switching aims to prevent this bone loss.

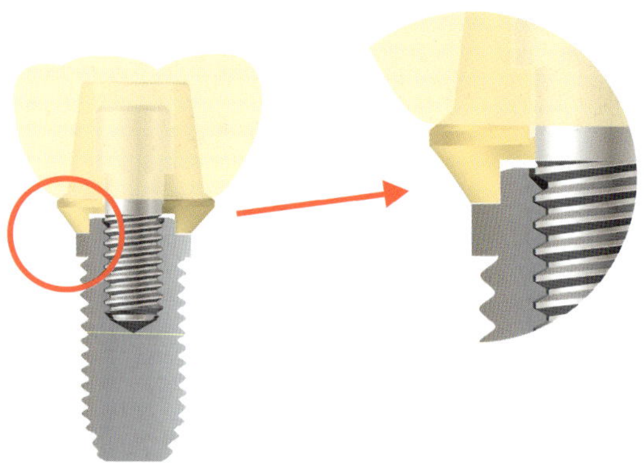

7-24

A micro-gap exists between the implant (fixture) and the abutment.

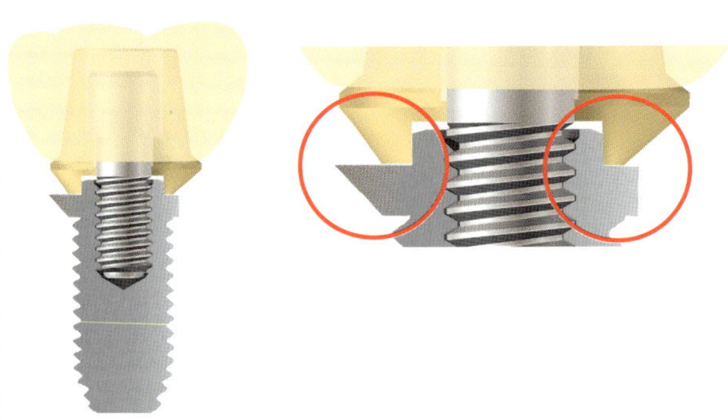

7-25

The concept of platform switching is to move the location of bacteria released from the micro-gap away from the alveolar bone, thereby preventing bone loss due to bacterial invasion. To achieve this, two methods can be employed: either increasing the platform size of external connection implants or decreasing the diameter of the abutment **(Figure 7-25)**.

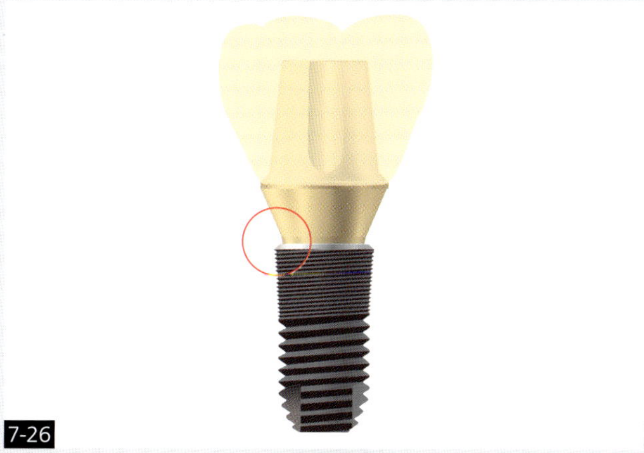

7-26

In Astra-type implants, bone loss is less common, and, as seen in the author's cases, both the quantity and quality of bone may increase. There are claims that this positive bone response is due to platform switching; however, actual observations suggest otherwise **(Figure 7-26)**.

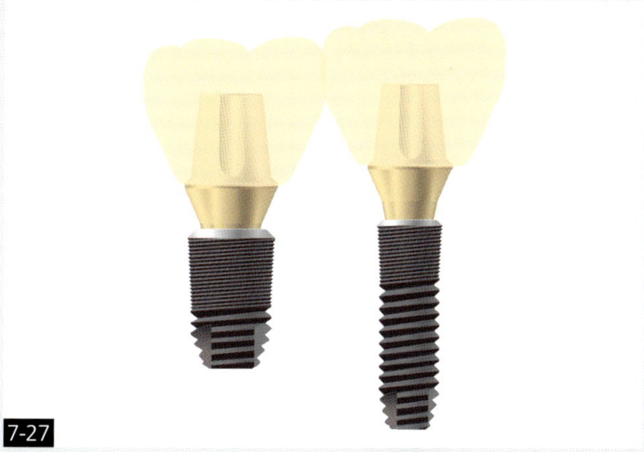

7-27

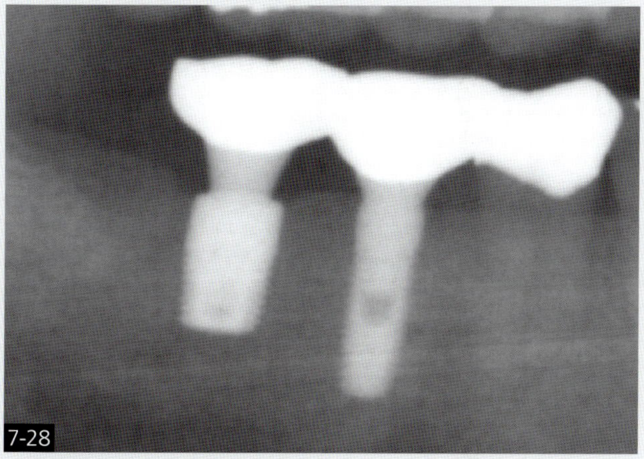

7-28

In **Figure 7-27**, the left side shows a thicker implant, while the right side shows a thinner implant. The thicker implant has relatively more platform switching, while the thinner implant has less. Theoretically, one would expect less bone resorption around the thicker implant and more around the thinner one. However, radiographic images of actual clinical cases **(Figure 7-28)** demonstrate a bone response that contradicts the concept of platform switching.

Based on the discussed cases, it becomes evident that the platform switching theory cannot adequately explain the bone response observed in Astra-type implants. According to this theory, implant 47, which exhibits significant platform switching, should have the alveolar bone located closer to the fixture-abutment connection. Conversely, implant 46, with less platform switching, should have the alveolar bone positioned further away from the connection. However, clinical observations reveal the opposite response, indicating that platform switching does not account for all alveolar bone reactions, particularly in Astra-type implants.

Chapter 8

Conclusion of Part 1.

Bone loss can lead to the loss of gingiva or the formation of periodontal pockets, which are primary contributors to peri-implantitis. It is essential to summarize the reasons behind alveolar bone loss and identify the necessary conditions that dentists, products, and patients must meet to ensure the long-term prognosis of implants.

The theory that alveolar bone recedes a certain distance from the fixture-abutment interface is inadequate. I propose that "alveolar bone recedes a certain distance from the attacking factors." But what are these attacking factors? The following elements have been identified as contributors to marginal bone loss:

1. Micro-mobility
2. Abutment materials that do not allow for mucosal seal formation (failure of epithelial cell attachment)
3. Deep subgingival margins of prosthetic restorations
4. Absence or loss of attached gingiva, shallow vestibule, and frenum
5. Residual dental cement

The long-term prognosis of implant treatment is determined by three factors: the clinician, the product, and the patient. Below are the necessary considerations for each factor to prevent and treat peri-implantitis.

Clinician Factors

- Use products that do not allow screw loosening (select abutments that do not allow for movement).
- When using Astra-type implants, ensure multiple re-tightening sessions.
- During periodic patient visits, check for any loosening of screws and abutments. Additionally, gently press the gingiva to check for any drainage. If necessary, use a probe to measure the depth of periodontal pockets.
- Choose abutment materials that allow for mucosal seal formation (e.g., titanium, alumina, zirconia).
- Avoid repeatedly attaching and detaching the superstructure from the implant.
- Place the implant in the center of the gingiva (consider gingival grafting and vestibuloplasty if needed).
- When treating peri-implantitis, perform surgery to clean the contaminated implant surface while reducing the periodontal pocket (consider bone grafting as an adjunct).

Product Factors

- Ensure there is no screw loosening or abutment movement.
- The product should not be prone to mechanical fracture.
- Screws should extend to the top of the fixture.

Patient Factors

- Maintain thorough oral hygiene.
- Attend regular dental check-ups to monitor for drainage from periodontal pockets, gingival inflammation, abutment movement, and screw loosening.

P E R I - I M P L A N T I T I S

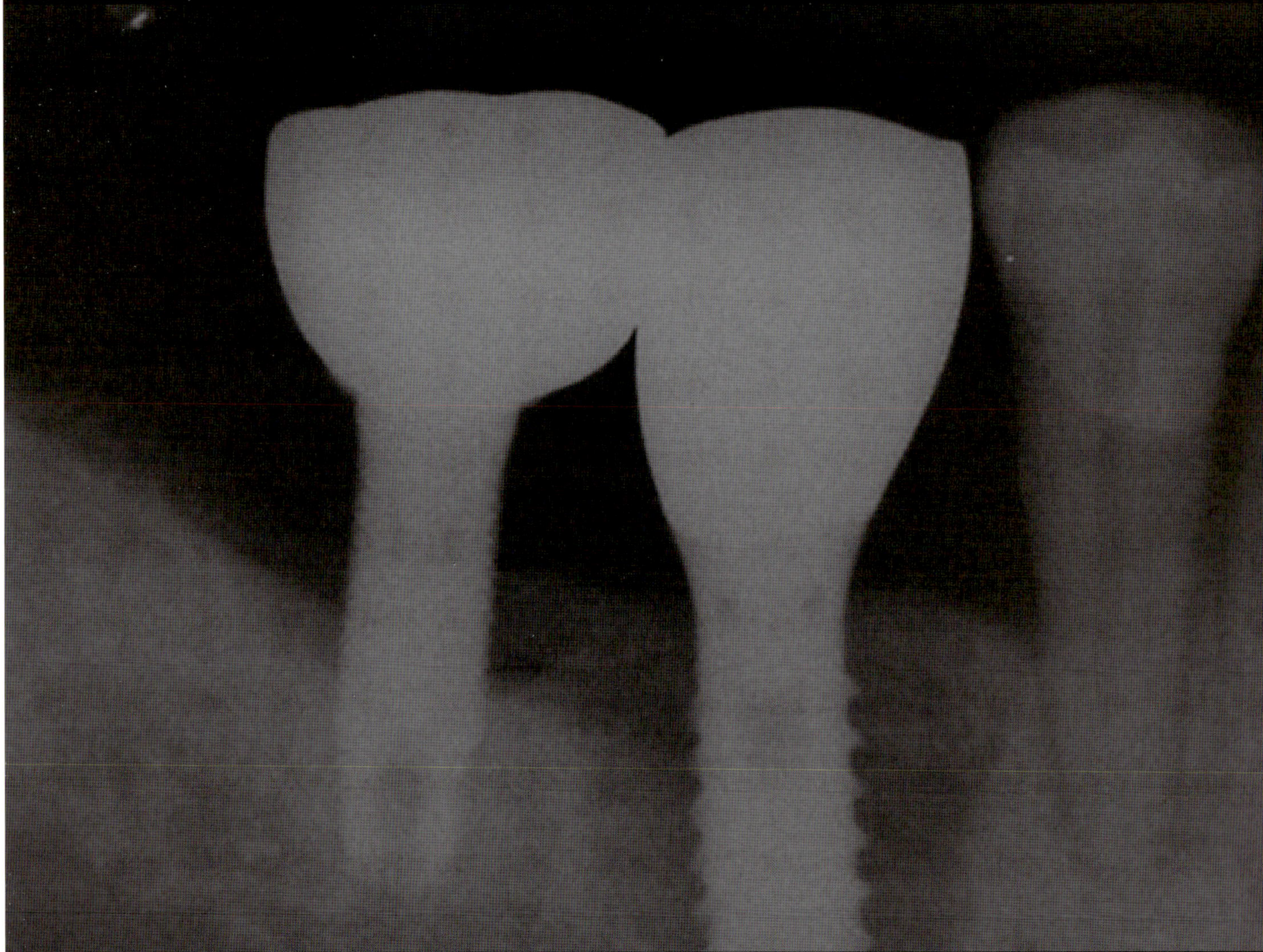

PART

2

PERI-IMPLANTITIS

Chapter 1 Longitudinal fracture of dental implants

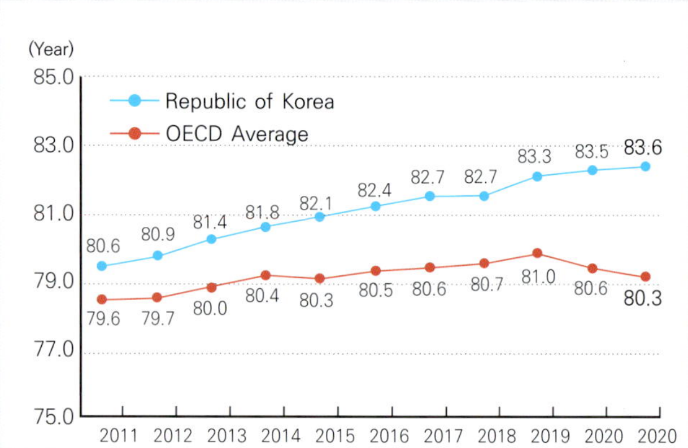

1-1

Life expectancy of Korean people (OECD health statistics 2023)

A dental implant is a prosthetic device intended to replace a missing natural tooth. Accordingly, it must function properly within the human body, and as human life expectancy continues to increase, it should also provide stable long-term outcomes consistent with contemporary clinical expectations.

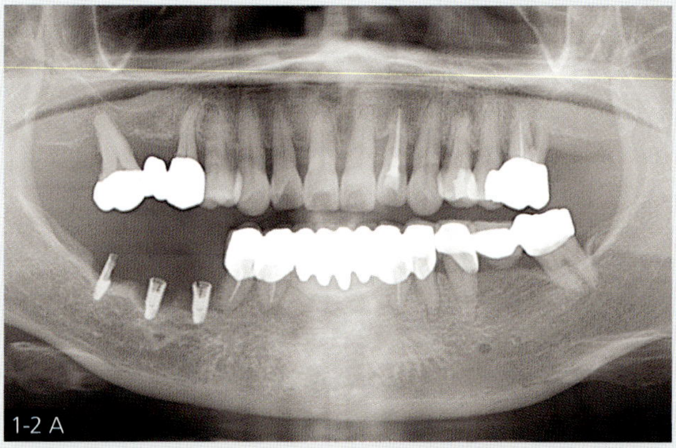

1-2 A

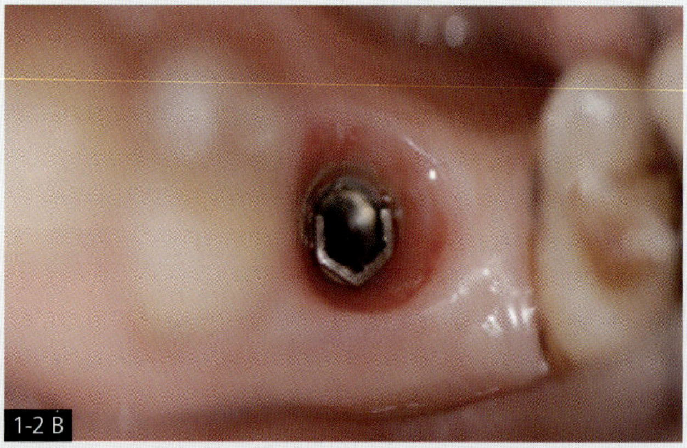

1-2 B

Orthopantomographic and clinical views of peri-implantitis (A) and fractured implants (A, B).

For an implant to maintain proper long-term function within the oral cavity, the surrounding hard and soft tissues must remain free from both biological and mechanical complications.

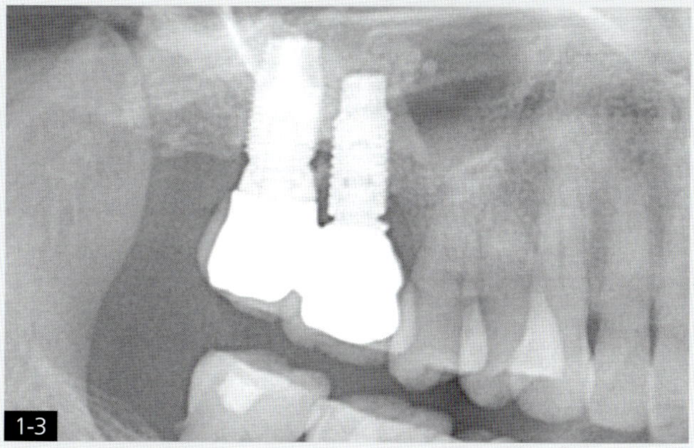
1-3

Peri-implantitis has developed at the implant placed in position #16, leading to observable alveolar bone loss.

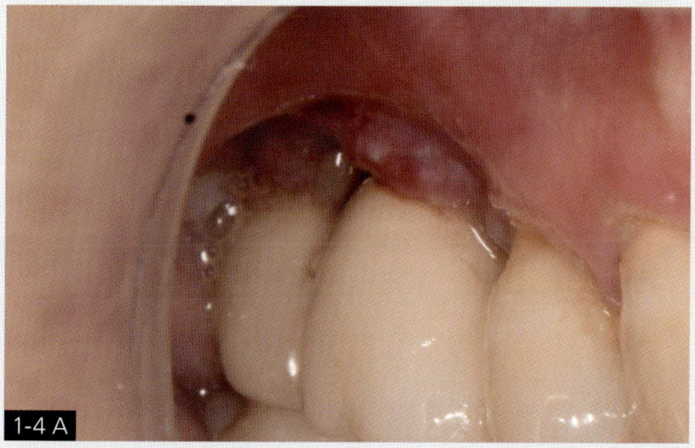
1-4 A

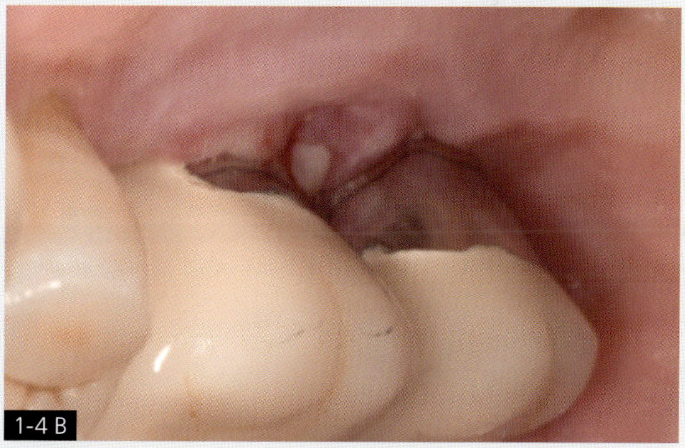
1-4 B

Peri-implantitis has developed, resulting in observable gingival inflammation. **Figure 1-4 A** shows the buccal aspect, and **Figure 1-4 B** shows the palatal aspect.

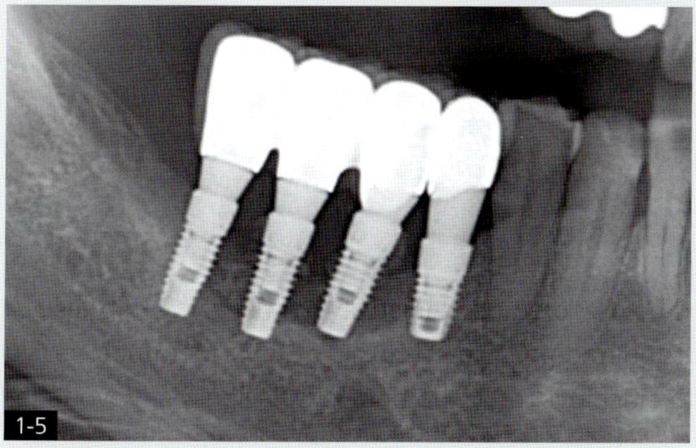
1-5

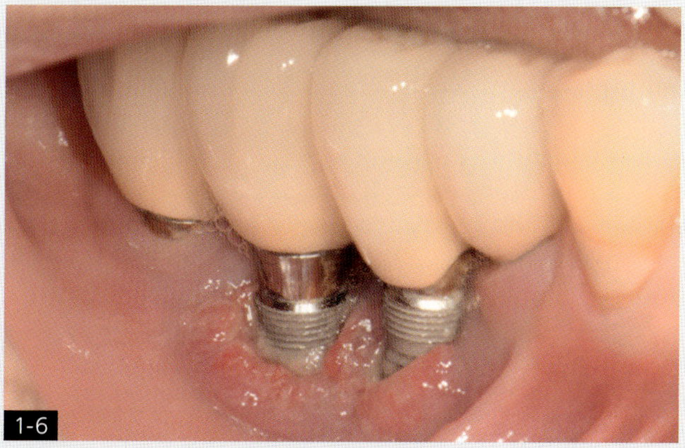
1-6

In another clinical case of peri-implantitis, excessive gingival inflammation and alveolar bone loss are observed. The loss of alveolar bone leads to gingival recession, resulting in implant exposure.

The stability of the implant–abutment connection is a critical factor influencing the long-term clinical success of dental implants. To prevent complications arising from instability at this interface, it is essential to thoroughly investigate the biomechanics of the implant–abutment connection, both theoretically and through empirical testing.

Contemporary dental implants used daily in dental clinics can be broadly categorized into two primary types—internal friction connections and external hex connections—based on their implant–abutment interface design. Notably, the mechanical characteristics of the implant–abutment connection are closely related to the biological responses of the surrounding hard and soft tissues at the implant interface.

1. External hex connection

In an external hex connection, the abutment is attached to the implant by an abutment screw, and the stability of the implant–abutment interface is entirely dependent on the screw.
This configuration is often referred to as a "butt joint" interface, since the flat upper surface of the implant engages in a flat-on-flat contact with the abutment's flat underside.

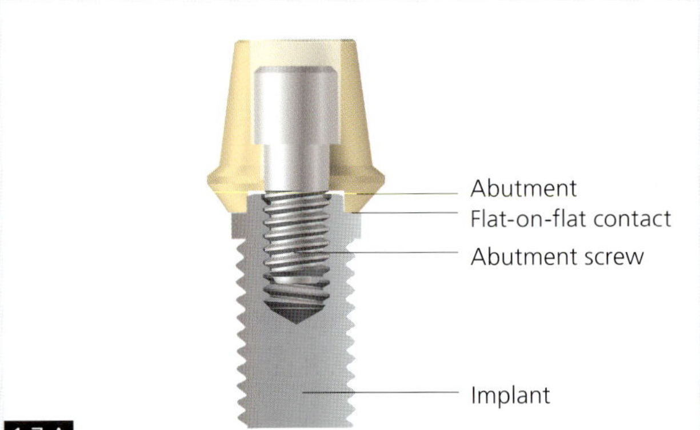

1-7 A

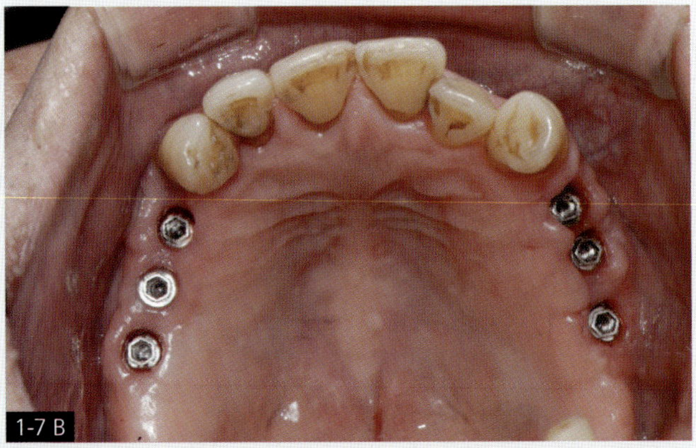

1-7 B

A schematic representation of the longitudinal section of an external hex connection (A) and an intraoral photograph illustrating external hex connection implants placed in the maxillary posterior region (B).

When torque is applied to tighten the abutment screw within the implant–abutment connection, the abutment screw undergoes elongation, thereby generating a preload.

Since this connection fundamentally depends on the clamping force (preload) produced by the abutment screw, the mechanics of the screw play a critical role. As previously mentioned, the preload acts as a tightening force that stabilizes the implant–abutment connection. When occlusal forces are applied to an implant with this type of connection, its flat top surface resists the vertical component of the occlusal load. The horizontal component of the load is transferred to both the hexagonal structure at the top of the implant and the abutment screw. Additionally, the hexagonal structure serves as an anti-rotational device, countering any torsional forces generated by the occlusal load.

The earliest screw-type implants featuring an external hex connection to be used clinically were exemplified by Brånemark implants **(Figure 1-8)**. Manufacturers of such external hex connection implants typically recommend an optimal tightening torque of 30–35 Ncm for the abutment screws.

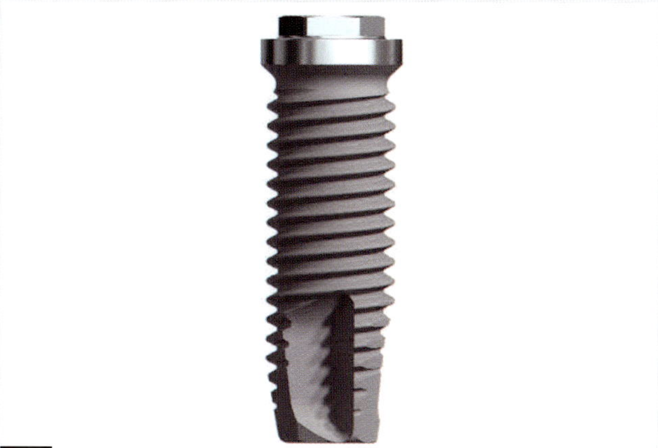

1-8

A Brånemark implant (TiUnite MkIII)

Figure 1-8 shows an implant that has undergone anodic oxidation for surface modification, although it originally featured a turned pure titanium surface without any treatment.

The key issue is that the recommended torque value does not generate sufficient clamping force to ensure a stable implant–abutment connection. Clinically achievable tightening torques cannot reliably prevent screw loosening. Moreover, even when an external hex connection is properly tightened to the recommended torque, transient abutment movement may occur during intraoral function due to the diverse vectors of masticatory forces.

Conclusively, the greatest disadvantage of the external hex connection lies in the fact that, although the implant–abutment connection is established through the tightening torque of the abutment screw, it does not guarantee adequate stability. These mechanical characteristics may contribute to various biological complications.

2. Internal friction connection

For internal friction connections, the stability of the implant–abutment interface is maintained not only by the preload exerted by the abutment screw, but also through the close contact between the abutment's external surface and the implant's internal surface **(Figure 1-9)**.

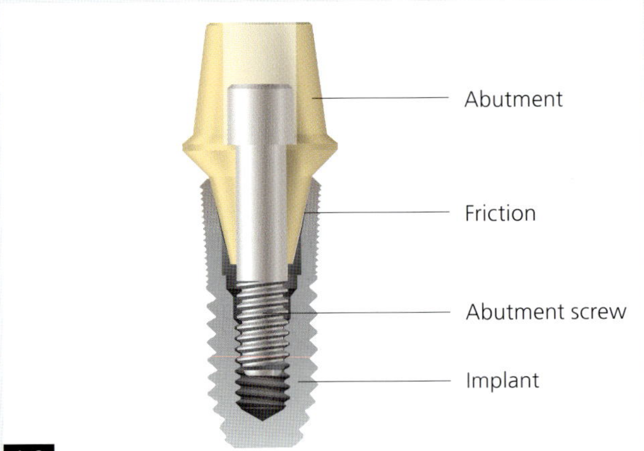

1-9

A longitudinal schematic diagram of an internal friction connection. In a two-piece abutment system, the frictional force generated by close contact along the inclined surfaces is depicted when the abutment is connected to the implant.

Close contact between the implant and abutment generates frictional forces, which play a significant role in enhancing the stability of the implant–abutment connection. Due to the critical function of these frictional forces, an internal friction connection is also sometimes referred to as a friction-screw-retained connection.

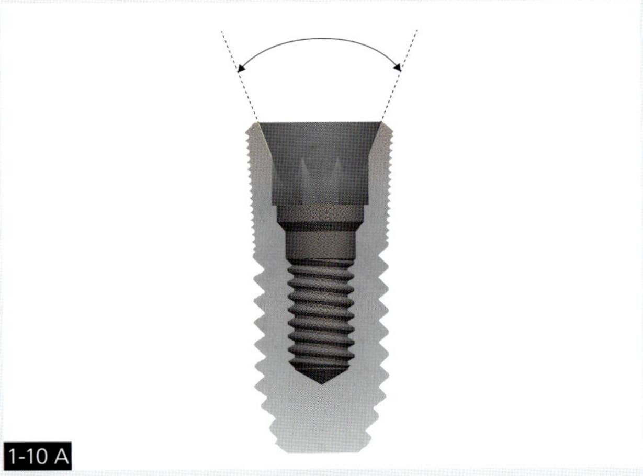

1-10 A

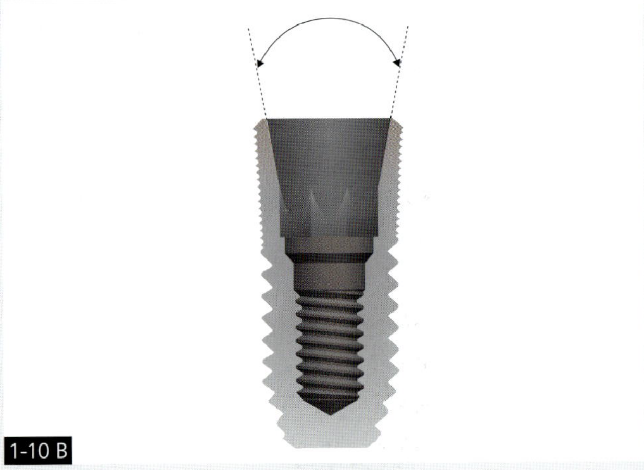

1-10 B

As the divergence angle, or the internal conical angle increases, the contact area between the implant and abutment decreases **(Figure 1-10 A)**, leading to greater instability of the implant–abutment connection.

Conversely, reducing the angle allows for increased contact depth, resulting in a broader contact surface **(Figure 1-10 B)** and thereby enhancing the stability of the implant–abutment connection.

The internal conical angle of the implant–abutment interface relative to the implant's long axis is a critical factor influencing abutment stability in internal friction connections. Although increasing this conical angle can reduce the incidence of implant fracture or tearing under functional loading, it also compromises the stability of the implant–abutment connection **(Figure 1-10)**.

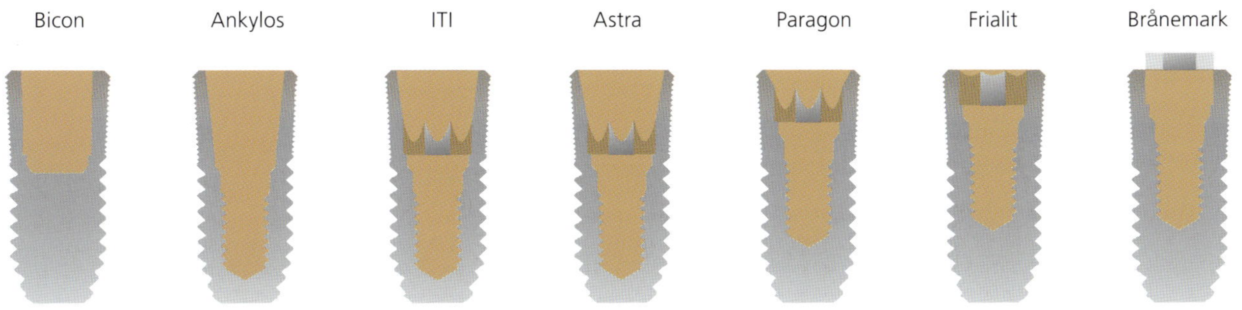

1-11

Internal conical angles observed in the implant–abutment connections of various implant systems.
As the internal conical angle increases toward the right, it eventually becomes similar to an external hex connection, such as that of the Brånemark implant system.

From a biomechanical standpoint, increasing the conical angle to reduce friction between the implant and the abutment results in the implant–abutment connection's stability relying more heavily on the preload of the abutment screw. Consequently, the structural characteristics of the connection increasingly resemble those of an external hex connection **(Figure 1-11)**.

Since around the year 2010, there has been a growing tendency in the field of dental implantology to classify implant-related complications into mechanical and biological categories, aiming to investigate their respective causes and outcomes.

Among the many variables influencing clinical outcomes, focusing on a single variable can simplify the examination of causal relationships. By doing so, the influence of other variables need not be considered, which can facilitate drawing clearer conclusions. However, this classification is merely a conceptual tool designed to improve clarity of thought; it does not reflect an inherent division in nature.

If dental researchers and clinicians investigate mechanical complications while completely disregarding biological factors, or investigates biological complications without considering mechanical aspects, critical errors may occur in interpreting the overall clinical phenomenon **(Figure 1-12)**.

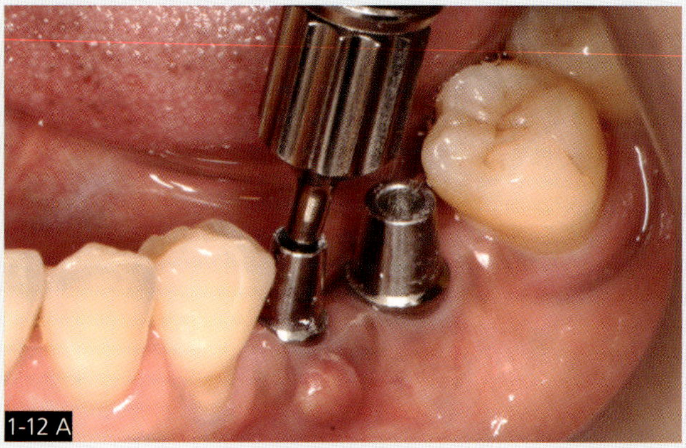
1-12 A

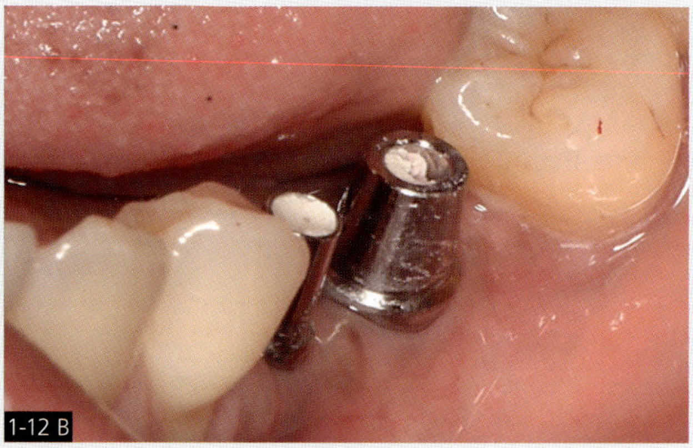
1-12 B

Resolution of screw loosening, a mechanical complication (A), leading to the treatment of gingivitis, a biological complication (B).

Dental implants are surgically placed into the bone, specifically the maxilla or mandible, and are functionally connected to external inputs, such as food, within the oral cavity. The abutment serves as an intermediary structure that interfaces with the gingiva, acting as a conduit between the intraoral (outside of the body) and systemic (inside of the body) environments. Consequently, the bone-implant interface, gingiva-abutment interface, and implant-abutment interface are simultaneously exposed to both oral and systemic conditions. When considered holistically, it becomes evident that an issue at one of these interfaces can readily influence and lead to complications in the others.

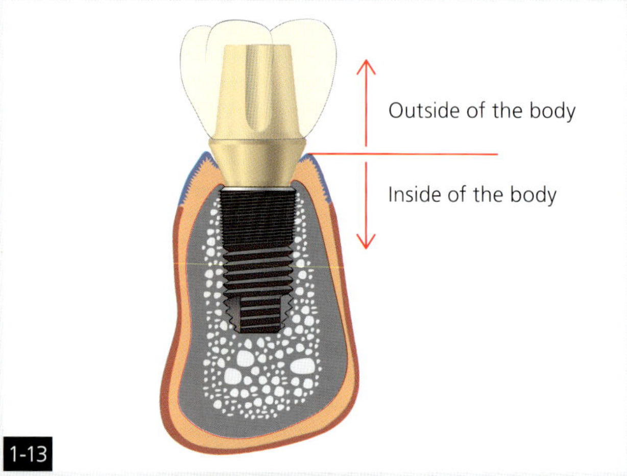

1-13

Screw loosening compromises the attachment of periodontal epithelial cells, which serve as a barrier between the internal and external environments. This disruption facilitates the invasion of external bacteria into the internal tissues.

When abutment screw loosening occurs, compromising the stability of the implant–abutment connection—a major mechanical complication—the gingival tissues previously attached around the abutment become detached. This detachment leads to the formation of a periodontal pocket, where plaque and calculus can accumulate. The accumulation of these deposits can cause bone loss at the bone–implant interface, ultimately progressing to peri-implantitis, a major biological complication.

Recent clinical studies have reported findings based on these mechanisms. This illustrates that categorizing implant complications into mechanical and biological categories is an artificial construct created for conceptual clarity. In clinical practice, however, such complications should be evaluated comprehensively, highlighting the importance of a holistic approach to implant-related issues.

Both the internal conical angle of the implant–abutment interface relative to the implant's long axis and the tightening torque of the abutment screw are significant factors influencing the implant–abutment connection.

These factors should be comprehensively examined, considering both mechanical and biological aspects.

When implants are designed with an increased conical angle to reduce friction, the stability of the implant–abutment connection becomes dependent on the tightening torque of the abutment screw. Consequently, if the screw loosens, the abutment can immediately lose stability and become wobbly. In both internal friction connections and external hex connections, the majority of occlusal forces are concentrated on the abutment screw within this structural design, thereby increasing the risk of abutment screw fracture. In such cases, the fractured screw can be removed intraorally, and a new implant-supported restoration can be fabricated while replacing the abutment screw. This procedure is generally considered clinically feasible and relatively straightforward.

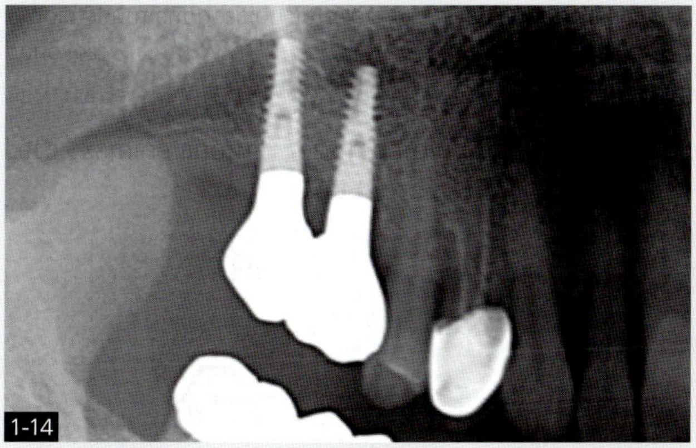
1-14

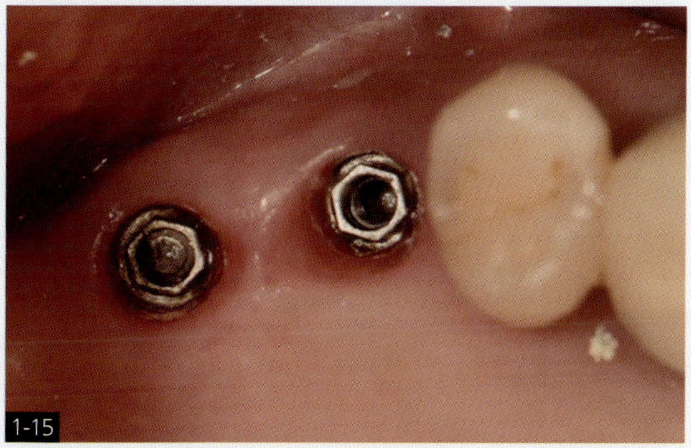
1-15

A complication occurred with the external hex connection **(Figures 1-14 and 1-15)**. The abutment screw has been fractured **(Figure 1-15)**.

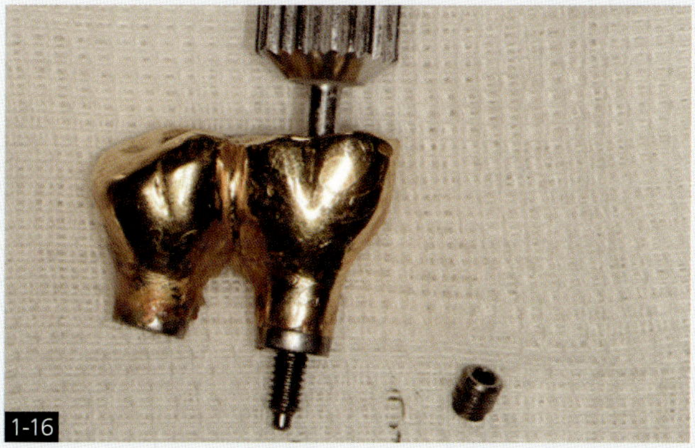
1-16

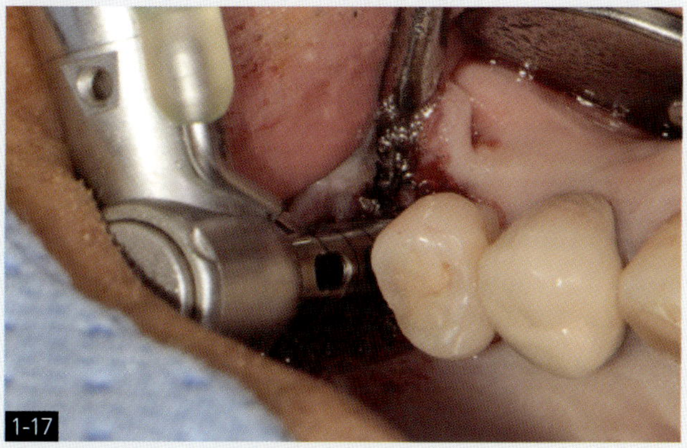
1-17

As shown in **Figure 1-16**, the abutment screw repeatedly loosened over time, eventually resulting in the fracture of the screw head. After replacing the abutment screw and re-tightening it, the screw loosened again within three months. It was concluded that further tightening would not resolve the issue, leading to the decision to replace the implant. A trephine drill was typically used for implant removal **(Figure 1-17)**.

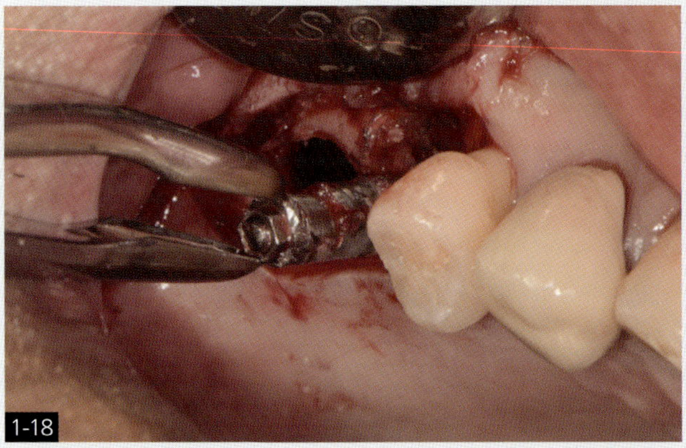
1-18

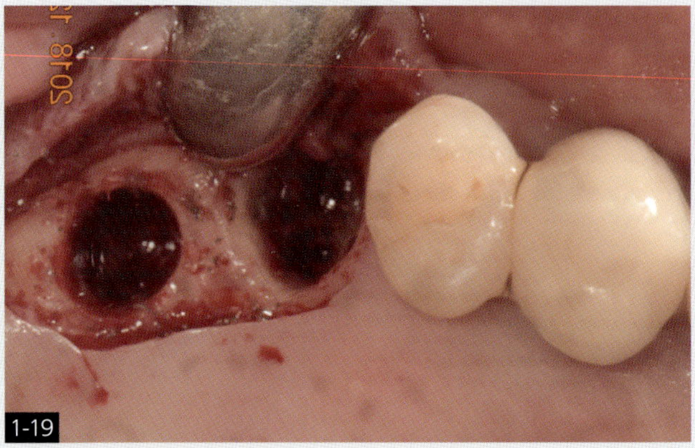
1-19

Figures 1-18 and 1-19 illustrate the implant removal procedure and the site condition following removal, respectively.

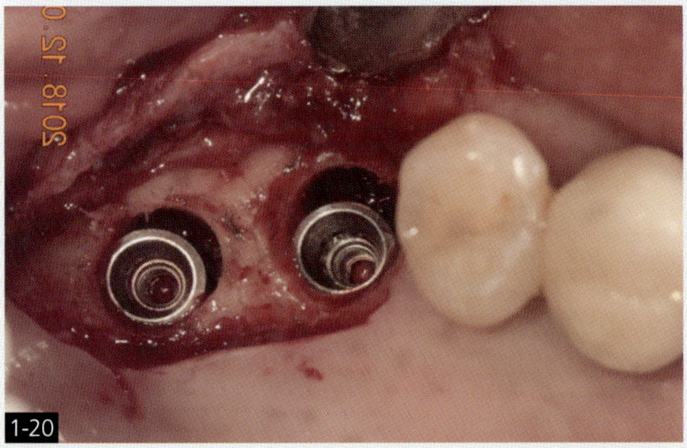
1-20

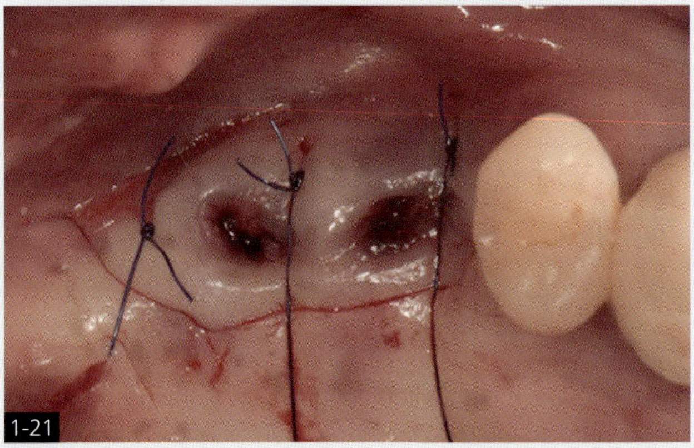
1-21

The implant was replaced with a product that minimizes screw loosening and fracturing **(Figures 1-20, 21 and 22)**.

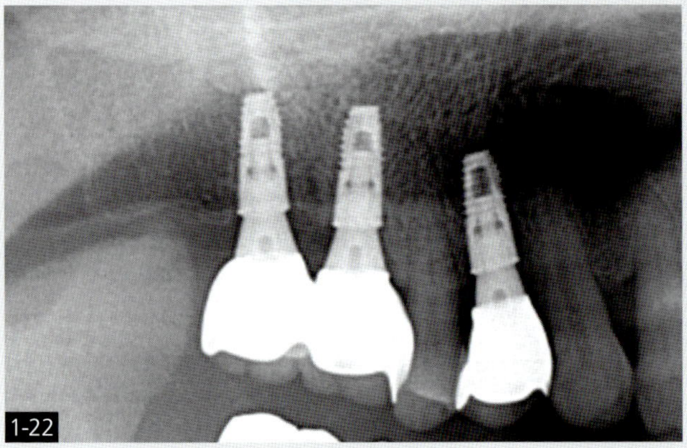
1-22

The patient experienced no instances of screw loosening during the 18 months following the implant replacement.

While it may be assumed that re-tightening a loosened screw will resolve the issue, in practice, the screw often continues to loosen. This persistence occurs because the underlying cause is not related to the screw itself. When the contribution of interface friction to the stability of the implant–abutment connection in an internal friction connection is reduced, the abutment screw can loosen, similar to what occurs in an external hex connection. This loss of stability increases the risk of biological complications, such as soft tissue attachment loss and subsequent peri-implantitis.

Conversely, reducing the internal conical angle of the implant–abutment interface relative to the implant's long axis to enhance frictional stability allows occlusal forces to be distributed across the implant–abutment interface rather than being concentrated on the abutment screw. In these cases, mechanical complications are more likely to involve abutment fractures or implant tearing rather than screw fractures. Clinically, these types of complications are often more challenging to manage.

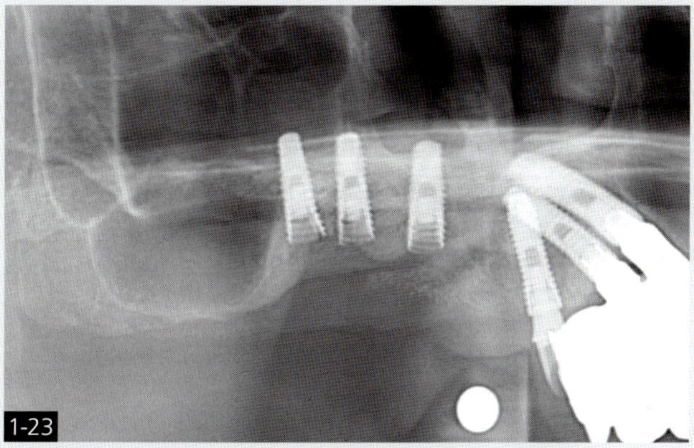

1-23

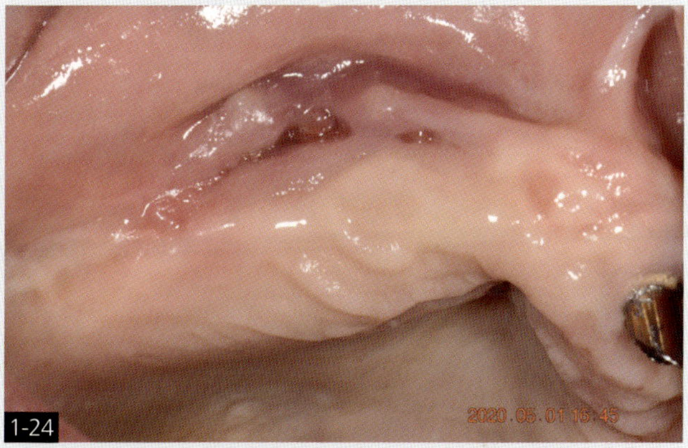

1-24

Three implants in the patient's tooth #10 region have fractured **(Figures 1-23, 24)**. The original implants fractured three years ago and were subsequently replaced with new implants; however, these replacements have also fractured.

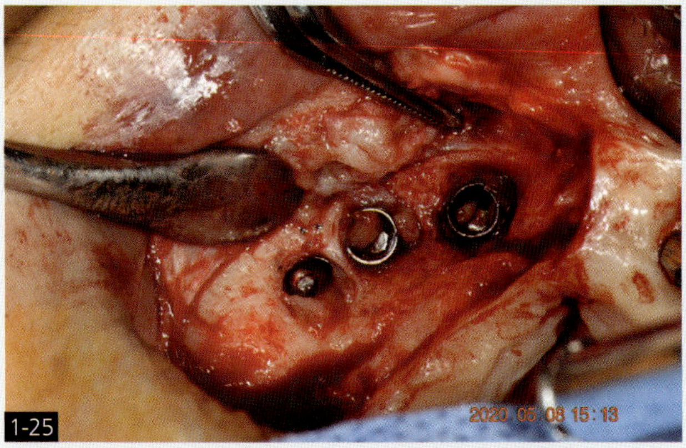

1-25

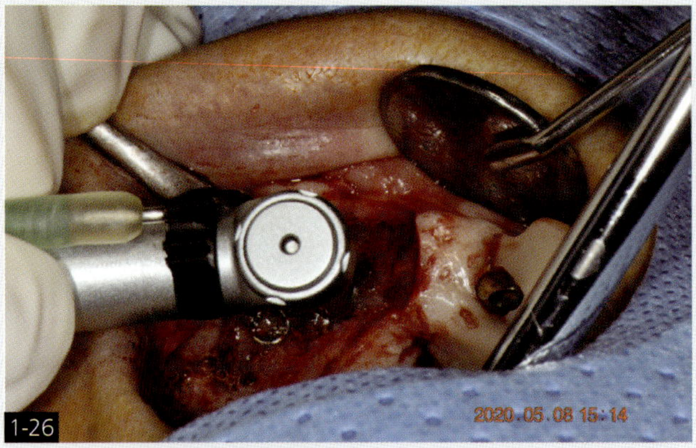

1-26

After reflecting the mucosal flap, the fractured implant was identified **(Figure 1-25)** and subsequently removed **(Figures 1-26 and 27)**.

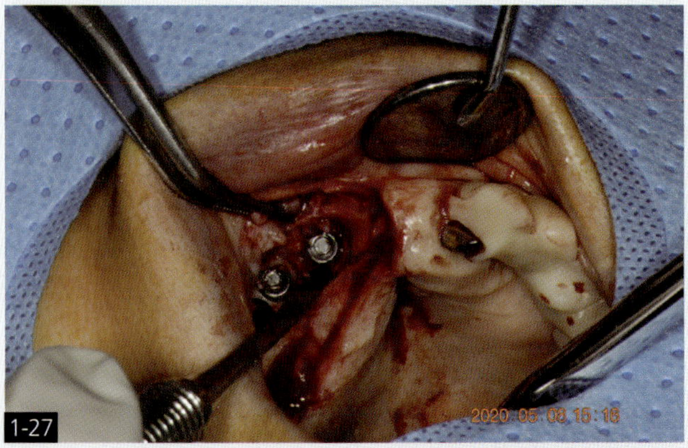

1-27

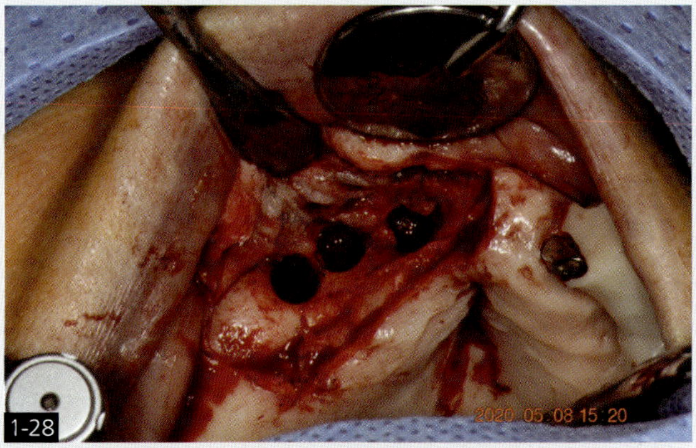

1-28

After removing the fractured implant, the resulting bone defect is observable **(Figure 1-28)**.

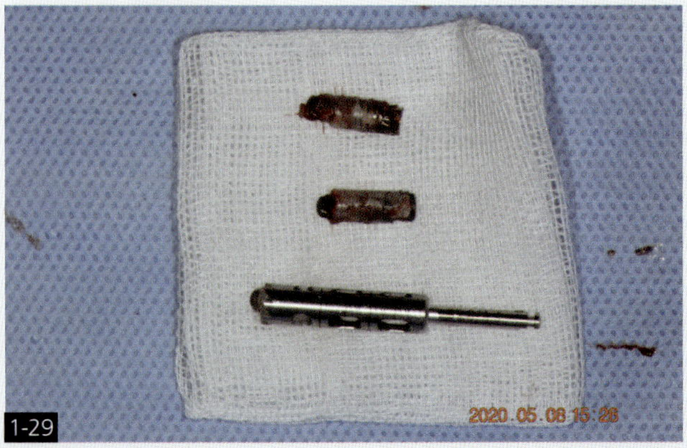

1-29

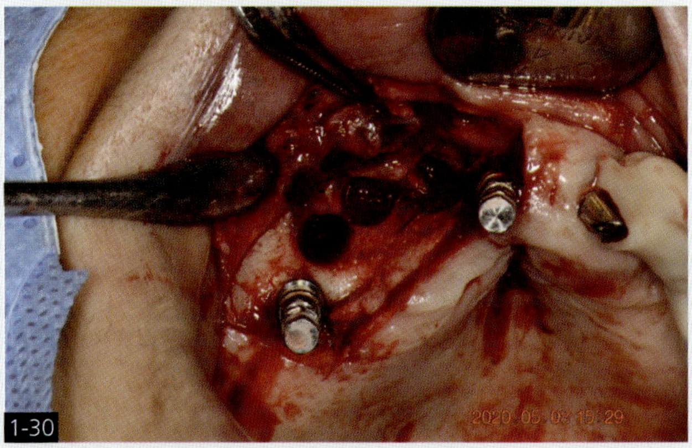

1-30

Figure 1-29 displays the removed implant. Due to the presence of a bone defect, it was not possible to place an implant in that specific area. Consequently, implants were positioned adjacent to the defect on either side, as shown in **Figure 1-30**.

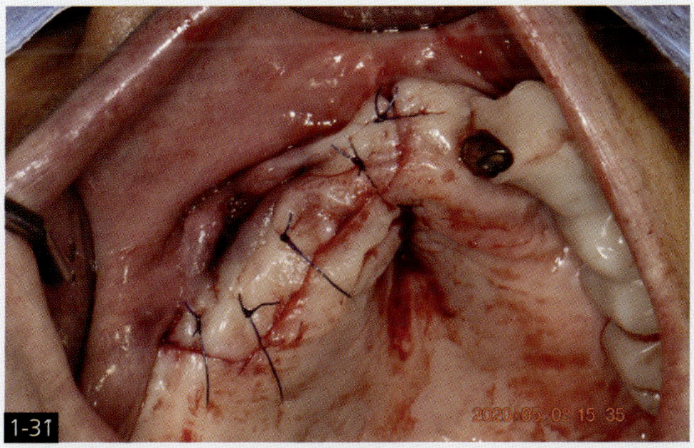

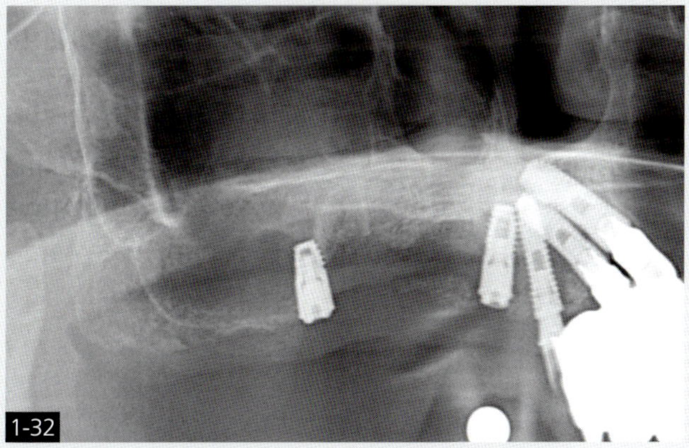

Figure 1-31 depicts the site following surgery, and **Figure 1-32** shows the radiographic image.

Dental implants featuring an internal friction connection are prone to fracture as a postoperative complication. After removing the fractured implant, it was replaced with a product less susceptible to fracturing than the original. However, in implant–abutment connection structures with high friction, the connection's stability can be preserved even if the abutment screw loosens. This sustained stability helps prevent soft tissue attachment loss and subsequent biological complications, representing a significant clinical advantage.

The mechanical structure of the implant–abutment connection is closely associated with biological complications, such as peri-implant mucositis and peri-implantitis.

Another crucial point is that complications such as implant fractures and tearing ultimately originate from screw loosening, which can be viewed as a natural consequence of the mechanical design. Therefore, it is essential for dental clinicians to thoroughly understand the biomechanics of screw loosening in order to provide effective and reliable implant-supported prosthetic treatments for their patients.

Chapter 2

Biomechanics of screw loosening and clinical interpretation

The clinical success of implant treatment depends on numerous factors affecting not only the bone–implant and gingiva–abutment interfaces but also the implant–abutment interface.

Abutment screw loosening, one of the most common complications in implant dentistry, can lead to peri-implantitis and ultimately implant failure (Figures A and B).

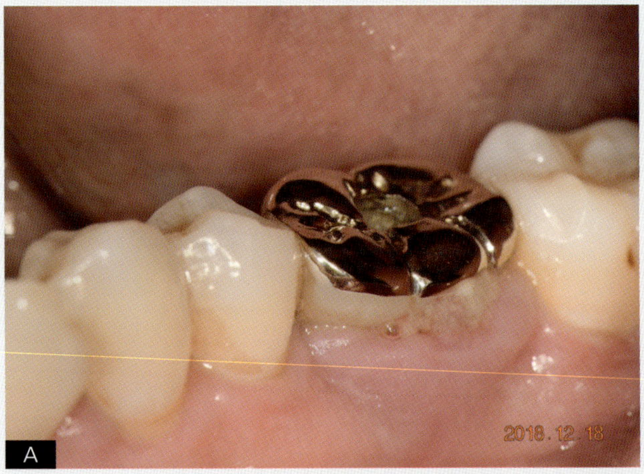

A

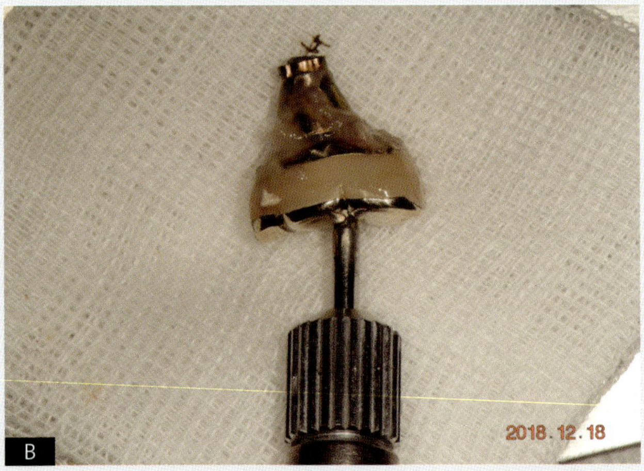

B

Therefore, it is essential for dental clinicians to have a comprehensive understanding of the implant–abutment interface, which encompasses the implant, abutment, and abutment screw.

1. Biomechanics of implant-abutment interface

The stability of the implant–abutment connection is a critical factor for the long-term clinical success of dental implants. To address complications caused by unstable implant–abutment connections—commonly observed in clinical practice—it is essential to thoroughly understand the biomechanics at the implant–abutment interface. Currently, implants used in clinical practice feature one of two connection types: the external hex connection or the internal friction connection. Accordingly, this section will examine in detail the biomechanical characteristics of the screw-retained connection (external hex connection) and the friction-screw-retained connection (internal friction connection)

1) Screw-retained connection

A screw-retained connection is an implant–abutment connection maintained solely by tightening the abutment screw. In this arrangement, the abutment is secured to the implant by the force applied through the tightened abutment screw.

This connection type is known as an external hex connection because the topmost portion of the implant exhibits a hexagonal geometry when viewed from above (Figure 2-1).

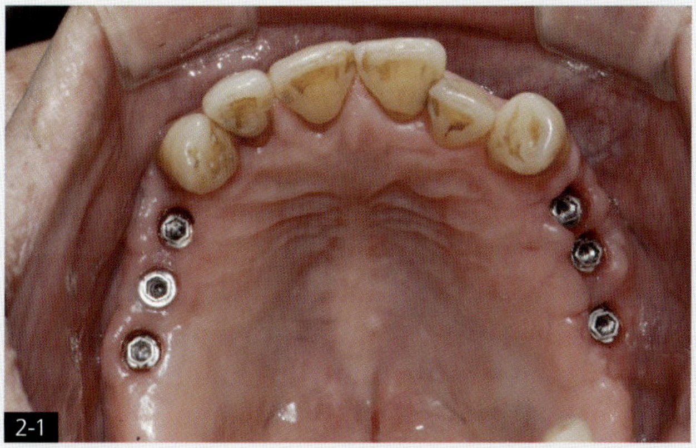

2-1

The dental implants with an external hex connection are shown. Notice the hexagonal geometry on top of the implants.

The flat surface at the top of the implant comes into direct contact with the flat surface at the bottom of the abutment, forming a butt joint interface.

A screw-retained connection is stabilized solely by the tightening force of the abutment screw. As the abutment screw is tightened, it elongates, thereby generating preload. Because the stability of the implant–abutment connection depends on this preload, it is considered a critical factor in screw mechanics (Figure 2-2). Preload, defined as the tension created in a fastener when it is tightened, serves as the tightening force within the implant–abutment connection and provides stability to the interface.

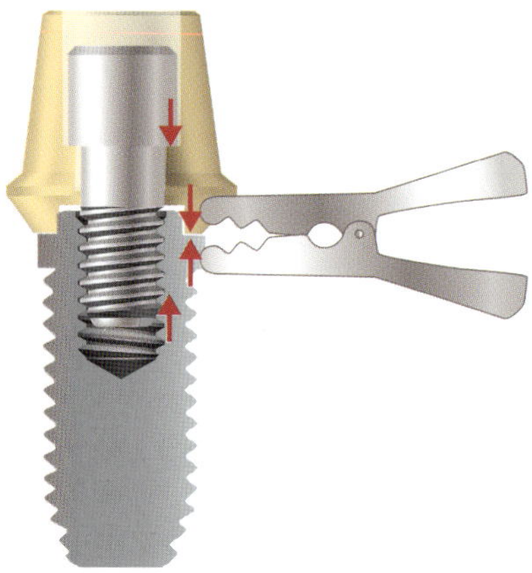

2-2

Schematic diagram illustrating the preload (also referred to as clamping force) generated by screw tightening.

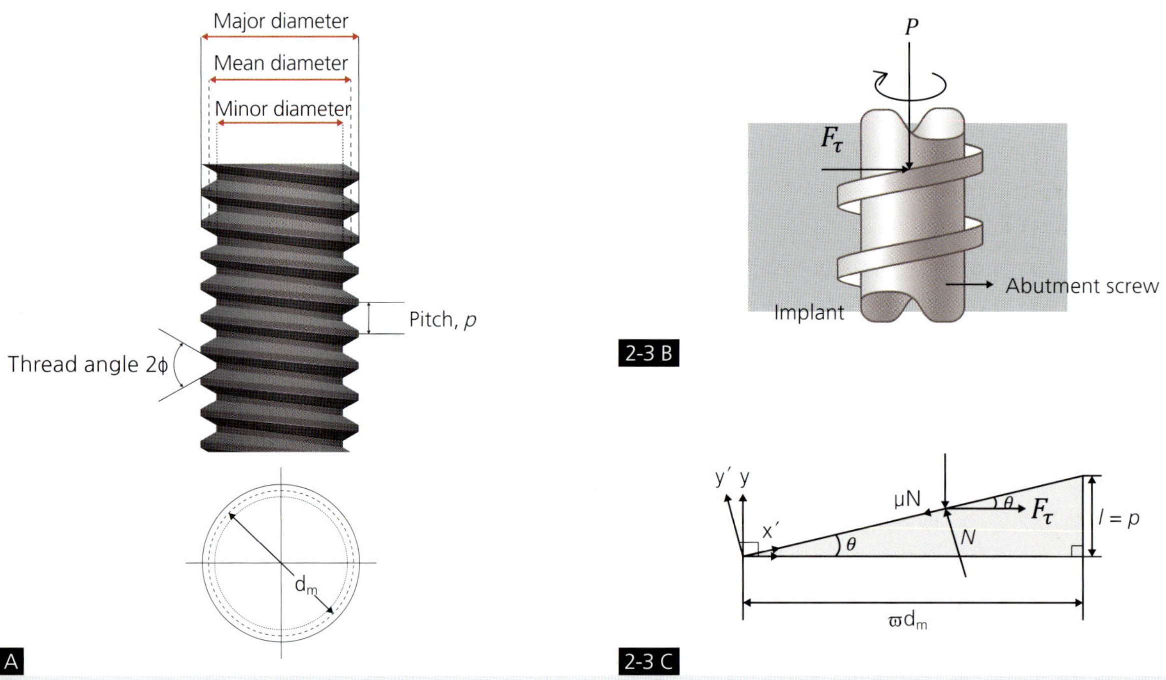

2-3 A 2-3 B 2-3 C

Terms and schematic diagrams used in screw mechanics.
(A) The major diameter refers to the largest diameter of the screw thread, while the minor diameter represents the smallest diameter. The mean diameter (dm) can be considered the screw's average diameter, although it is not strictly the arithmetic mean of the major and minor diameters. Notably, when discussing the diameter of a threaded implant, dental clinicians and researchers typically refer to the major diameter, whereas professionals in fields such as mechanical engineering often consider the mean diameter. (B) Tightening the abutment screw generates preload (P). (C) A free body diagram for force analysis, illustrating the state depicted in (B).

As shown in **Figure 2-3**, a screw is composed of several critical components. The structure presented here is a single-thread design, featuring identical lead (*l*) and pitch (*p*).

Screw joint structures can be theoretically analyzed based on the principles of screw mechanics. Assuming zero acceleration until just before the screw begins to rotate under the applied torque, the force equilibrium in the x'-axis direction can be expressed as follows.

$$① \quad F_{x'} = -P\sin\theta + F_\tau\cos\theta - \mu N = 0$$

P represents preload, and F_τ denotes the transitional force generated by torque. N is the normal force, the force that the two contact surfaces exert to prevent solid objects from passing through each other. μ is the friction coefficient between the screw threads, and θ is the lead angle of the screw. Since the normal force can be expressed as $N = P\cos\theta + F_\tau\sin\theta$, combining this with Equation ① allows for the calculation of the tightening torque (τ_t) as follows:

$$② \quad \tau_t = \frac{d_m}{2}F_\tau = \frac{d_m}{2}P\frac{\tan\theta+\mu}{1-\mu\tan\theta} \quad (d_m\text{: mean diameter})$$

When the implant's screw thread is V-shaped (as is the case with most abutment screws used in dental clinics) and the thread angle is 2φ, the friction coefficient μ is divided by $\cos\varphi$. Therefore, the tightening torque is calculated as follows:

$$③ \quad \tau_t = \frac{d_m}{2}P\frac{l+\pi\mu d_m\sec\varphi}{\pi d_m-\mu l\sec\varphi}$$

Regarding loosening torque, the direction of the forces is opposite. By reversing the signs of the transitional force and frictional force, the equation can be rearranged as follows:

$$④ \quad \tau_l = \frac{d_m}{2}P\frac{\pi\mu d_m\sec\varphi-l}{\pi d_m+\mu l\sec\varphi}$$

Although the coefficients of static friction and kinetic friction differ, this analysis considers the conditions at the end of tightening and the onset of loosening, where the forces are in equilibrium. Therefore, the friction coefficient is assumed to be identical in both scenarios. Since θ and $\mu\sec\varphi$ are very small values, the difference between tightening torque and loosening torque can be represented as a linear function.

$$⑤ \quad \Delta\tau = \tau_t - \tau_l = P\frac{l}{\pi}$$

Abutment screws are predominantly manufactured from grade 5 titanium alloy, which has a yield strength of approximately 827 MPa.

It is established that screws subjected to a preload exceeding 75% of the yield strength do not experience loosening. Based on this, the minimum preload required to prevent screw loosening is calculated to be 620 MPa. In clinical settings, abutment screws typically have a thread depth of about 0.2 mm and a major diameter of approximately 2.0 mm, with approximately three to five threads engaging and being tightened with the internal screw portion of the implant.

Therefore, by referencing these findings and applying the aforementioned equation with the manufacturer-recommended tightening torque values of 30–35 Ncm, the calculated preload reaches a maximum of approximately 125 MPa, which is significantly lower than the minimum preload of 620 MPa required to prevent screw loosening.

In practice, using Equation ⑤ to determine the tightening torque needed to achieve this minimum preload in a linear model results in a value exceeding 200 Ncm. Applying such high tightening torques in a clinical setting would likely cause abutment screw fractures or disrupt implant osseointegration.

In conclusion, the clinically recommended tightening torque of 30-35 Ncm is insufficient to prevent complications associated with screw loosening.

Implant–abutment connections that rely solely on screw-connection structures are inherently prone to loosening. Therefore, it is necessary to implement a clinical protocol in which abutment screws are periodically re-tightened to the manufacturer-recommended torque values during patient visits to maintain connection stability.

Another important aspect of the aforementioned biomechanical analysis is that when the implant–abutment connection depends exclusively on screw torque, as seen in screw-based structures, various factors inherent to screw mechanics naturally increase structural instability. Consequently, additional mechanisms beyond the screw are required to maintain stability.

One such mechanism is the utilization of interface friction. Through biomechanical analysis, it is possible to determine the extent to which friction contributes to the stability of the implant–abutment connection, even when the screw loosens.

2) Friction-screw-retained connection

The implant–abutment connection, classified as a friction-screw-retained connection, is stabilized by both the frictional forces at the interface and the tightening torque of the abutment screw. While the tightening torque of the abutment screw contributes to the connection's stability, it is also maintained through the close contact between the implant's inclined inner and the abutment's inclined outer surface.

This close contact generates the normal force, which in turn produces frictional forces, thereby enhancing the stability of the connection structure. In implant dentistry, this type of joint is observed in internal friction connections, where the abutment is inserted into the interior of the implant, forming a frictional interface between the implant and abutment.

A one-piece abutment integrates both the frictional interface and the screw components into a single unit, whereas a two-piece abutment comprises two separate components: the abutment forming the frictional interface and the abutment screw **(Figure 2-4)**.

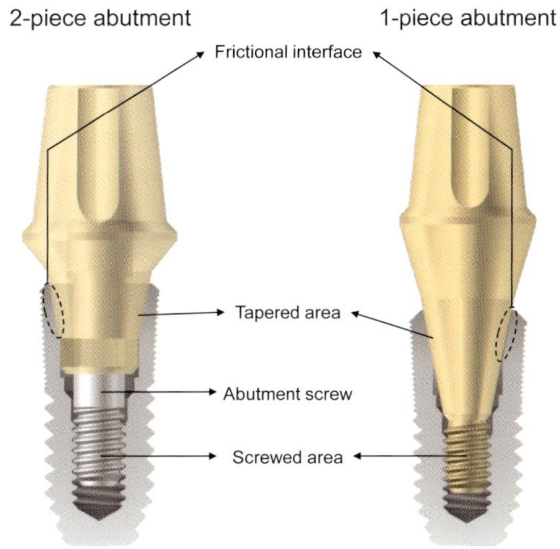

2-4

Cross-sectional schematic diagram illustrating the structural differences between two-piece abutment (left) and one-piece abutment (right).

As shown in **Figure 2-4**, when a tightening force is applied between the implant and abutment, resistance occurs at the taper region, where significant friction is generated, leading to the development of preload as the screw advances. Assuming the implant and abutment are made of the same material, the taper region and the screw portion can be biomechanically analyzed as distinct components within this type of friction-screw-retained connection.

In clinical practice, implants are often made of Grade 4 commercially pure titanium, whereas abutments and abutment screws are typically manufactured from Grade 5 titanium alloy. Because these materials exhibit different chemical properties, their interactions may produce biomechanical outcomes that differ from those of components made of identical materials. Nonetheless, this variation is primarily a matter of interpretation, given that the underlying mechanisms remain fundamentally the same.
The total tightening torque can be calculated as the sum of the torque applied to the taper region and the screw portion.

① $\tau_{t,sum} = \tau_{t,T} + \tau_{t,S}$ (T: Tapered area, S: Screwed area)

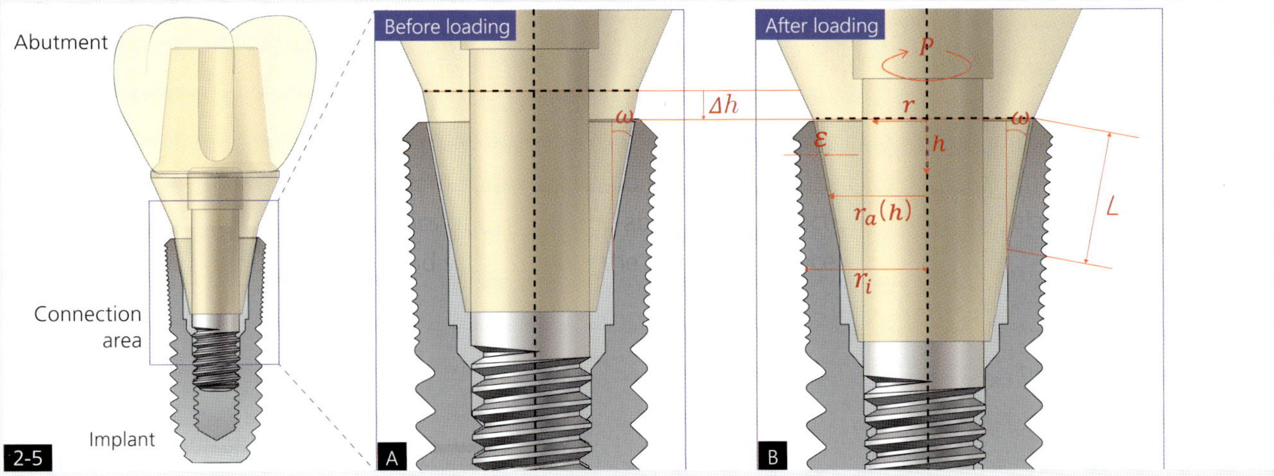

2-5

(A) Cross-sectional schematic diagram showing an enlarged view of the connection area in a friction-screw-retained connection. (B) Illustration of the system when the abutment screw is tightened, generating torque and preload. The abutment advances by Δh along the implant's long axis ($\varepsilon = \Delta h \tan \omega$). In this two-dimensional cross-section, the contact between the abutment's external surface and the implant's internal surface is represented as a length L. Together with the angle ω formed between the taper and the implant's long axis, these two variables predominantly govern the stability of the implant–abutment connection.

Figure 2-5 schematically shows the taper portion of an abutment inserted into a dental implant with a friction-screw-retained connection.

Similar to the screw-retained connection, the friction-screw-retained connection is assumed to achieve a stable equilibrium state after final tightening. By applying the same coefficient of friction for both tightening and loosening, calculations can be performed with relative ease. As shown in Figure 2-5A, there is initially no resistance. However, as tightening is applied, the normal force is generated, causing the implant to strongly resist the insertion of the abutment, as depicted in Figure 2-5B.

Consequently, when the vertical height at which the abutment is inserted from the uppermost surface of the implant is defined as h, the contact pressure $p(h)$ generated at the contact interface between the two structures during the tightening of the abutment to the implant is calculated as follows:

② $$p(h) = \frac{E\varepsilon\left[r_i^2 - r_a^2(h)\right]\cos\omega}{2r_a(h)r_i^2}$$

(E: Young's modulus of implant and abutment materials, ε: dimensional difference between implant and abutment generating resistance, r_i: radius of the implant, $r_a(h)$: radius of the abutment as a function of height, ω: taper angle, the angle between the inclined plane and the implant's long axis)

Differential of the normal force, dN, resulting from the insertion and tightening of the abutment into the implant, and the abutment's external radius as a function of insertion height, $r_a(h)$, are related by the following equation:

③ $dN = p(h) \times 2\pi r_a(h)dh$

By combining the equation derived from the section, '1) Screw-retained connection,' with the tightening torque calculated at the friction interface of the taper portion discussed herein, an approximate relationship can be established as follows:

$$④\quad \tau_{t,sum} = \frac{d_m}{2} P \frac{l+\pi\mu d_m \sec\varphi}{\pi d_m - \mu l \sec\varphi} + \int r_a(h)\mu dN \cos\theta$$

$$= \frac{d_m}{2} P \frac{l+\pi\mu d_m \sec\varphi}{\pi d_m - \mu l \sec\varphi} + AL^4 + BL^3 + CL^2 + DL$$

(2φ: thread angle of the abutment screw, θ: lead angle of the abutment screw. A, B, C, and D are all constants)

Here, the preload, P, represents the force opposing the direction of progression when the abutment is tightened by the abutment screw. Similarly, the total loosening torque can be calculated by considering only the sections where the vector directions in the screw portion are opposite. Notably, the calculation for the taper portion ultimately results in a value equivalent to the tightening torque.

$$⑤\quad \tau_{l,sum} = \tau_{l,S} + \tau_{l,T} = \frac{d_m}{2} P \frac{\pi\mu d_m \sec\varphi - l}{\pi d_m + \mu l \sec\varphi} + (AL^4 + BL^3 + CL^2 + DL)$$

It is important to note that the scenario described by Equation ⑤ represents the moment just before loosening occurs. When the screw portion subsequently becomes loose, the preload disappears ($P = 0$), resulting in $\tau_{l,S} = 0$ in Equation ⑤. Consequently, the stability of the implant–abutment connection relies solely on the taper portion. Considering a one-piece abutment makes this biomechanical scenario easier to understand.

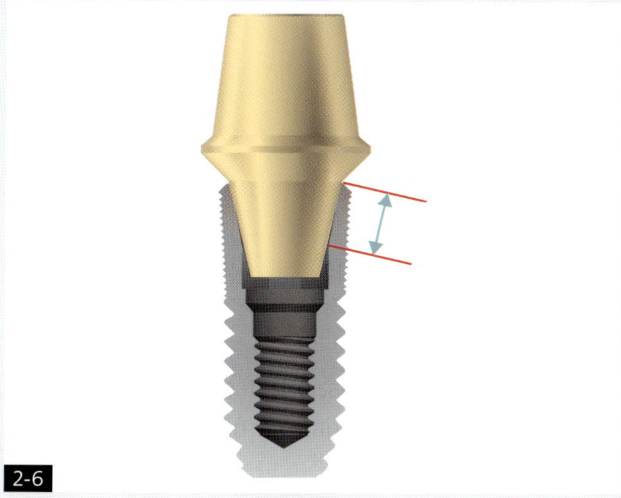
2-6

The contact occurs between the implant's inner surface and the abutment's outer surface in the arrow-marked region shown in **Figure 2-6**. The stability of the implant–abutment connection is proportional to the fourth power of this contact length.

Equations ④ and ⑤ reveal several biomechanical characteristics of the friction-screw-retained connection.

It is particularly important to understand that torque is proportional to the fourth power of the contact length between the implant's inner surface and the abutment's outer surface. In other words, in an internal friction connection, even a slight increase in contact length can significantly enhance the loosening torque value, which is clinically interpreted as highly beneficial for maintaining the stability of the implant–abutment connection.

When considering a two-piece abutment, this phenomenon becomes even more apparent. In clinical settings, when implant-supported restorations are subjected to cyclic loading—such as during mastication—screw loosening may occur, resulting in the loss of preload. Despite this, the taper portion of the implant–abutment connection can maintain stability, preventing abutment movement. This helps avoid soft tissue attachment loss around the implant, the subsequent formation of periodontal pockets, and the progression to peri-implantitis, at least until the abutment screw is retightened during routine follow-up visits.

The space at the arrow-marked region **(Figure 2-7)** results from repeated (cyclic) loading, eliminating the preload. However, abutment movement may not be observed clinically, because the friction between the implant's inner surface and the abutment's outer surface maintains stability. If the contact area of the implant–abutment connection decreases, the connection stability is significantly reduced, thereby diminishing its effectiveness in preventing such clinical complications.

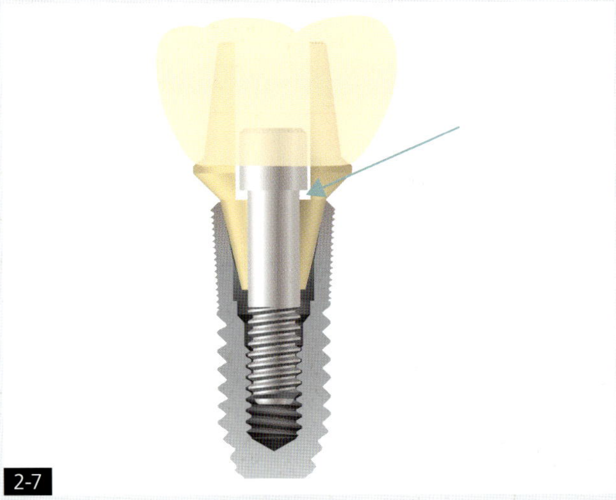

2-7

In a friction-screw-retained connection, the proportion of torque contributed by the taper portion to the total torque can be calculated. As shown in **Figure 2-7**, the smaller the taper angle ω formed between the oblique line (inclined plane) and the implant's long axis, the greater the proportion of torque contributed by the taper portion. When ω is 11° or less, the taper portion accounts for more than 70% of the total torque. More importantly, in cases of screw loosening, where preload is lost, the entire torque is exerted solely by the taper portion, resulting in the taper's contribution reaching 1 (100%).

2. Stability of the implant-abutment connection: a mechanical factor contributing to peri-implantitis

To ensure the long-term success of implant-supported restorations, it is essential to minimize complications involving the abutment, abutment screw, and prosthetic superstructure. A thorough evaluation of both the mechanical and biological aspects of these restorations, coupled with accurate clinical interpretation, is crucial for the implant to function effectively in the patient's oral cavity over an extended period.
Mechanical complications include implant tearing or fracture, abutment screw loosening or fracture, and detachment or fracture of the prosthodontic superstructure.

Let us examine clinical cases of these complications.

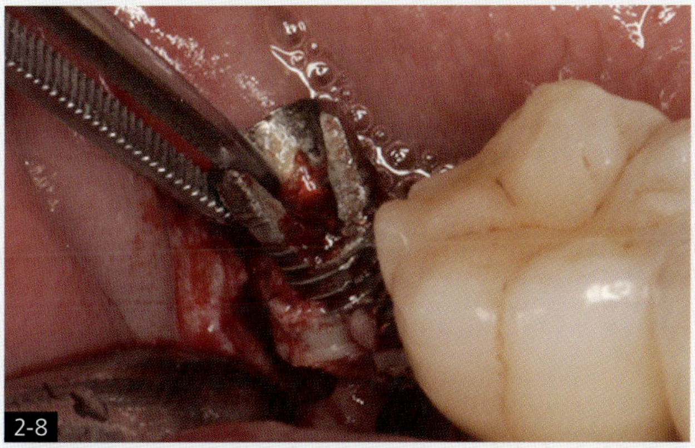
2-8

In Figure 2-8, a relatively thick implant tore unexpectedly, illustrating implant fracture.

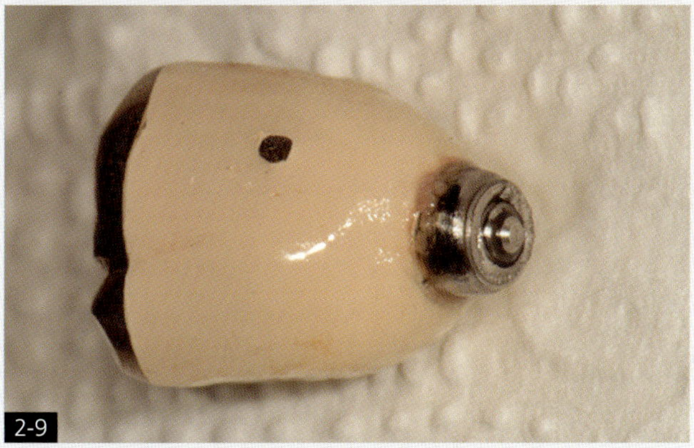
2-9

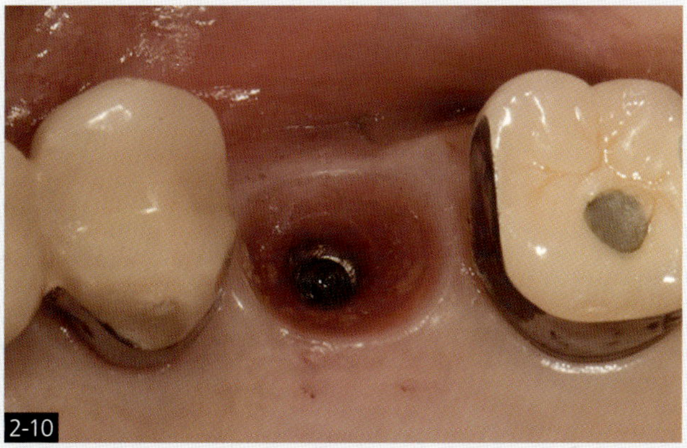
2-10

Figures 2-9 and 2-10 depict an internal friction connection implant in which both the abutment and the screw fractured simultaneously.

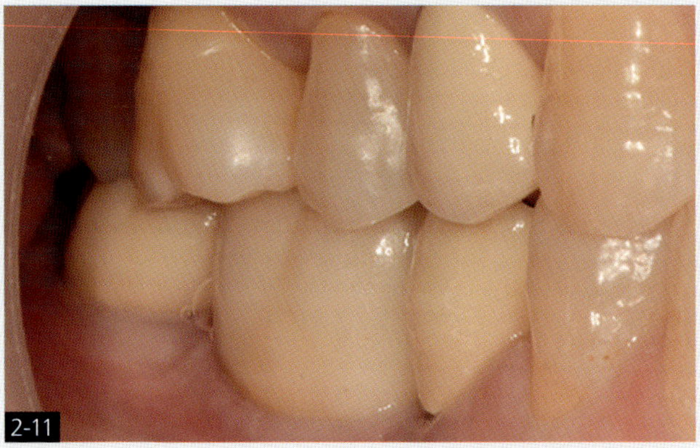
2-11

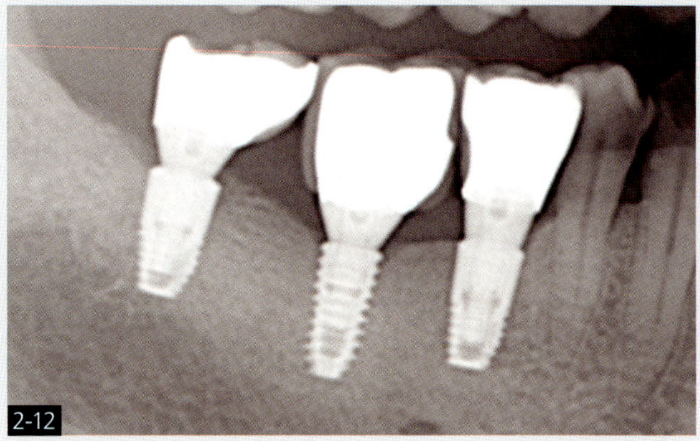
2-12

Three implants were placed, and each was restored with a prosthesis.

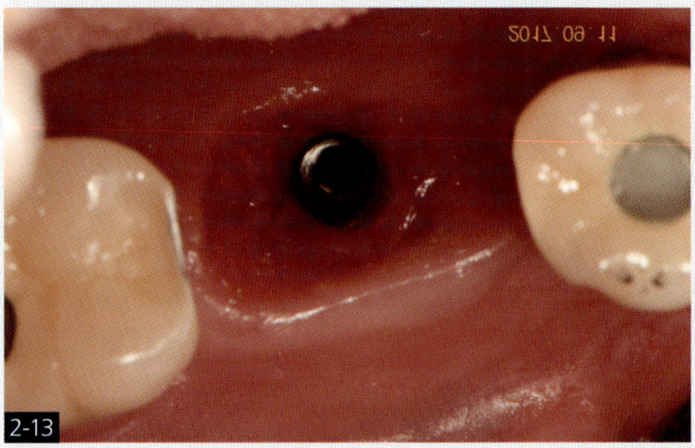
2-13

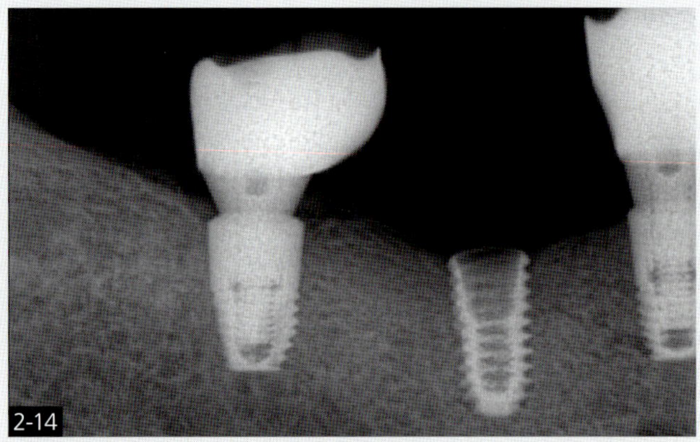
2-14

On a later visit, the patient presented with the prosthesis detached, as the abutment screw had loosened.

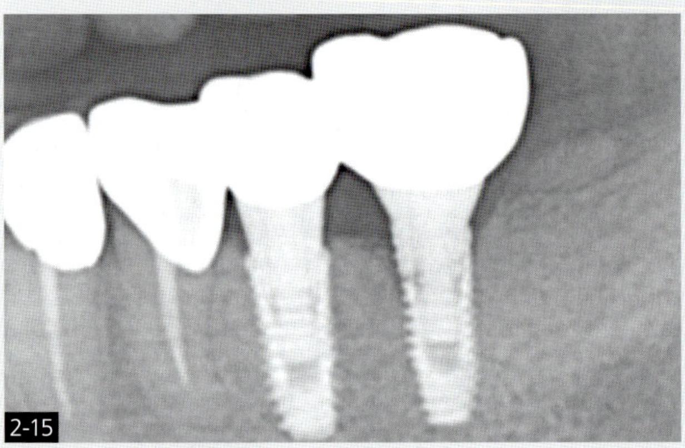
2-15

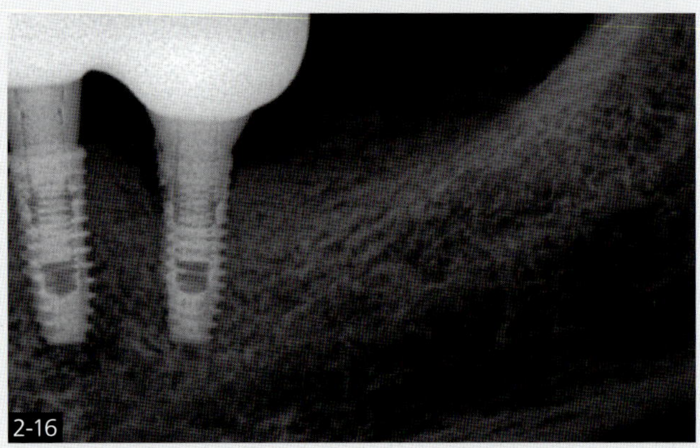
2-16

Let us examine another clinical case.
A fracture in the #37 implant was noted on a panoramic radiograph and subsequently confirmed on a periapical radiograph.

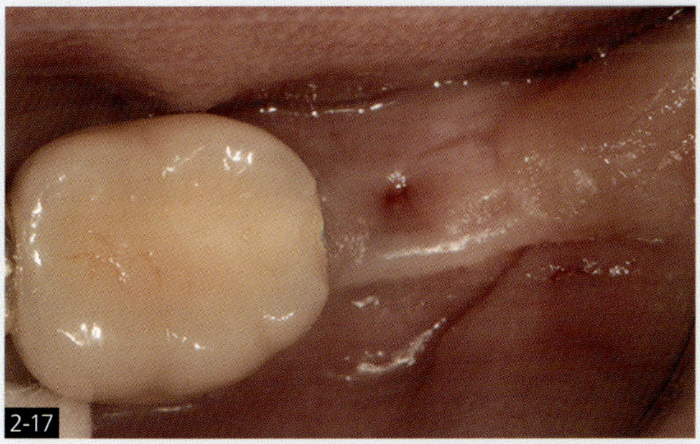

2-17

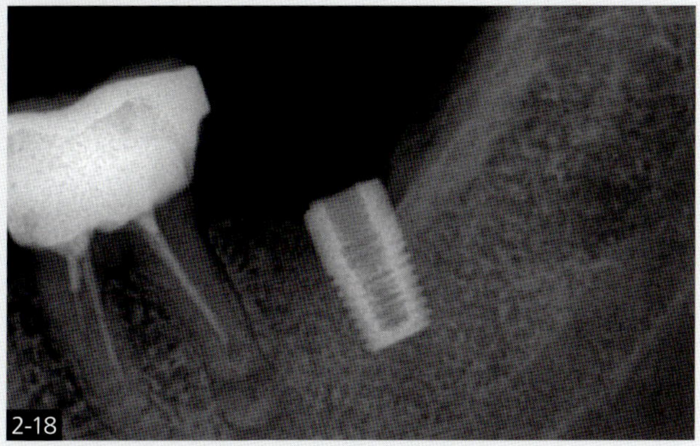

2-18

After definitive restoration, the abutment fractured, the screw became loosened and separated from the implant, prompting the patient to return for care **(Figures 2-17 and 18)**.

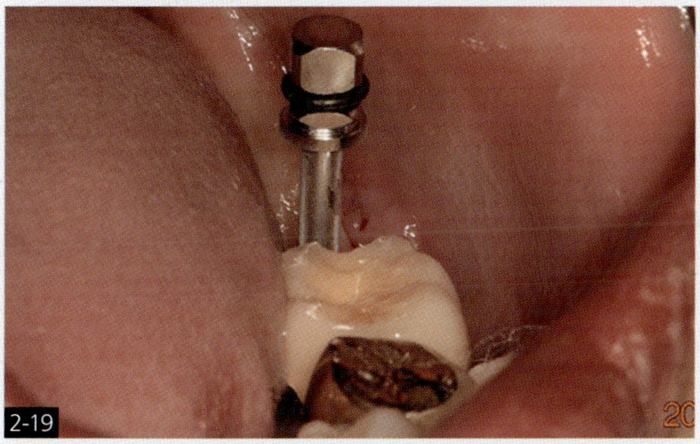

2-19

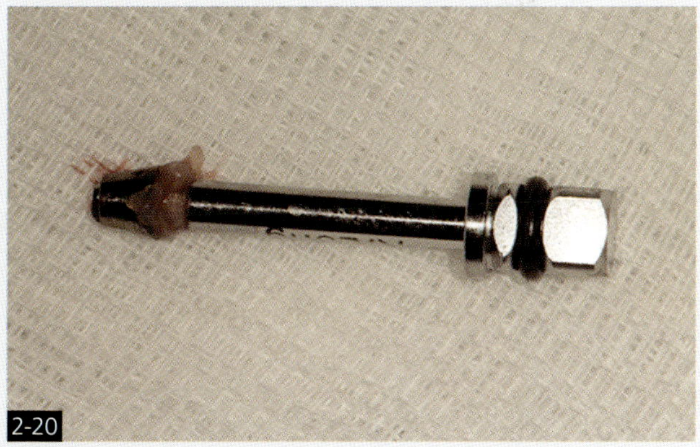

2-20

Using a removal tool produced by an implant manufacturer, the fractured abutment was removed with ease **(Figures 2-19 and 20)**.

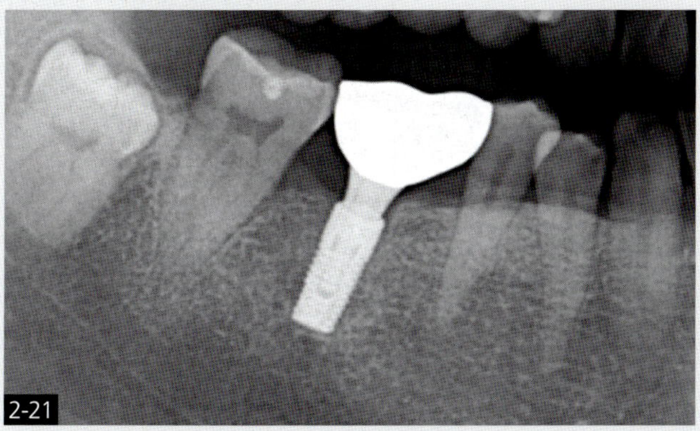

2-21

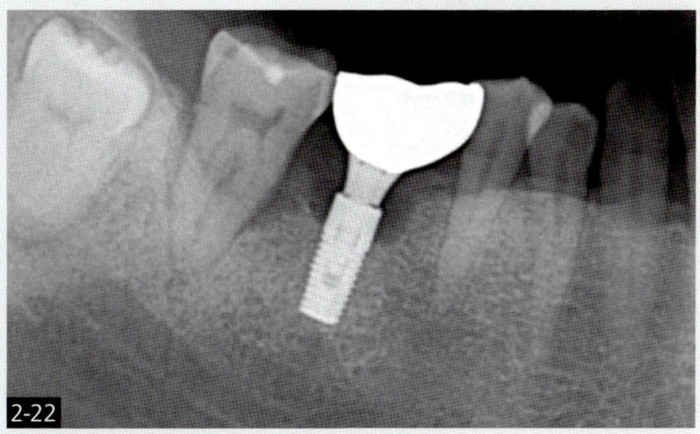

2-22

Peri-implantitis suddenly developed around the #46 implant, and radiographs confirmed the abutment fracture **(Figures 2-21 and 22)**. The mobility resulting from the fractured abutment disrupted the mucosal seal, allowing bacterial infiltration and leading to alveolar bone loss.

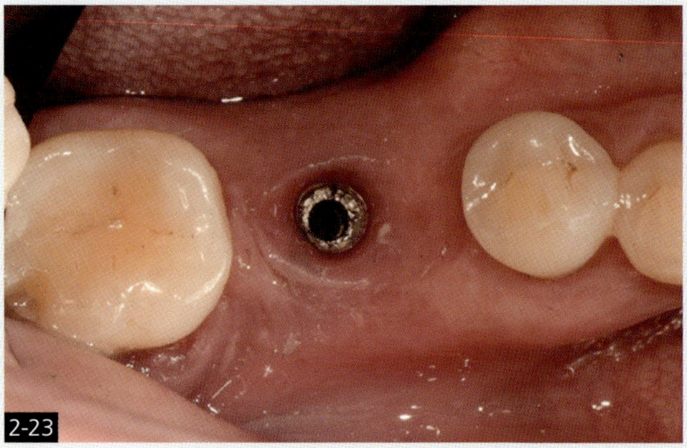
2-23

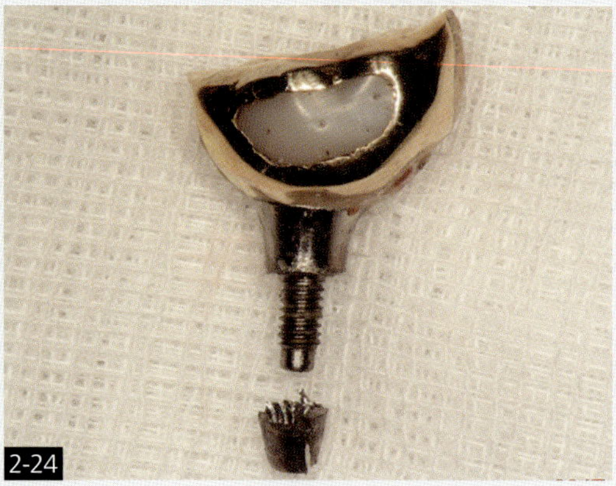
2-24

We removed the fractured abutment (Figures 2-23 and 24). If an implant-supported crown becomes mobile, abutment fracture should be considered in addition to screw loosening. Furthermore, abutment fracture or instability can lead to peri-implantitis.

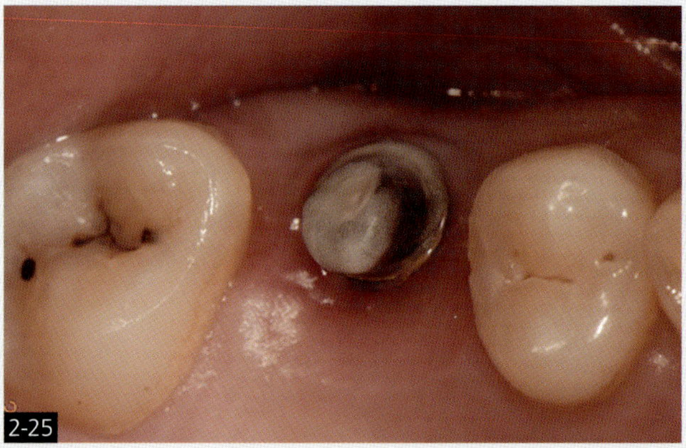
2-25

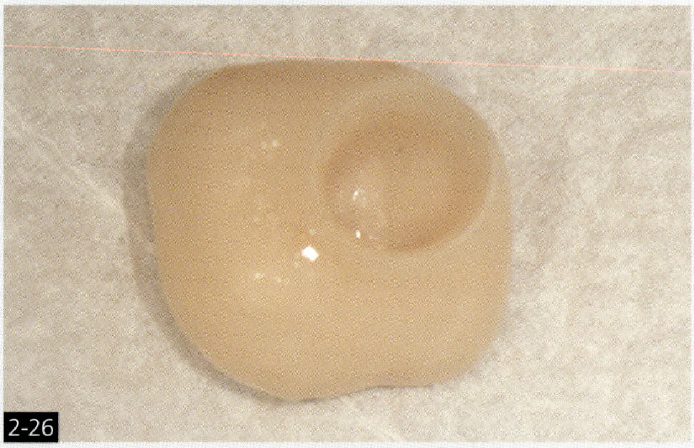
2-26

A patient presented with a chief complaint of a dislodged crown. While the abutment surface retained some cement (Figure 2-25), the internal surface of the prosthesis had no residual cement (Figure 2-26).

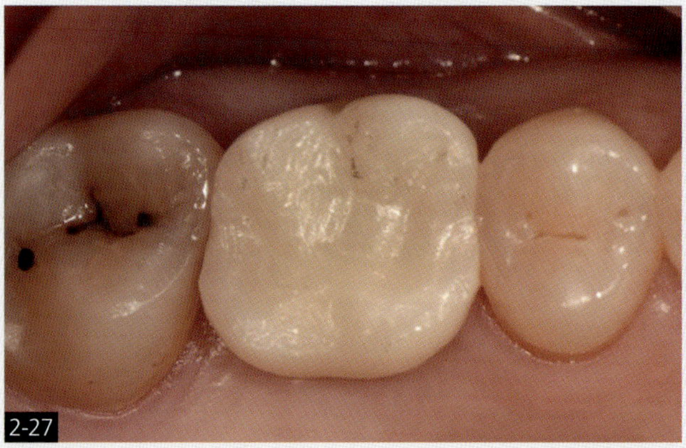
2-27

Although the crown was re-cemented, it is expected to become dislodged again (Figure 2-27).

In an artificial crown supported by one implant, loss of cement typically results in the crown dislodging; however, in a prosthesis supported by multiple implants, as demonstrated in the following cases, the situation can become more complicated.

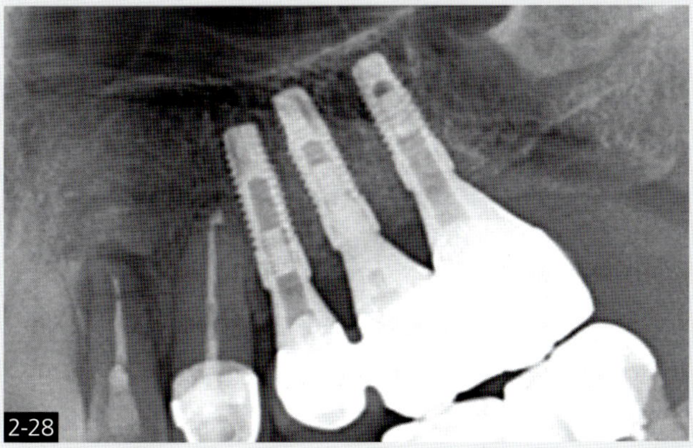

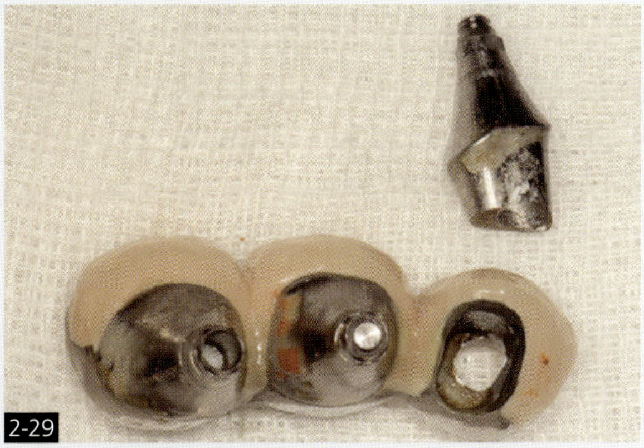

This patient was referred by a senior colleague. The abutment screws in implants #25 and #27 have fractured, leaving remnants inside the implants **(Figure 2-28)**. The internal surface of the prosthesis on tooth #24 shows loss of cement **(Figure 2-29)**, which appears to be directly related to the screw fracture.

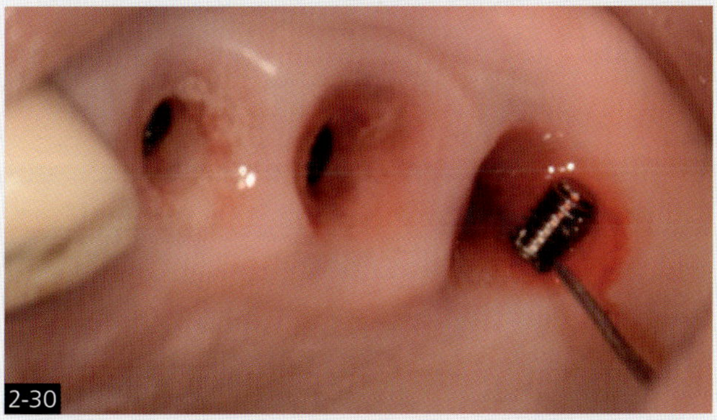

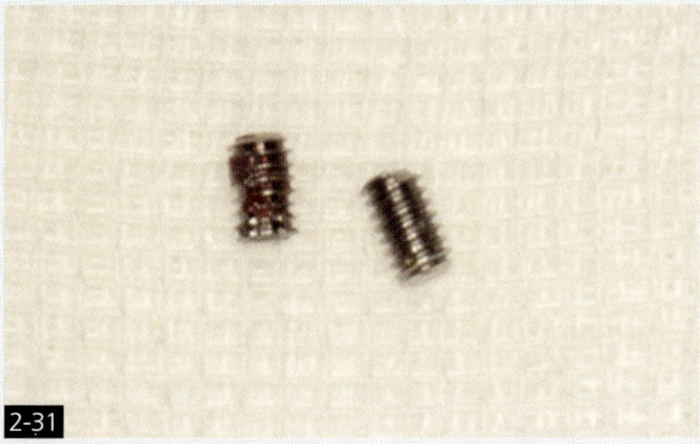

The fractured abutment screw remnants are removed by rotating them counterclockwise with a dental probe **(Figures 2-30 and 31)**.

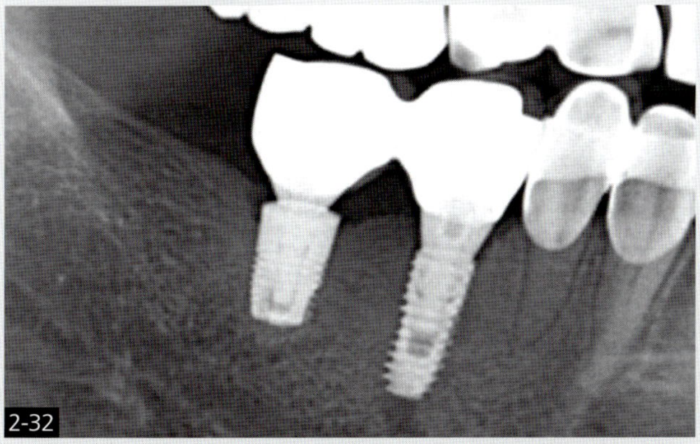

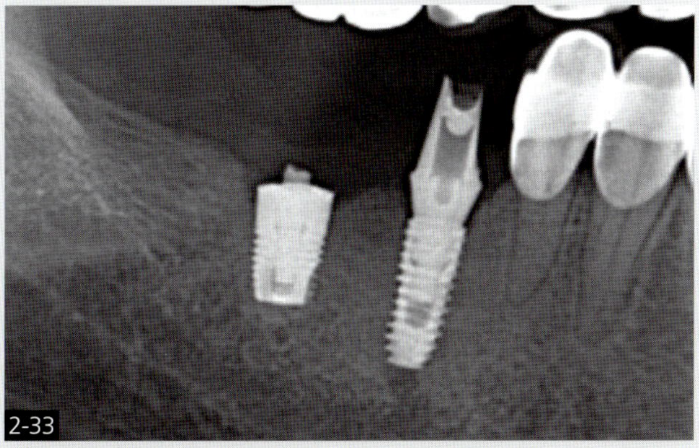

When the prosthesis dislodged from the implant at tooth #45, the abutment and abutment screw at tooth #46 subsequently fractured **(Figures 2-32 and 33)**.

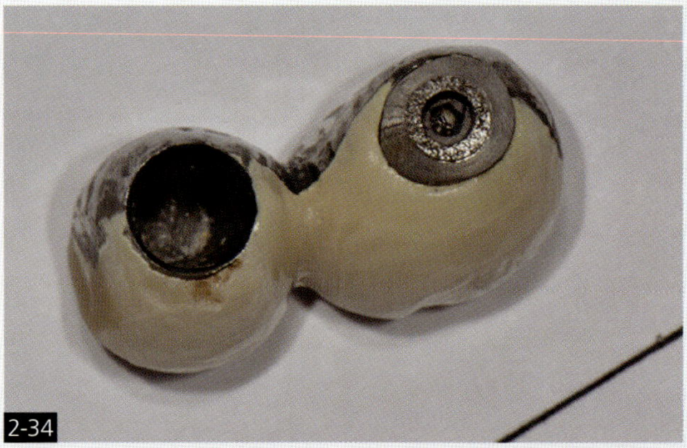
2-34

The inner surface of the prosthesis at tooth #45 shows a loss of cement, causing all masticatory forces to concentrate on tooth #46, which is believed to have led to the mechanical complication. The poor quality of the prosthesis is considered a contributing factor to the fracture of the implant components.

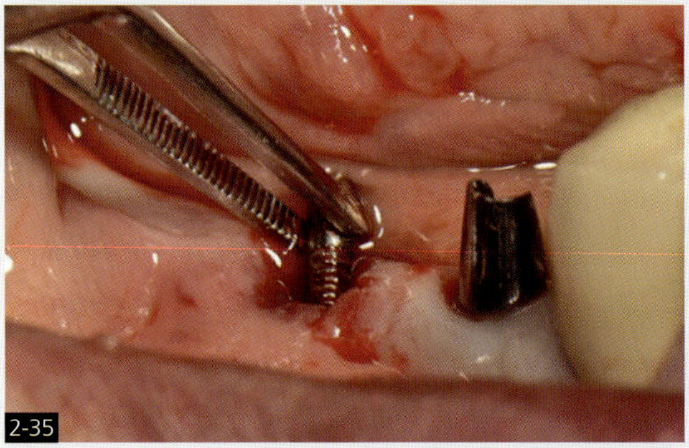
2-35

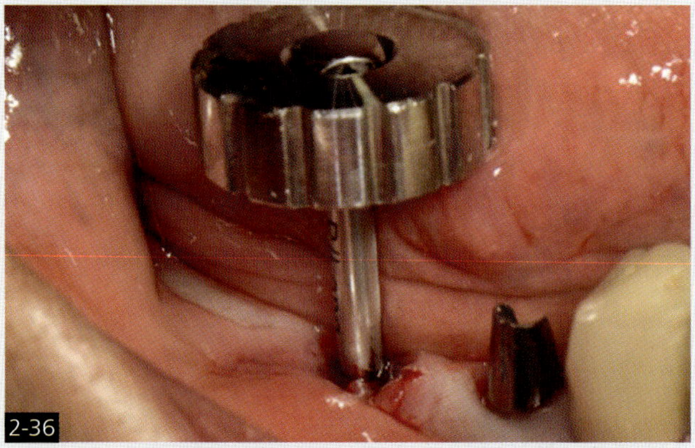
2-36

The fractured screw is removed **(Figure 2-35)**, and the remaining abutment fragments are extracted **(Figure 2-36)**.
Numerous issues can arise at the implant connection interface due to various factors.

Biological complications primarily refer to issues affecting the peri-implant tissues, with bacterial invasion identified as a major cause. These complications can be categorized into peri-implant mucositis and peri-implantitis, corresponding to gingivitis and periodontitis in natural teeth, respectively. Peri-implantitis and periodontitis are known to share similar initiation and progression patterns, as well as bacterial profiles.

Historically, mechanical complications and bacteria-induced biological complications were considered independent phenomena. However, recent studies have demonstrated a close relationship between these two types of complications. This relationship underscores that the disruption of the soft tissue seal can lead to peri-implantitis. When the soft tissue seal is lost, it permits bacterial colonization and invasion, ultimately resulting in peri-implantitis.

The loss of soft tissue attachment can occur due to factors such as a lack of attached gingiva, a shallow vestibule, or a high frenum. However, in implant-supported restorations, this loss is primarily caused by abutment movement resulting from an unstable implant–abutment

When the stability of the implant–abutment connection is compromised, abutment movement can occur. Consequently, the mechanical connection between the implant and abutment becomes a critical factor in determining the longevity of implant-supported restorations.

Once the prosthetic superstructure is installed, three types of forces act on the implant–abutment interface: vertical forces, lateral forces, and rotational forces **(Figure 2-37)**.

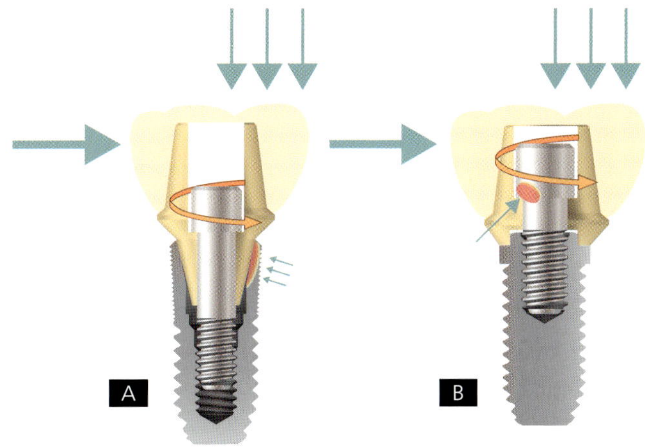

2-37

Schematic diagram illustrating the vertical, lateral, and rotational forces acting on the implant–abutment interface during masticatory loading (indicated by the light blue arrow).
The friction-screw-retained connection (A) demonstrates greater resistance due to its frictional interface compared to the screw-retained connection (B). In the screw-retained connection (B), micromovement of the abutment, where it momentarily separates from the implant under masticatory forces, can be observed.

Most implants are structurally strong against vertical forces but are weaker against lateral forces, which significantly contribute to the loosening of the abutment screw. Generally, the implant–abutment connection area incorporates a hexagonal anti-rotational structure at the junction to resist rotational forces. To ensure the long-term success and functionality of implant-supported restorations, the implant–abutment connection must effectively resist these three types of forces—vertical, lateral, and rotational—while adequately distributing the loads in conjunction with the abutment screw and hexagonal structure.

The Brånemark implant, the first commercially available screw-shaped implant in modern dentistry, is a classic example of a screw-retained connection (external hex connection). Vertical forces are well-supported by the robust platform where the implant and abutment meet, while the abutment screw and hexagonal structure at the top of the implant resist lateral forces. Additionally, the hexagonal structure is designed to withstand rotational forces.

Issues arise when masticatory forces are applied to the implant, as all forces concentrate on the abutment screw. Due to the structure's relative weakness in resisting lateral and rotational forces, the implant–abutment connection area tends to exhibit movement under load. This instability disrupts the soft tissue attachment, or mucosal seal, allowing routine bacterial infiltration and increasing the likelihood of peri-implant tissue inflammation. To prevent abutment movement, the height of the hexagonal structure at the top of the implant should ideally be increased. However, clinically, increasing the height of this hexagonal structure complicates procedures such as soft tissue flap closure. Consequently, the hexagonal structure is typically maintained at a height of 0.7 mm, functioning more as a tool for implant placement rather than as a design optimized for resisting masticatory forces. To enhance the stability of the implant–abutment connection, several approaches can be considered, such as manufacturing abutment screws from materials with higher strength, widening the implant platform, or applying greater torque during tightening. However, these methods face significant clinical limitations. In conclusion, implant systems utilizing the external hex connection, which is representative of screw-retained connections, cannot fundamentally prevent abutment movement.

Although friction-screw-retained connections also incorporate abutment screws, the abutment screw plays a less critical role than in screw-retained connections. In friction-screw-retained connections, the stability of the implant–abutment connection is more dependent on the frictional forces between the two components. Some implant manufacturers have developed systems that rely exclusively on these frictional forces. These systems are designed to secure the abutment to the implant without the use of an abutment screw by adjusting the taper angle of the abutment to as little as 1.5°, approaching 0°.

The close contact between the internal surface of the implant and the external surface of the abutment provides effective resistance to vertical, lateral, and rotational forces generated during mastication, without causing abutment movement. Consequently, this minimizes soft tissue attachment loss and helps prevent marginal bone resorption.

As explained in the biomechanical analysis section, the taper angle formed between the contact surface of the abutment and the implant's long axis is a critical factor in determining the stability of a friction-screw-retained connection. A larger taper angle reduces stability and increases reliance on the abutment screw. Although not explicitly considered in theoretical calculations, an important feature from clinical and engineering perspectives in friction-screw-retained connections must be accounted for: when the abutment initially engages with the implant via friction, contact is limited to the uppermost portion of the implant. Over time, as functional loads such as masticatory forces are applied, the contact area gradually increases to encompass the entire internal surface of the implant. This phenomenon occurs due to the slight expansion of the upper part of the implant under repeated loading, resulting in the abutment becoming progressively more deeply engaged within the implant.
Therefore, as the preload on the abutment screw decreases, screw loosening occurs, making it essential to perform retightening procedures during regular follow-up visits in clinical practice. If this retightening process is skipped, it may eventually lead to abutment movement, resulting in soft tissue attachment loss and peri-implant tissue diseases.

Although all implant manufacturers claim to have unique connection designs, almost all connection structures can be categorized into one of two types: screw-retained connections or friction-screw-retained connections. Dental clinicians must have a thorough understanding of the mechanisms associated with implant–abutment connection structures. This knowledge is critical for selecting appropriate implant systems and managing them effectively in the oral environment to prevent peri-implant diseases by ensuring the stability of the abutment and preventing its movement.

3. Hard and soft tissue responses surrounding the implant-abutment interface

Implant-supported dental restorations must effectively replace the function of lost natural teeth and ensure long-term durability. As human life expectancy continues to increase, the longevity of these artificial replacements becomes increasingly critical.

Mechanical issues inherent to the implant system, as well as complications involving the surrounding soft and hard tissues, can limit the long-term use of implant-supported restorations in the oral cavity and, therefore, must be avoided.

The anatomical structures surrounding the implant include the alveolar bone, alveolar mucosa, and gingiva. The alveolar bone transmits occlusal forces applied to the implant, while the alveolar mucosa and gingiva protect the alveolar bone from oral bacteria, with the gingiva primarily fulfilling this protective role.

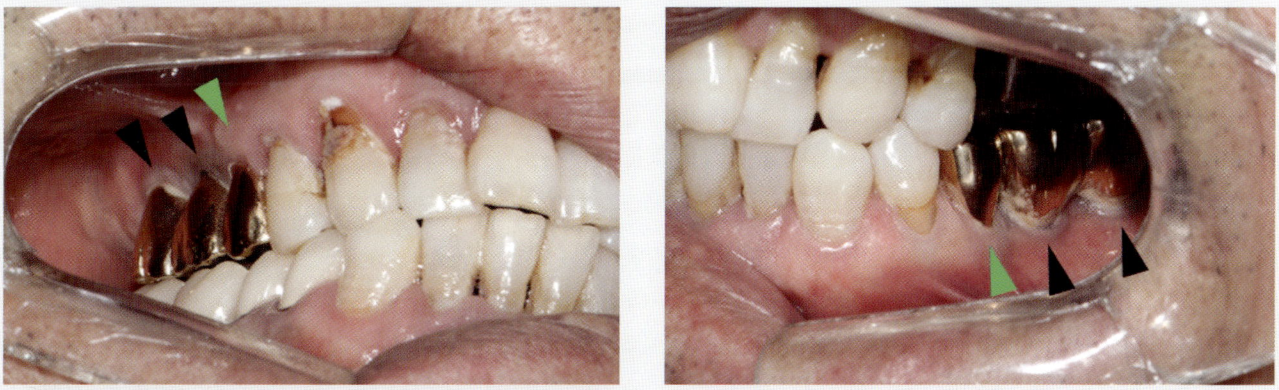

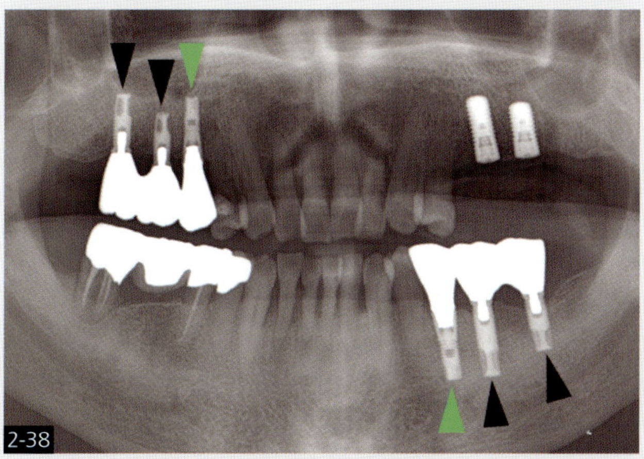

2-38 A case demonstrating the differences in clinical outcomes between friction-screw-retained and screw-retained connections

The alveolar bone and gingiva are mutually supportive. The health of the gingiva is maintained by the underlying alveolar bone, while the alveolar bone remains healthy under the protective cover of the gingiva. Generally, peri-implant alveolar bone undergoes resorption of 1–1.5 mm within the first year of occlusal loading, with subsequent annual resorption typically limited to 0.2 mm.

However, such research findings are based on the long-term clinical outcomes of the Brånemark implant system, which features a screw-retained connection structure with an unstable implant–abutment connection.
Implant systems with friction-screw-retained connections demonstrate relatively less bone resorption, and some clinical studies have even shown an increase in alveolar bone following occlusal loading **(Figure 2-38)**.

Implants with friction-screw-retained connections (indicated by green arrowheads in Figure 2-38) show maintenance or an increase in alveolar bone height, as well as a relative preservation of bone volume. In contrast, implants with screw-retained connections (indicated by black arrowheads in Figure 2-38) exhibit a gradual decrease in alveolar bone height and significant bone resorption.

If alveolar bone resorption occurs within normal physiological limits after the application of occlusal forces, the use of longer implants is generally advantageous for ensuring the long-term success of implant-supported restorations. Additionally, performing bone grafting after implant placement is recommended to compensate for this physiological bone resorption.

However, surgery with longer implants and bone grafting are more invasive procedures for the patient and pose greater challenges for the dental clinician. In some cases, longer implants may encroach upon the patient's anatomical structures, potentially causing complications such as nerve damage.

Therefore, using implant systems with friction-screw-retained connections, which minimize bone resorption, allows for the placement of shorter implants and reduces the need for extensive bone grafting. This approach lessens the surgical burden on the clinician and facilitates the implementation of minimally invasive techniques for the patient. Consequently, implant treatment is increasingly shifting toward methods that preserve alveolar bone height following functional loading in the oral cavity.

Alveolar bone is preserved when teeth are present. However, in cases of periodontitis, the alveolar bone is irreversibly destroyed. In the absence of periodontitis, most alveolar bone maintains its original volume and quality when dental function is properly maintained. When teeth are subjected to occlusal forces, these forces are transmitted through the periodontal ligament, which adequately stimulates the alveolar bone to preserve its volume and quality.

This relationship between teeth and alveolar bone provides insight into how alveolar bone may respond to implants.
If peri-implantitis is absent and the peri-implant alveolar bone is appropriately stimulated, it can similarly maintain its volume and quality. Astra Tech was among the first to design and supply implants incorporating this concept, demonstrating clinically that a properly designed implant–abutment connection can effectively stimulate alveolar bone, leading to increased bone volume and quality.

Frost's hypothesis supports this mechanism, proposing that strain applied to alveolar bone activates osteoblasts, which helps maintain bone volume and quality.

Despite the widespread use of implants in the oral cavity over recent decades, many have failed to sustain their initial healthy state.

Many studies report a survival rate exceeding 85% after 10 years of implant use. However, implants that remain in a healthy state without complications account for less than 30%. This indicates that implant-supported restorations frequently experience biological or mechanical complications over time in clinical settings.

In the 1980s, reports demonstrating that Brånemark implants achieved a clinical survival rate exceeding 90% after more than 10 years were groundbreaking and had a global impact. At that time, most cylindrical implants were failing, and the success of screw-shaped implants over extended periods in the oral cavity led to an oversight of issues such as soft tissue attachment loss, peri-implantitis, and the implant–abutment connection structure.

The high survival rate of Brånemark implants can be attributed to the incorporation of a threaded structure in their design. Unlike cylindrical implants, which were unable to effectively transmit occlusal forces to the alveolar bone, the threaded design of Brånemark implants allowed for better force transmission. Specifically, the threaded structure converts shear stress—forces that bone poorly tolerates—into compressive stress, which bone resists effectively. This ability to mitigate stress was a critical factor in supporting the long-term functionality of the prosthetic superstructure within the oral cavity **(Figure 2-39)**.

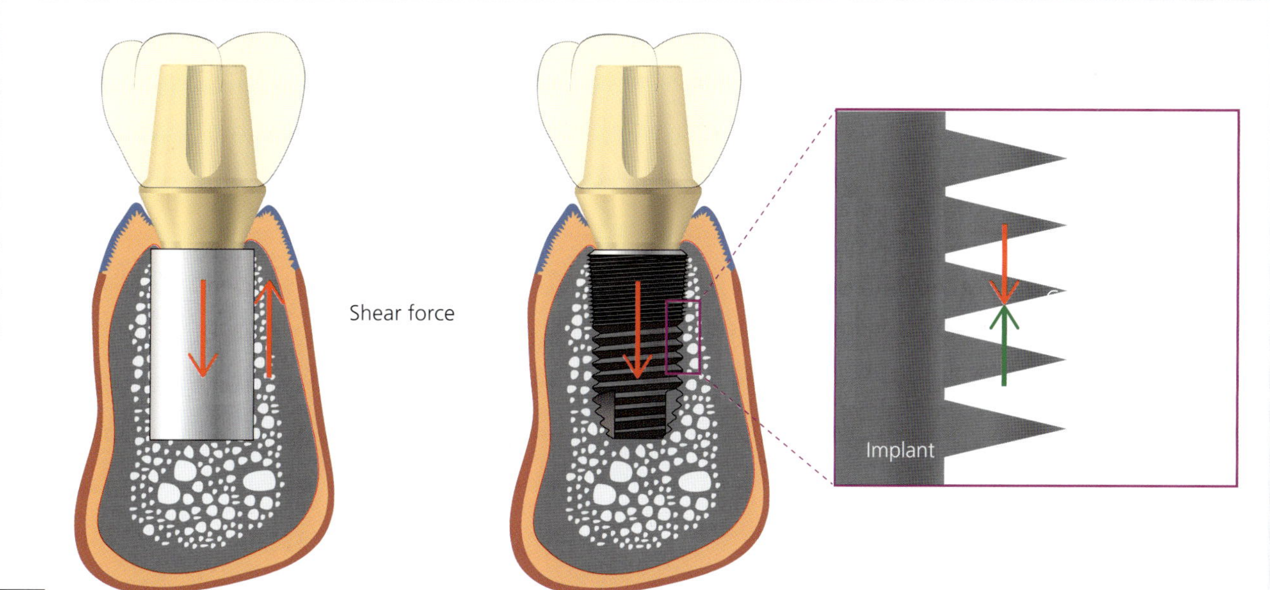

2-39

The screw-shaped design of the implant effectively converts vulnerable shear forces into compressive forces, significantly contributing to the clinical success.

The converted compressive forces induce appropriate strain in the alveolar bone, stimulating biological responses that help maintain bone volume and quality.

However, the implant–abutment structure of Brånemark implants, which features an external hex connection, causes abutment micromovement under masticatory forces. This mechanical instability leads to the loss of soft tissue attachment, ultimately resulting in marginal bone resorption.

Compared to other implant systems of its time, the Brånemark implant system exhibited a superior survival rate, which made the marginal bone resorption, resulting from the instability of its implant–abutment connection, be interpreted as a physiological phenomenon. Consequently, both dental clinicians and patients faced the additional burdens of bone grafting procedures and the use of longer implants.

Alveolar bone resorption occurs when bacterial infiltration takes place due to the loss of soft tissue attachment or when the bone fails to receive appropriate strain stimulation from mechanical stress. The introduction and clinical application of the Astra Tech implant system prompted a closer examination of these factors.

The Astra Tech implant features a conical implant–abutment connection structure.

This design allows the upper portion of the implant to be appropriately thin, creating a slight expansion effect when occlusal forces are transmitted through the prosthetic superstructure. This expansion effectively stimulates the alveolar bone, promoting its health and maintenance **(Figure 2-40)**.

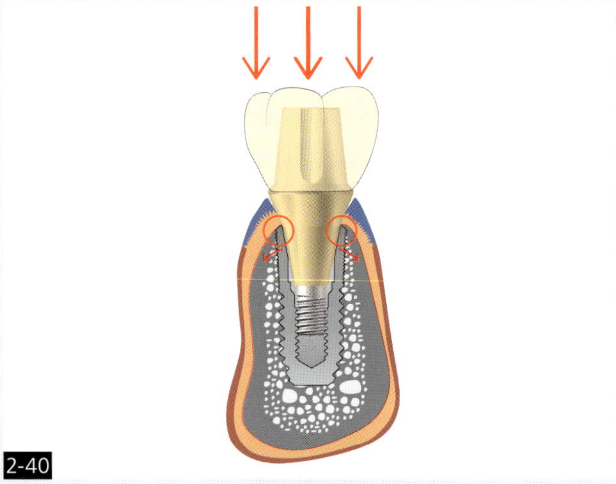

2-40

Schematic diagram illustrating the mechanism of strain generation in the alveolar bone surrounding an implant with the conical connection

In a friction-screw-retained connection, the thickness of the implant's upper portion gradually decreases, allowing for some degree of deformation (red circles in **Figure 2-40**) . Mechanical cyclic loading experiments reveal that the upper portion of the implant undergoes slight expansion, sometimes referred to as coronal expansion. In biomechanical analyses of friction-screw-retained connections, a smaller abutment taper angle increases connection stability. However, this also thickens the implant's upper portion, reducing its capacity to stimulate the alveolar bone. Achieving a balance between these two effects is therefore essential.

Clinically, when the taper angle is too large, the implant's upper portion becomes excessively thin, leading to a higher incidence of complications such as implant fractures (tearing). Conversely, if the taper angle is too small, the implant becomes rigid and does not allow for deformation, failing to stimulate the alveolar bone effectively. In addition, the narrower abutment connection area can result in frequent abutment fractures.

Under repeated masticatory forces, the abutment is driven downward toward the implant, causing the implant to expand slightly. This expansion induces strain in the marginal bone that contacts the expanding implant, triggering a remodeling process that increases or maintains bone quantity and quality.

The ability to preserve or even increase peri-implant bone volume carries significant clinical implications. In particular, concerns about bone grafting—often raised due to the bone resorption patterns observed in Brånemark implants—can frequently be avoided. Additionally, instead of relying on long implants justified by assumptions of physiological bone resorption, shorter implants can be placed according to the patient's anatomical structure, achieving long-term stability without bone loss. This approach significantly reduces the procedural burden for both dental clinicians and patients, simplifying the implant procedure and enhancing clinical outcomes.

The gingiva maintains the health of the alveolar bone by resisting bacterial invasion through its attachment. In natural teeth, the gingiva is divided into free gingiva and attached gingiva. Attached gingiva adheres to both the tooth root and the alveolar bone in natural teeth. However, in implants, the attached gingiva adheres only to the alveolar bone, with very weak attachment around the abutment. Therefore, only the attached gingiva adhering to the alveolar bone performs a role comparable to that in natural teeth.

Marginal bone resorption around implants presents a significant issue from a periodontal perspective. When abutment loosening occurs due to screw loosening or structural weaknesses in the screw-retained implant–abutment connection, soft tissue attachment is lost. This leads to the formation of periodontal pockets, allowing bacterial infiltration and subsequent marginal bone resorption. Such resorption alters the characteristics of the attached gingiva supported by the resorbed marginal bone, causing it to exhibit properties similar to free gingiva. When the characteristics of the gingiva change, bacterial infiltration becomes easier, thereby exacerbating peri-implantitis. To ensure long-term stable outcomes, dental clinicians must closely monitor the condition of the marginal bone to adequately support gingival health.

Conversely, if the gingiva around the abutment is frequently stretched due to a shallow vestibule or a high frenum, it can lead to the loss of soft tissue attachment around the abutment, resulting in similar adverse outcomes.

Considering these aspects, selecting an appropriate implant system to maintain a stable implant–abutment connection is critical. Clinicians must also address mechanical complications, particularly screw loosening, and ensure that the attached gingiva around the abutment remains healthy to prevent it from reverting to the characteristics of free gingiva due to other conditions.

As human life expectancy continues to increase, dental implants in modern dentistry are expected to function in the oral cavity for extended periods. To meet these demands, it is essential to eliminate or minimize alveolar bone loss caused by occlusal forces and to enhance the health of the attached gingiva to prevent bacterial infiltration resulting from soft tissue attachment loss. To achieve this, dental clinicians must prioritize the management of the transitional area where the implant system connects the internal and external environments. This includes focusing on the abutment and the surrounding hard and soft tissues, guided by biomechanical analyses and clinical interpretations of the implant–abutment connection structure discussed earlier.

4. Clinical cases related to management of interfacial issues at implant-abutment connection

The implant–abutment interface is subject to various complications, including abutment screw loosening, abutment screw fracture, abutment fracture, and simultaneous fractures of the abutment and screw. Although screw loosening is often considered a minor issue and fractures are deemed severe, these complications are clinically comparable in their impact. This is because screw loosening is frequently attributed to the screw itself, leading to the assumption that replacing the screw will resolve the problem. However, in practice, loosening often recurs after a certain period, even after screw replacement.

1) Abutment screw loosening

Fractured screws are a common occurrence for dental clinicians with extensive experience in implant procedures. Many clinicians are well-versed in removing broken screws and replacing them with new ones.

As previously mentioned, screws do not loosen due to counterclockwise rotation; rather, they are already loose, allowing for counterclockwise rotation. The general principle for removing a fractured screw is to first loosen it. Once loosened, the screw can be rotated counterclockwise and removed.

Loosening the screw is typically achieved using ultrasonic vibration, which can also be performed with a piezoelectric device. Ultrasonic vibrations help loosen the broken screw, enabling counterclockwise rotation.

The authors use a pointed instrument, often an endodontic probe, to apply counterclockwise rotation while transmitting ultrasonic vibrations to the screw **(Figure 2-41)**. During this process, the probe is positioned in the space between the broken screw and the internal threading of the implant. Excessive force must be avoided, as it can deform the internal threading of the implant, impeding counterclockwise rotation and making screw removal impossible.

Screw removal kits provided by some implant manufacturers are designed to facilitate the counterclockwise rotation of fractured screws. However, based on the authors' experience, successful removal using these kits is rare. This highlights the importance of the loosening process over the counterclockwise rotation action itself.

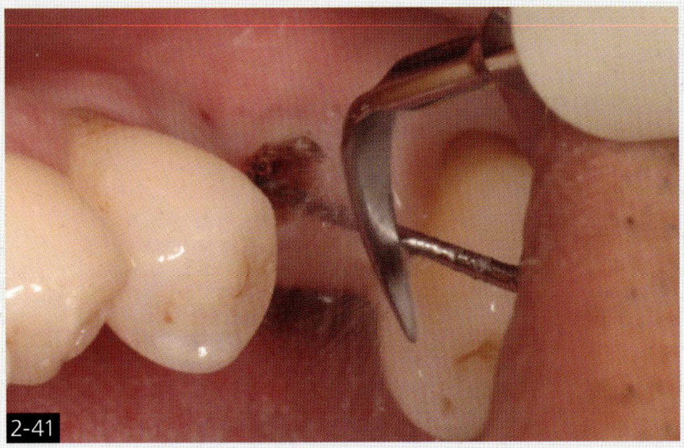

2-41

Application of ultrasonic vibrations to the periodontal probe

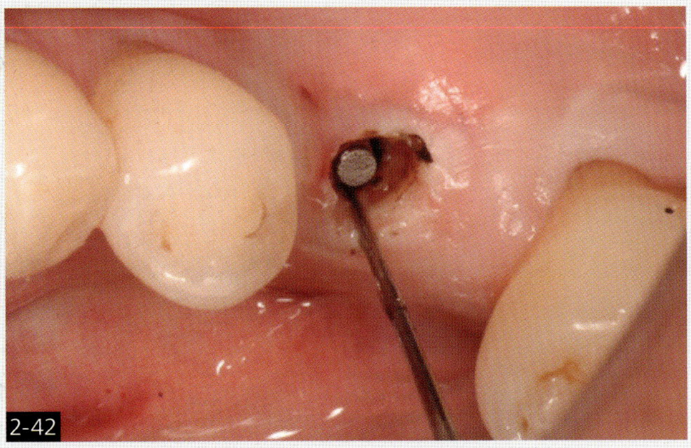

2-42

The screw fragment is loosened, rotated counterclockwise, and removed

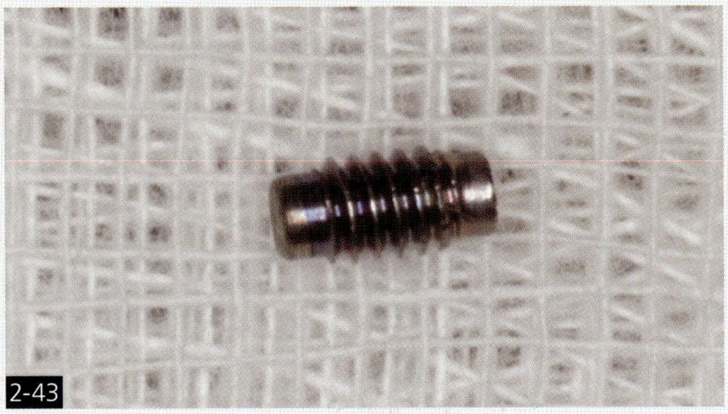

2-43

The removed abutment screw fragment.

2) Abutment fracture

In implants with a friction-screw-retained connection, the screw plays a minimal role, and the stability of the connection is primarily maintained by the frictional forces between the implant's internal surface and the abutment's external surface. In such cases, even if the screw becomes loosened or entirely loose, the abutment often remains stable.

However, when the screw is completely loose, lateral pressure can lead to abutment fractures. If a patient presents with complaints of prosthetic mobility and the mobility recurs within a day or two after tightening the screw, clinicians should suspect an abutment fracture in addition to screw loosening, rather than attributing the issue solely to screw loosening.

In these cases, the authors occasionally use a #330 bur to make three incisions inside the fractured abutment to facilitate its removal. Extreme caution is necessary to avoid damaging the implant's internal structure, as overly deep cuts can cause harm. Additionally, making only one or two cuts is often insufficient. By carefully making three cuts at approximately equal intervals and alternating between them, the fractured abutment can eventually be dislodged.

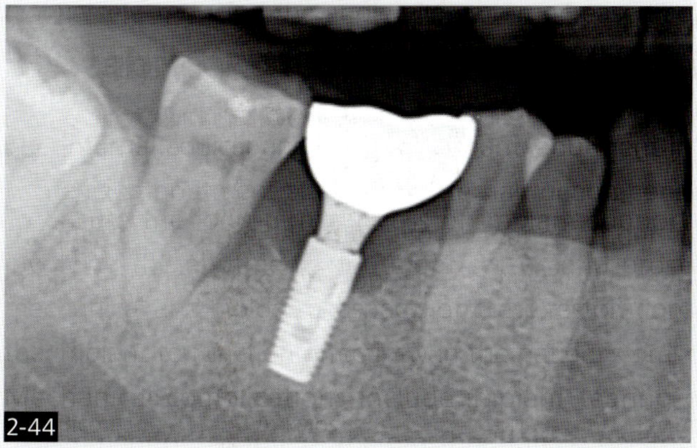
2-44

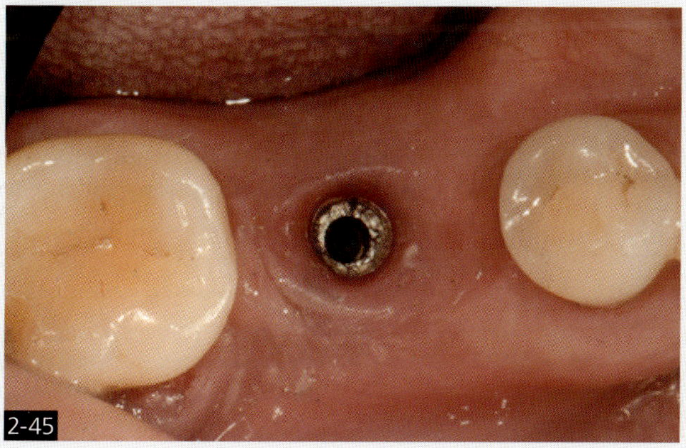
2-45

The patient presented with complaints of prosthetic mobility. Although the screw was tightened, the prosthetic mobility recurred the following day, prompting another visit. Upon removing the prosthesis, it was revealed that the issue was not merely screw loosening but an abutment fracture **(Figure 2-44)**. Accessing the site through the occlusal surface, a high-speed #330 bur was employed to create approximately three partial cuts in the upper portion **(Figure 2-45)**, facilitating the removal of the fractured abutment.

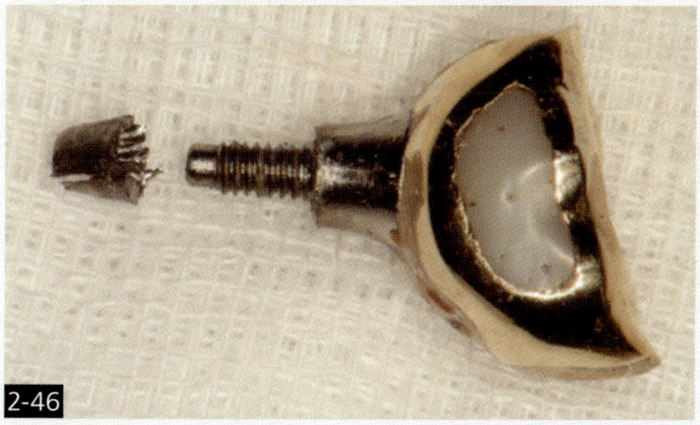
2-46

The removed abutment is shown **(Figure 2-46)**.

When the screw is loosened and the abutment is fractured, if the patient delays seeking treatment, soft tissue may grow over the implant area. In such cases, a surgical incision is necessary to expose the fractured abutment.

The following case illustrates a patient who presented after a significant delay following the detachment of the prosthesis **(Figures 2-47 and 48)**.

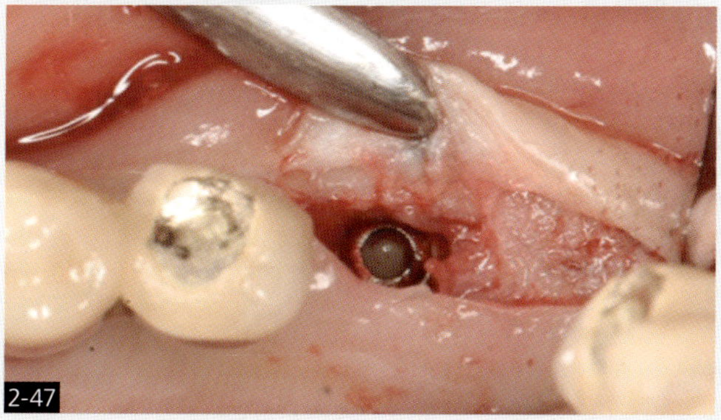
2-47

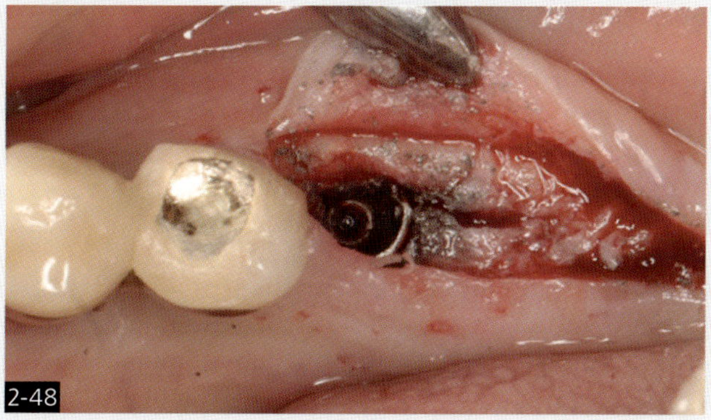
2-48

The soft tissue covering the implant was incised **(Figure 2-47)**, and the fractured abutment was removed using a #330 bur **(Figure 2-48)**.

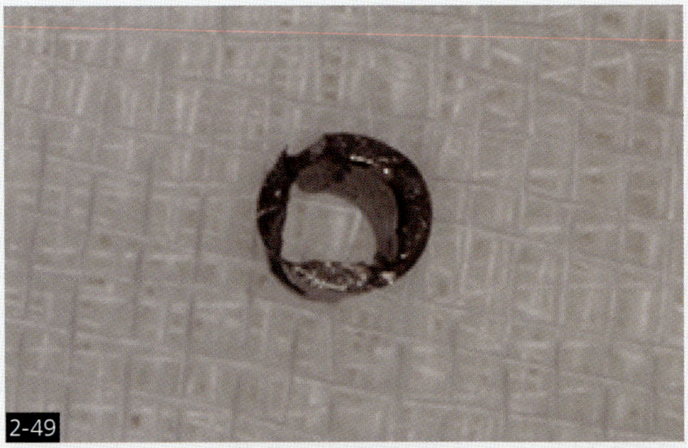
2-49

Figure 2-49 shows the abutment after three partial cuts were made using a #330 bur.

Due to the high incidence of clinical cases involving abutment fractures in Korea, most domestic implant manufacturers now provide dedicated kits for their removal. When the screw is intact or a fractured screw has already been removed, using an abutment removal kit offers a significantly more convenient solution.

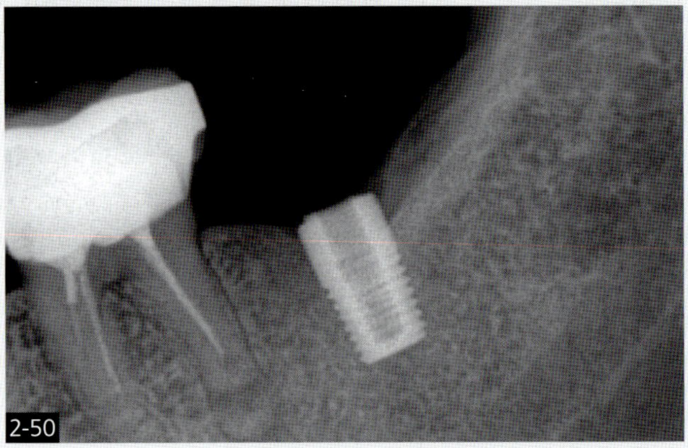
2-50

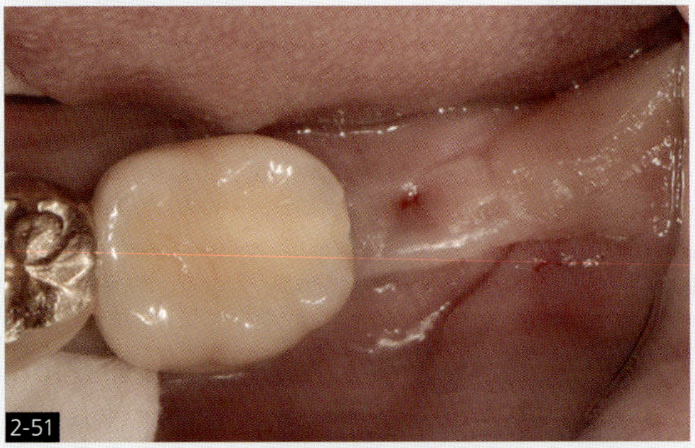
2-51

The radiographic image reveals a fracture of the abutment, accompanied by the detachment of both the prosthesis and the abutment screw **(Figure 2-50)**. Following the detachment of the prosthesis, the gingiva rapidly re-epithelialized the area, as observed in the patient who returned one day after the prosthetic loss **(Figure 2-51)**.

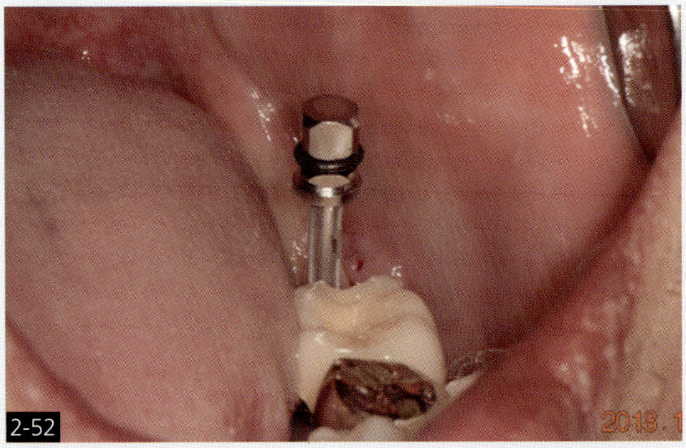
2-52

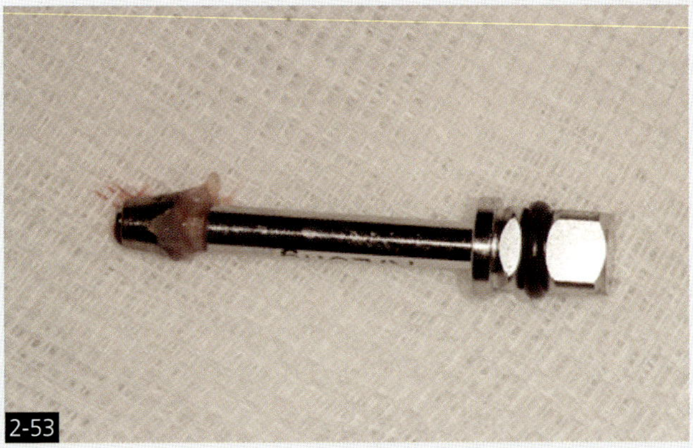
2-53

A fractured abutment has been successfully removed using an abutment removal kit provided by a Korean implant manufacturer **(Figures 2-52 and 53)**.

3) Simultaneous fracture of abutment and abutment screw

Occasionally, both the abutment and the screw may fracture simultaneously. In such scenarios, the recommended approach is to first remove the screw before attempting to extract the abutment.

The screw is removed by applying ultrasonic vibrations to a probe, whereas the abutment is typically extracted using a specialized removal kit.

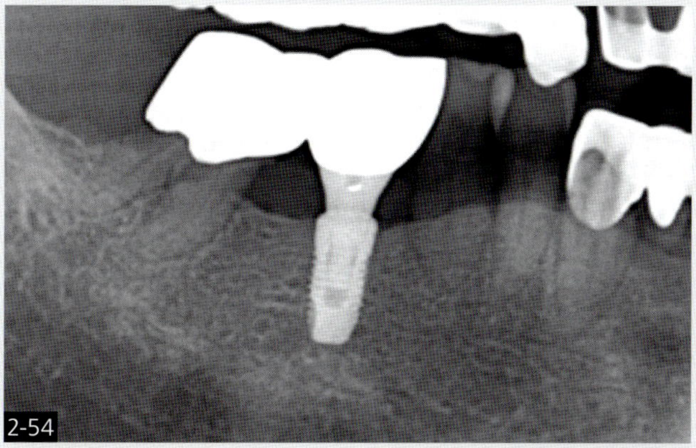

2-54

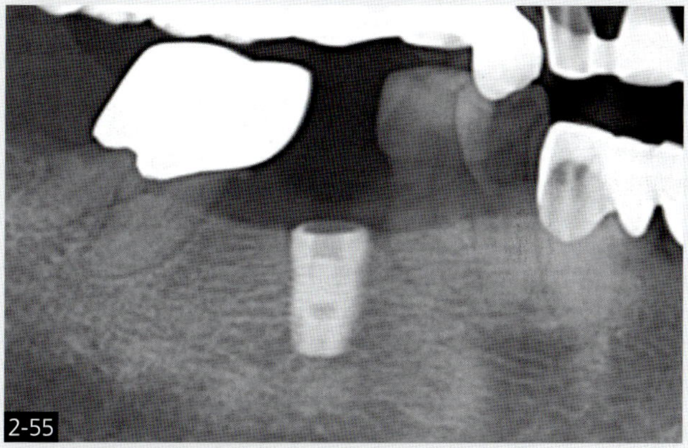

2-55

A patient presented with simultaneous fractures of the abutment and screw. Radiographic imaging confirmed the concurrent fractures (Figures 2-54 and 55).

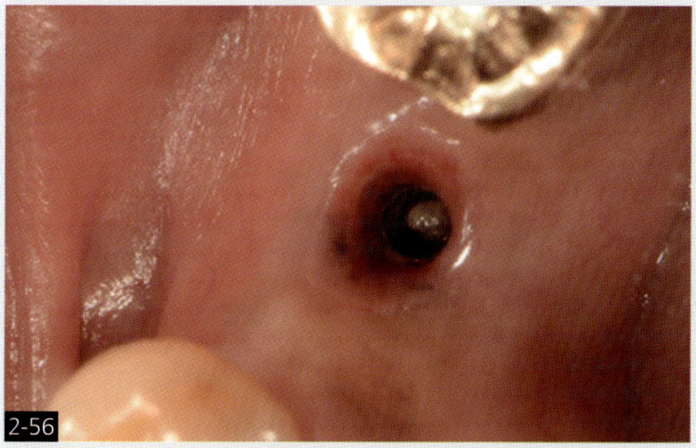

2-56

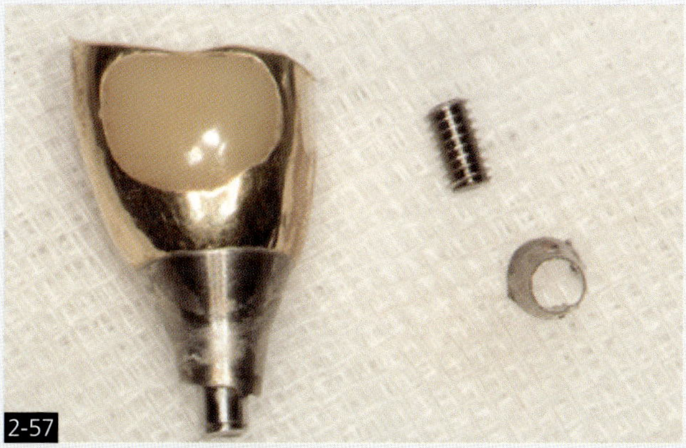

2-57

Figure 2-56 displays an intraoral photograph of the fractured abutment and screw, while Figure 2-57 shows the individually removed abutment and screw. In some instances, removing a fractured screw using a probe with ultrasonic vibrations proves challenging. In such cases, the authors occasionally employ a high-speed #330 bur, despite the associated risks. The #330 bur is utilized not only for abutment removal but also for extracting fractured screws.

The removal technique involves briefly and lightly contacting the side of the fractured screw with the rotating #330 bur. The #330 bur rotates clockwise; when it contacts the side of the fractured screw, it induces a counterclockwise rotation in the screw, facilitating its removal. This counterclockwise rotation effectively loosens and extracts the broken screw.

Excessive rotation applied deep within the implant can damage its internal structure and deform the internal threading, potentially making it impossible to remove the fractured abutment screw. Therefore, this technique must be performed with extreme caution.

This method may also be employed in cases where both the screw and abutment have fractured simultaneously. The following case illustrates an instance where using a probe with ultrasonic vibration proved ineffective, necessitating the use of this alternative approach as an extreme measure.

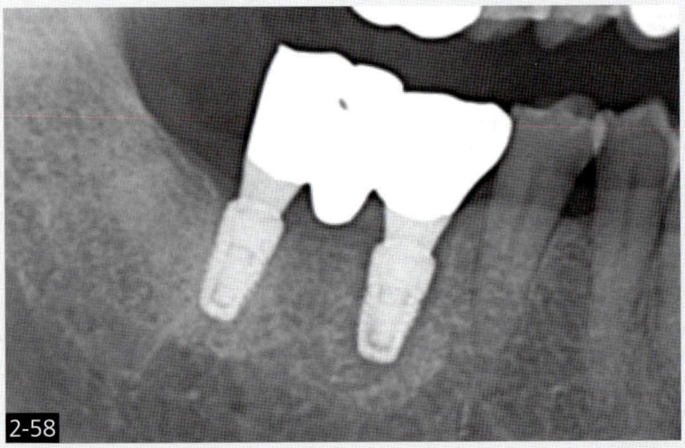

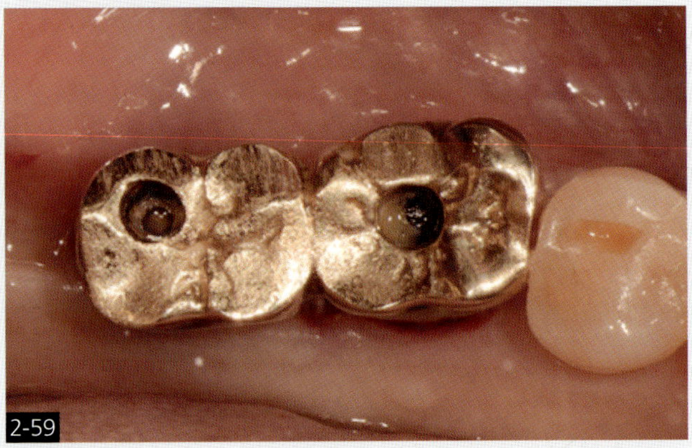

The failure of #46 implant is evident in radiographic image **(Figure 2-58)**. The implant exhibits signs of mobility **(Figure 2-59)**, and the patient presented with complaints of discomfort.

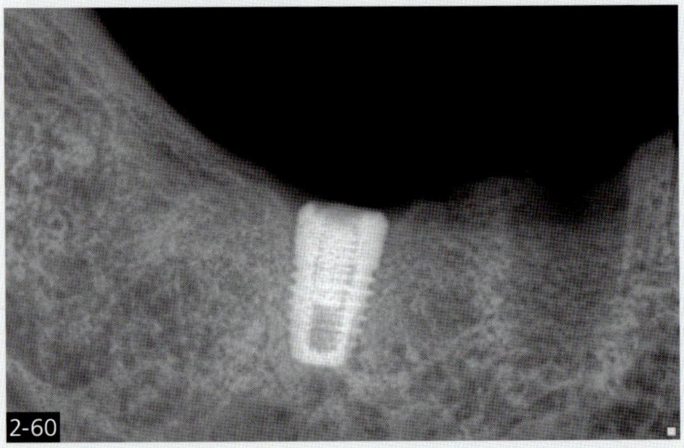

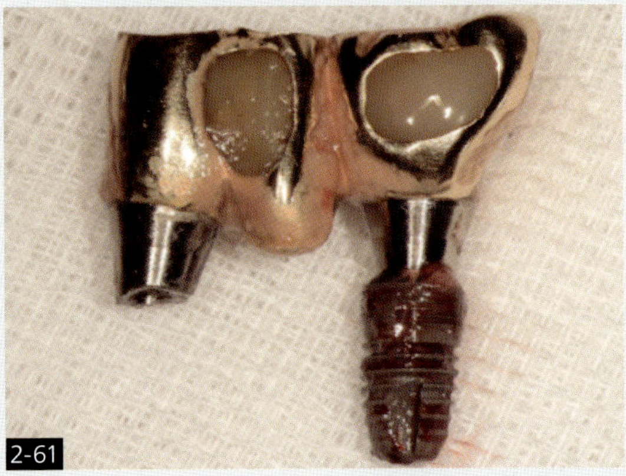

The implant in position #47 exhibits simultaneous fractures of the abutment and screw **(Figure 2-60)**. **Figure 2-61** illustrates the removed failed implant along with the fractured abutment and screw.

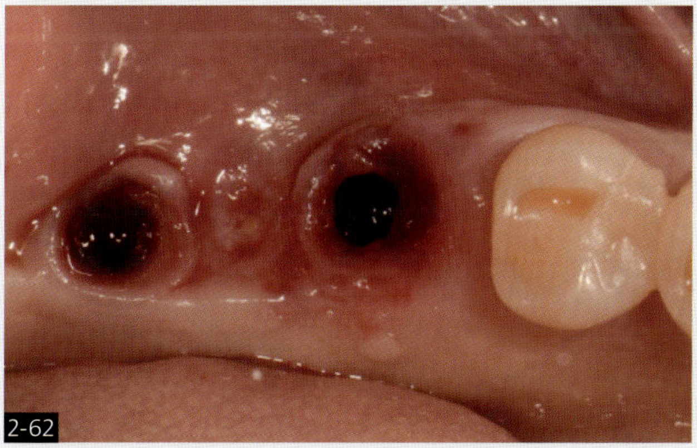

2-62

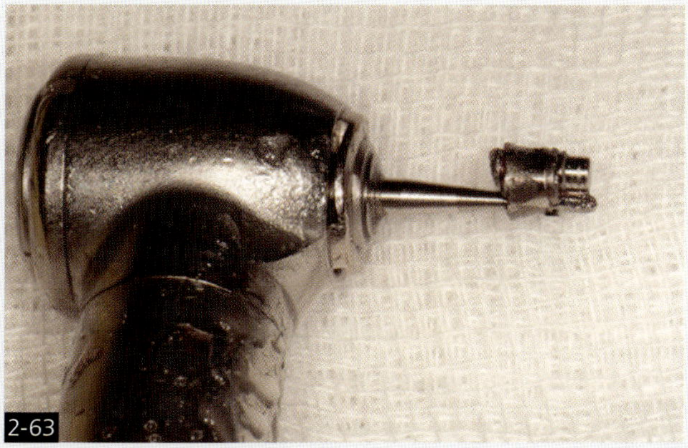

2-63

The intraoral photograph following the removal of the failed implant is shown in **Figure 2-62**, while **Figure 2-63** depicts the removal of the fractured screw and abutment using a #330 bur. In this case, the #330 bur was rotated and carefully inserted between the fractured abutment and screw. The fractured abutment acted as a protective barrier, preventing damage to the internal structure of the implant. In the absence of the fractured abutment, there would be a risk of internal damage to the implant. Therefore, this technique must be applied with the utmost caution.

4) Fracture of one-piece abutments

In the implant systems with a friction-screw-retained connection, 1-piece abutments, also known as solid abutments, are sometimes employed. These abutments lack internal voids for abutment screws, leading to the perception that they are stronger than 2-piece abutments. Particularly in cases where multiple implants are connected as a single prosthetic unit, it was previously believed that screw loosening could not occur with 1-piece abutments.

During a period when it was widely assumed that abutment screws loosened due to counter-rotation, there was a prevailing belief that connecting two or more implants with 1-piece abutments into a single prosthetic structure would completely eliminate screw loosening and associated issues. The authors also adhered to this misconception and performed restorations based on this erroneous understanding.

A patient returned after 10 years with fractures in a prosthesis supported by two implants using 1-piece abutments connected as a single unit **(Figure 2-64)**. While it may be argued that 10 years represents the expected lifespan of such restorations, the authors believe that using 2-piece abutments could have prevented these complications. This case exemplifies the unfortunate consequences of misunderstandings surrounding 1-piece abutments.

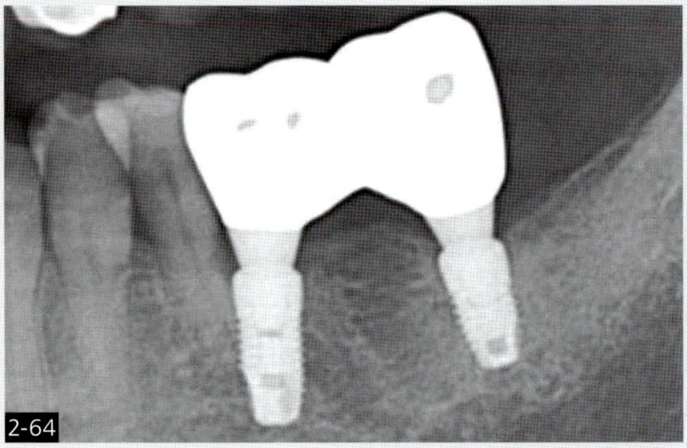

2-64

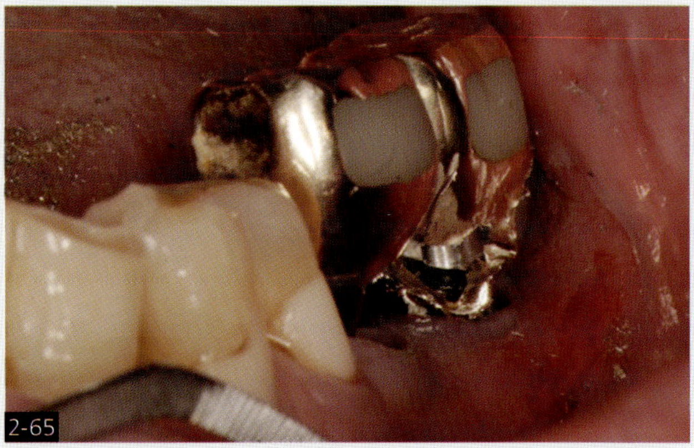

2-65

The patient presented with complaints of prosthetic mobility. Radiographic examination, as depicted in **Figure 2-64**, revealed a screw fracture in the 1-piece abutment of the #36 implant.

In such cases, the authors horizontally cut the intact #37 abutment. Using a #330 bur, this procedure can typically be completed within five minutes. Conventional methods of cutting the prosthesis are time-consuming, particularly when working with non-metallic or ceramic materials such as zirconia, which require significant effort and consume a substantial number of burs.

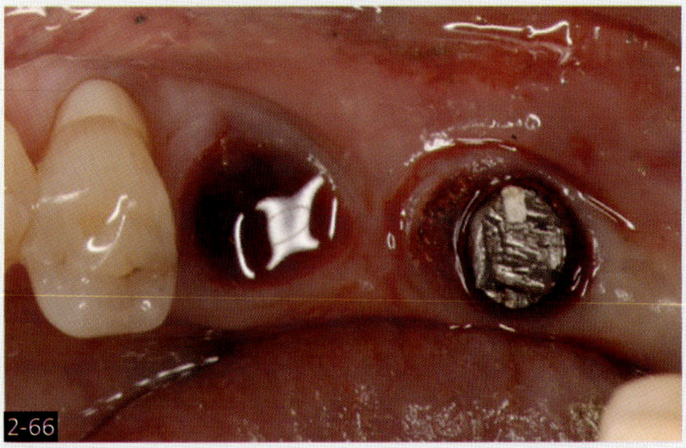

2-66

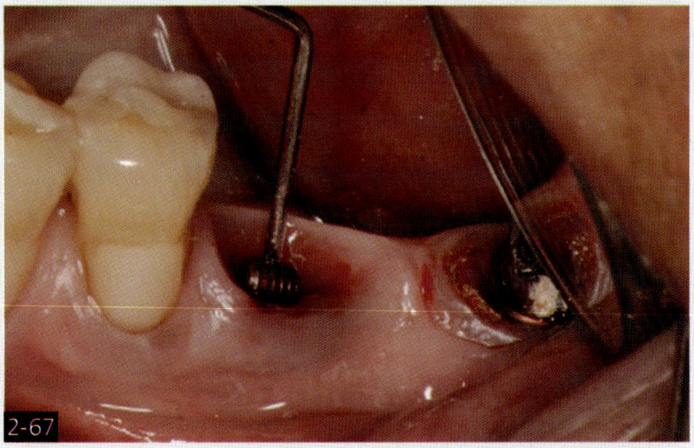

2-67

The prosthesis was easily removed by horizontally sectioning the #37 abutment **(Figure 2-66)**, and the fractured screw was subsequently extracted without difficulty using a probe with ultrasonic vibrations **(Figure 2-67)**. The horizontally sectioned #37 abutment can be easily unscrewed by securely gripping it with pliers and applying counterclockwise rotation.

If the pliers slip due to the abutment's cylindrical shape, the side of the abutment can be filed to create flat surfaces for better grip. Alternatively, a groove can be carved into the top of the abutment to facilitate the use of a flathead screwdriver.

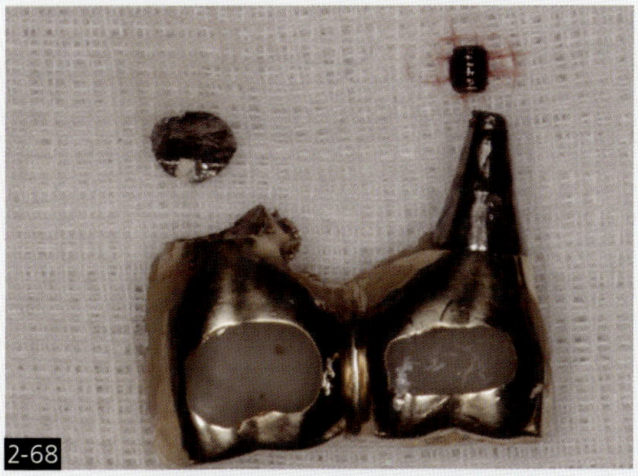

Figure 2-68 illustrates the fragmented 1-piece abutments and prosthesis removed using the aforementioned approaches.

Another patient presented with complaints of prosthetic mobility, and a fracture of the 1-piece abutment was identified.

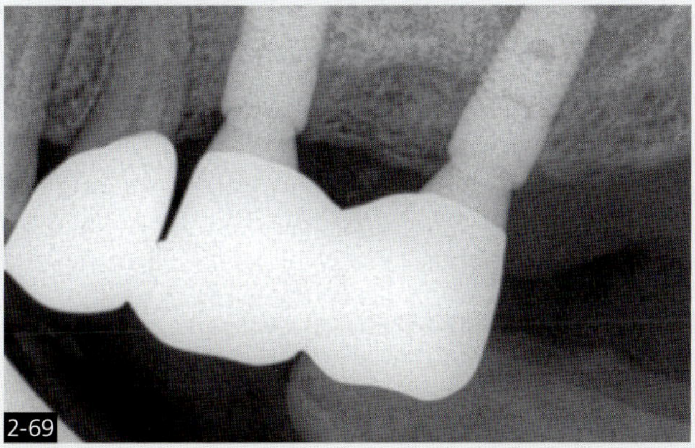

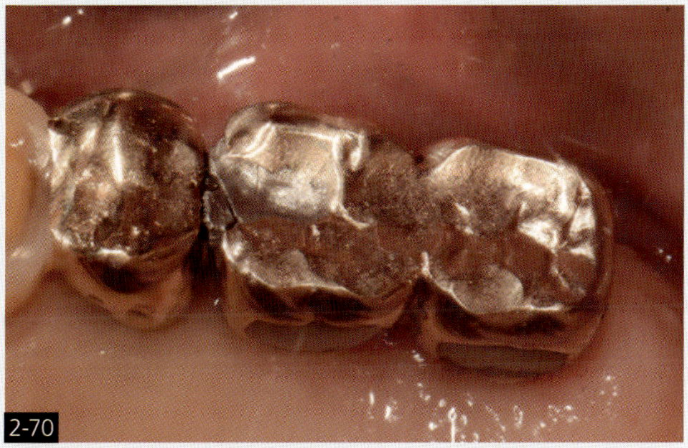

The radiographic image reveals a fracture in the screw portion of the 1-piece abutment at #27 (Figure 2-69). Figure 2-70 provides an intraoral view of the affected area.

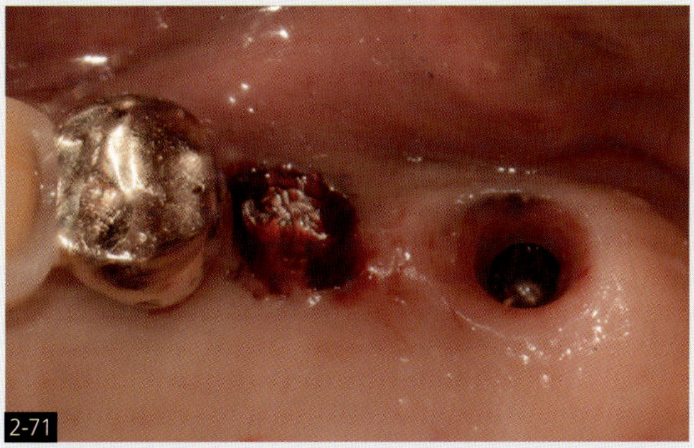

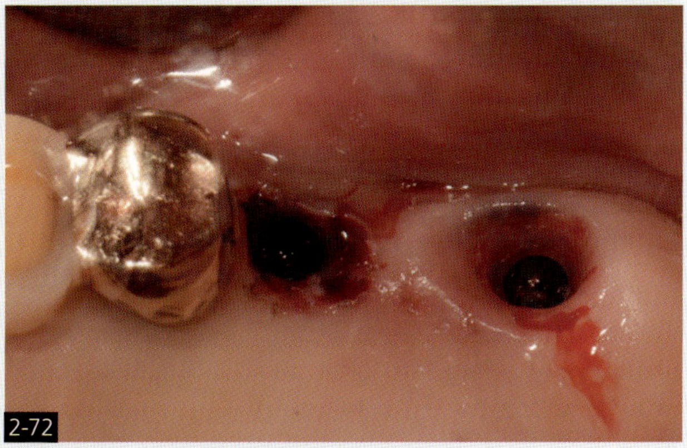

Horizontal sectioning of the 1-piece abutment was performed at #26 (Figure 2-71). The horizontally sectioned 1-piece abutment and the fractured screw were subsequently removed (Figures 2-72 and 73).

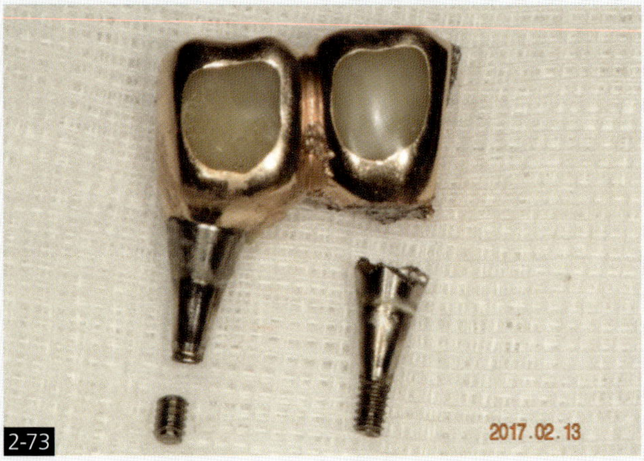

2-73

The removed 1-piece abutments and prosthesis.

This section has explored clinical tips for effectively managing fractures of 1-piece abutments. Misconceptions, such as the erroneous belief that implant screws loosen due to counterclockwise rotation, have resulted in procedures that impose unnecessary challenges for both clinicians and patients. In friction-screw-retained connection implants, occlusal forces—particularly lateral forces—cause expansion of the implant's upper portion. This expansion leads to the loss of preload, generating bending stresses at the screw portion of the 1-piece abutment. Consequently, these bending stresses cause fractures in the 1-piece abutment.

5) Practical solutions to address issues with abutments and abutment screws

Problems related to abutment screws are often classified as screw-related issues, while those involving abutments are considered abutment-specific concerns. However, the primary consideration is identifying which part of the implant system bears the occlusal forces applied to the implant-supported restoration.

When occlusal forces predominantly act on the abutment screw, screw loosening or fractures can occur. Conversely, if these forces concentrate on the abutment, it can lead to abutment fractures. Therefore, addressing these issues necessitates a holistic perspective; a fragmented approach will not provide fundamental solutions.

Currently, dental clinicians worldwide utilize friction-screw-retained implants. Accordingly, solutions should be tailored to this specific implant type.

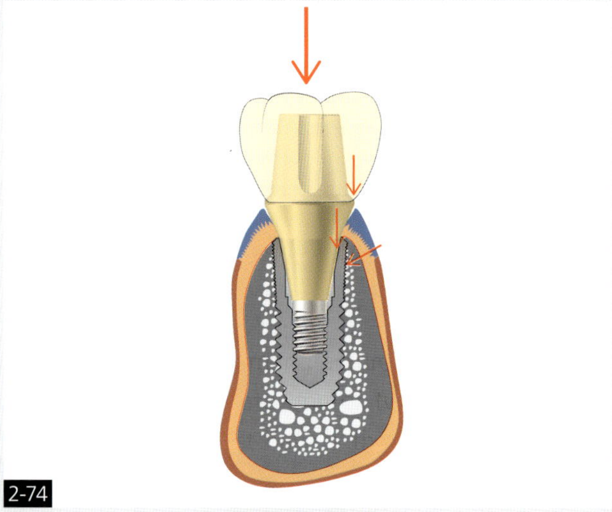

2-74

As illustrated in Figure 2-74, occlusal forces are applied to the crown but are ultimately transmitted to the alveolar bone through various implant components. In terms of long-term implant prognosis, these forces tend to concentrate on the weakest parts of the structure, resulting in complications. Among the various components, dental clinicians most frequently observe issues at the screw level, rendering it the most vulnerable part of the implant system.

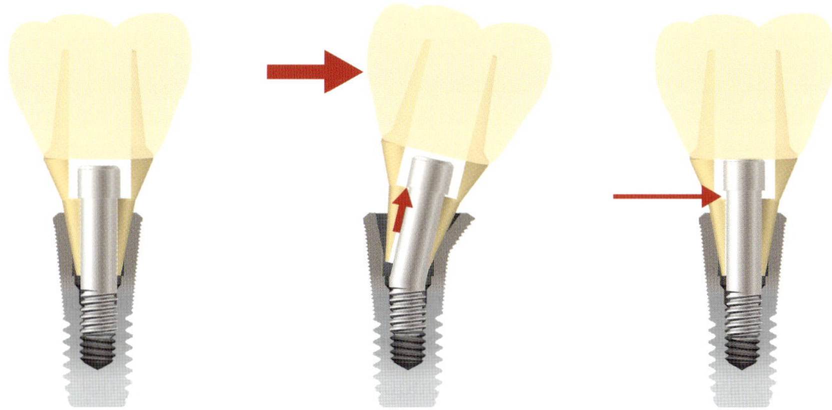

2-75

Schematic diagram illustrating the mechanism by which lateral forces applied to the implant-supported crown eliminate preload. The diagram demonstrates how the bending moment on the abutment screw causes screw elongation, leading to the loss of preload.

All forces applied to the screw and abutment ultimately act on the internal conical walls located in the upper portion of the implant, as shown in **Figure 2-75**. If these internal walls effectively withstand occlusal forces, the screw remains unaffected, and no issues arise. However, if the internal walls fail to adequately resist these forces, the stress is transmitted to the screw, leading to problems such as loosening or fracture.

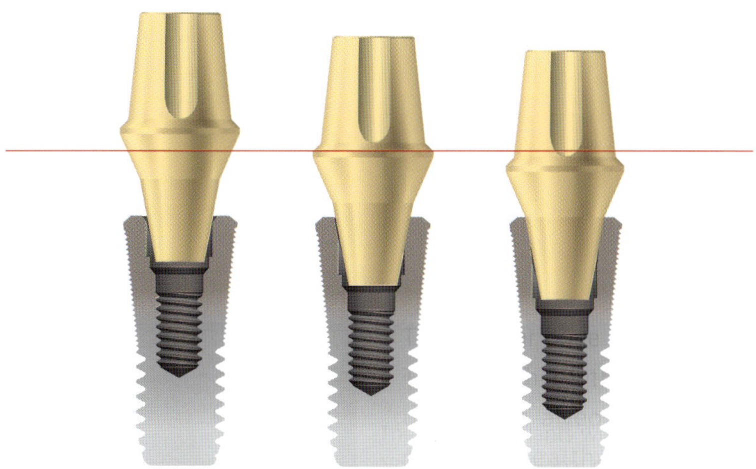

2-76

In implants with a friction-screw-retained connection, the frictional interface can be classified into three depths, as shown in **Figure 2-76**.

The stability of the connection is proportional to the fourth power of the contact length between the abutment and the implant. Therefore, as the abutment extends deeper into the implant, the connection stability increases. This enhanced stability reduces the external forces exerted on the screw, thereby lowering the likelihood of screw loosening or fracture.

Additionally, abutment fractures typically occur at the uppermost portion of the implant. When the diameter of the abutment at this critical location is larger, the risk of abutment fracture is significantly diminished.

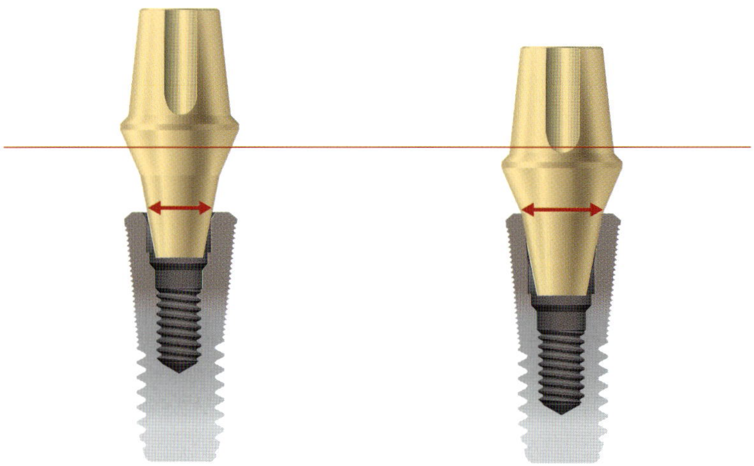

2-77

As shown in **Figure 2-77**, enhancing the depth and width of the implant-abutment connection significantly decreases the likelihood of complications, including screw loosening and abutment fractures.

Chapter 3

Conclusion of Part 2.

- Abutment mobility disrupts the mucosal seal, thereby leading to peri-implantitis.
- Abutment screw loosening is caused by the loss of preload due to masticatory forces, particularly lateral forces.
- In friction-screw-retained implants, the stability of the connection is proportional to the fourth power of the implant-abutment interfacial contact length.
- A deep connection, which increase the internal contact surface area, reduces the likelihood of screw loosening, screw fracture, and abutment fractures, thereby contributing to the prevention of peri-implantitis.

References

Bozkaya D, Müftü S. Mechanics of the tapered interference fit in dental implants. J Biomech. 2003 Nov;36(11):1649-58. doi: 10.1016/s0021-9290(03)00177-5.

Bozkaya D, Müftü S. Mechanics of the taper integrated screwed-in (TIS) abutments used in dental implants. J Biomech. 2005 Jan;38(1):87-97. doi: 10.1016/j.jbiomech.2004.03.006.

Frost HM. Perspectives: bone's mechanical usage windows. Bone Miner. 1992 Dec;19(3):257-71. doi: 10.1016/0169-6009(92)90875-e.

Hermann JS, Buser D, Schenk RK, Cochran DL. Crestal bone changes around titanium implants. A histometric evaluation of unloaded non-submerged and submerged implants in the canine mandible. J Periodontol. 2000 Sep;71(9):1412-24. doi: 10.1902/jop.2000.71.9.1412.

Hermann JS, Schoolfield JD, Schenk RK, Buser D, Cochran DL. Influence of the size of the microgap on crestal bone changes around titanium implants. A histometric evaluation of unloaded non-submerged implants in the canine mandible. J Periodontol. 2001 Oct;72(10):1372-83. doi: 10.1902/jop.2001.72.10.1372.

Jeong CG, Kim SK, Lee JH, Kim JW, Yeo IS. Clinically available preload prediction based on a mechanical analysis. Arch Appl Mech. 2017 Dec;87(12):2003-9. doi: 10.1007/s00419-017-1307-0.

Kim JC, Lee M, Yeo IL. Three interfaces of the dental implant system and their clinical effects on hard and soft tissues. Mater Horiz. 2022 May 10;9(5):1387-1411. doi: 10.1039/d1mh01621k.

Kim JJ, Lee JH, Kim JC, Lee JB, Yeo IL. Biological responses to the transitional area of dental implants: Material- and structure-dependent responses of peri-implant tissue to abutments. Materials (Basel). 2019 Dec 22;13(1):72. doi: 10.3390/ma13010072.

Lang LA, Kang B, Wang RF, Lang BR. Finite element analysis to determine implant preload. J Prosthet Dent. 2003 Dec;90(6):539-46. doi: 10.1016/j.prosdent.2003.09.012.

Lee JH, Kim JC, Kim HY, Yeo IL. Influence of connections and surfaces of dental implants on marginal bone loss: A retrospective study over 7 to 19 years. Int J Oral Maxillofac Implants. 2020 Nov/Dec;35(6):1195-1202. doi: 10.11607/jomi.8450.

Mishra SK, Chowdhary R, Kumari S. Microleakage at the different implant abutment interface: A systematic review. J Clin Diagn Res. 2017 Jun;11(6):ZE10-ZE15. doi: 10.7860/JCDR/2017/28951.10054.

Palmer RM, Palmer PJ, Smith BJ. A 5-year prospective study of Astra single tooth implants. Clin Oral Implants Res. 2000 Apr;11(2):179-82. doi: 10.1111/j.1600-0501.2000.tb00012.x.

Pjetursson BE, Heimisdottir K. Dental implants - are they better than natural teeth? Eur J Oral Sci. 2018 Oct;126 Suppl 1:81-87. doi: 10.1111/eos.12543.

Sahin C, Ayyildiz S. Correlation between microleakage and screw loosening at implant-abutment connection. J Adv Prosthodont. 2014 Feb;6(1):35-8. doi: 10.4047/jap.2014.6.1.35.

Sherif S, Susarla HK, Kapos T, Munoz D, Chang BM, Wright RF. A systematic review of screw- versus cement-retained implant-supported fixed restorations. J Prosthodont. 2014 Jan;23(1):1-9. doi: 10.1111/jopr.12128.

Budynas RG, Nisbett KJ. Shigley's mechanical engineering design: 2024 release ISE. 12th ed. New York:McGraw-Hill;2024 May. ISBN: 978-1266929892.

Simonis P, Dufour T, Tenenbaum H. Long-term implant survival and success: a 10-16-year follow-up of non-submerged dental implants. Clin Oral Implants Res. 2010 Jul;21(7):772-7. doi: 10.1111/j.1600-0501.2010.01912.x.

Tsuruta K, Ayukawa Y, Matsuzaki T, Kihara M, Koyano K. The influence of implant-abutment connection on the screw loosening and microleakage. Int J Implant Dent. 2018 Apr 9;4(1):11. doi: 10.1186/s40729-018-0121-y.

Yeo IL. Modifications of dental implant surfaces at the micro- and nano-level for enhanced osseointegration. Materials (Basel). 2019 Dec 23;13(1):89. doi: 10.3390/ma13010089.